Gene Therapy: Therapeutic Mechanisms and Strategies

Gene Therapy: Therapeutic Mechanisms and Strategies

Edited by Marvin Walker

STATES
ACADEMIC PRESS
www.statesacademicpress.com

States Academic Press,
109 South 5th Street,
Brooklyn, NY 11249, USA

Visit us on the World Wide Web at:
www.statesacademicpress.com

ISBN: 978-1-63989-236-5

Cataloging-in-Publication Data

Gene therapy : therapeutic mechanisms and strategies / edited by Marvin Walker.
p. cm.
Includes bibliographical references and index.
ISBN 978-1-63989-236-5
1. Gene therapy. 2. Therapeutics. 3. Genetic engineering. I. Walker, Marvin.
RB155.8 .G46 2022
616.042--dc23

Table of Contents

Preface

Gene therapy is a field of medical science that focuses on the genetic modifications of the cells to achieve a therapeutic effect for the treatment of a disease by repairing defective genetic material. The main objective of gene therapy is to fix a genetic disorder at its source. For example, if mutation in a certain gene occurs in an inherited disease which results in the production of a dysfunctional protein, then, gene therapy can be used to incorporate a copy of this gene that is normal and does not contain the mutation. Thus, it produces a functional protein. This strategy is used to treat inherited retinal diseases and is also known as gene replacement therapy. This book outlines the therapeutic management and strategies of gene therapy in detail. It traces the progress of this field and highlights some of its key concepts and applications. For someone with an interest and eye for detail, this book covers the most significant topics in the field of gene therapy.

This book unites the global concepts and researches in an organized manner for a comprehensive understanding of the subject. It is a ripe text for all researchers, students, scientists or anyone else who is interested in acquiring a better knowledge of this dynamic field.

I extend my sincere thanks to the contributors for such eloquent research chapters. Finally, I thank my family for being a source of support and help.

Editor

Preface

1

Modifiers of γ-Globin Gene Expression and Treatment β-Thalassemia

Anjana Munshi, Sneha Dadeech, M. Sai Babu and Preeti Khetarpal

Abstract

Beta thalassemia (β-thalassemia) is an autosomal recessive genetic disease with many genes involved. It is a heterogeneous disorder caused by variations in the inactivation mechanism of the Beta-globin (β-globin) genes. Despite seemingly similar genotypes, the patients with Beta-thalassemia have a remarkable variability in anaemia, growth development, and hepatospleenomegaly and transfusion requirements. The genetic factors may differ in each race or ethnic group for therapy and prevention. Despite remarkable successes in the treatment of Beta-thalassemia in the past decades, it is still the leading cause of death and premature disability in developed and developing countries. Possible factors that influence the severity of anaemia in thalassemia may be inherited or non-inherited. The inherited factors include the type of β-thalassemia, coinheritance of alpha thalassemia (α-thalassemia) and factors that stimulate fetal hemoglobin (HbF) production. In this chapter, respective contributions of known modifiers and also the pharmaceutical agents currently in use and under clinical trials for regulating the globin gene expression will be discussed.

Keywords: Hemoglobinopathies, gamma globin, fetal hemoglobin, modifier genes, drug discovery

1. Introduction

1.1. General introduction

The thalassemias are the commonest monogenic disorders in the world, and globally it is estimated that there are 270 million carriers, of which 80 million are carriers of β-thalassemia. β-thalassemia is widespread in the Mediterranean, Southeast Asian, African, and Middle East populations. The mean prevalence of this disease in India is 3.3%. It has become much more common recently in northern and central Europe, including Germany, due to immigration [1–

3]. The thalassemias refer to a diverse group of hemoglobin disorders characterized by a reduced synthesis of one or more of the globin chains (α, β, γ, δβ, γδβ, δ, and εγδβ). β-thalassemia occurs when there is a deficiency of β-globin, which is typically caused by a direct down-regulation in the synthesis of structurally normal b chains. However, a thalassemia phenotype can also arise from structural b chain variants if they are synthesized at a reduced rate. The most severe form of thalassemias is characterized by the complete absence of HbA ($\alpha_2\beta_2$) which results from the inheritance of two homozygous β-thalassemia alleles. This normally presents as a life-threatening anemia requiring blood transfusions from infancy. Inheritance of single β-thalassemia alleles is presented by a clinically asymptomatic condition, but may show a mild anemia [4].

More than 200 mutations of the β-globin gene which can lead to β-thalassemia major have been characterized worldwide [5–8]. Deletion mutations are rare; the majority of mutations are point mutations in important functional regions of the β-globin gene [9]. Splice mutations and those that occur in the promoter region tend to cause a reduction, rather than a complete absence of β-globin chains, and thus result in milder disease. Nonsense mutations and frameshift mutations tend not to produce any β-globin chains leading to severe disease (loss of function). The severity of anemia caused by β-thalassemia depends on which mutations are present and on whether they decrease beta-globin production (called beta$^+$ thalassemia) or there is complete elimination (called beta^0 thalassemia). A subset of common mutations is present in each ethnic group in which the disease is prevalent.

2. Clinical heterogenity in β-thalassemia

Clinical manifestations of β-thalassemia are extremely variable, ranging from nearly asymptomatic to severe and transfusion-dependant [10]. However, the marked variability of the clinical manifestations is not well-understood till date. The clinical picture in some patients may be a devastating course of acute and chronic events, resulting in severe organ damage. In other patients, the disease may be present with relatively mild clinical phenotype and minimal morbidity [11].

3. Factors influencing clinical severity

Various factors have been found to modulate the beta-thalassemia phenotype. These include the presence of alpha-thalassemia, elevated HbF levels, haplotypes that are linked to the beta-globin gene and chromosomal sites different from chromosome 11 [12]. Co-inheritance of a single alpha-globin (α-globin) gene deletion with β-thalassemia may have a milder phenotype, whereas deletion of both α-globin genes is typically associated with thalassemia intermedia [13]. Fetal hemoglobin is one of the most common and major modifiers of the disease severity in individuals with β-thalassemia. Because the severity of homozygous β-thalassemia is directly related to the imbalance between α- and β-globin chains, even the low levels of γ-globin in F cells reduce the relative excess of α-globin and provide a selective survival of cells making HbF at the time of ineffective erythropoiesis, in the most severe forms of β-thalassemia. Any factor that can reduce the degree of imbalance (by reducing α or increasing β and/or γ globin chains) may ameliorate the clinical phenotype [14]. Therefore, this selective survival might account for elevated levels of HbF in homozygous β-thalassemia. The presence of genetic variants that sustained fetal hemoglobin production have a strong impact on ameliorating the clinical phenotype.

4. Elevated levels of fetal hemoglobin (HbF)

HbF ($\alpha_2\gamma_2$) accounts for up to 90% of the total hemoglobin at birth. Its synthesis starts to decline during the third trimester, and over the first year of life, it is gradually replaced by adult Hb ($\alpha_2\beta_2$). An elevated level of HbF in an adult may result from a genetic disorder of hemoglobin production or from various acquired hematological conditions (such as placental insufficiency) in newborn infants of diabetic mothers, such as severe anemia, bronchopulmonary dysplasia (BPD), and congenital cyanotic heart (CCHD) [15–18]. Erythropoietic stress and hypoxemia has also been shown to increase the production of HbF [19–21]. Additional γ-globin chains bind with the excess of α-chains and decrease the imbalance between α- and β-globin chains caused because of absence of beta-globin chains, decreasing the deleterious effect of intracellular precipitation of unbound β-chains [22–23]. This reduces ineffective erythropoiesis and some functional HbF is produced in the red cell precursors which help red blood cells survive longer duration in the circulation. Induction of fetal haemoglobin expression in erythroid cells is an important therapeutic approach in patients with haemoglobin disease [24-25].

5. Genetic modifiers of γ-globin gene expression

To understand the clinical or molecular relationships, it is important to remember that the main pathophysiological determinant of the severity of beta-thalassemia is more than that of alpha/non-alpha-globin chain imbalance. Therefore, any factor capable of reducing the alpha/non-alpha-globin chain imbalance may have an ameliorating effect on the clinical picture [7]. Certain mutations within the β-globin promoter region are associated with increased γ-chain expression from the same chromosome [7]. These are known as primary modifiers. Recently, genetic variants that modulate HbF levels, but fall outside of the Hb genes (Secondary modifiers) have also been identified [26]. These modifiers, known as secondary modifiers, primarily act directly to alter the known pathophysiology of the disease.

5.1. Primary modifiers

Primary modifiers have been identified as different mutations within the β-globin gene resulting in varying severity. Severity of β-thalassemia ranges from the mutations (β0) causing complete absence of β-globin production to those in which β-globin is produced but to a small extent (β+). Inheritance of two β+ genes such as -28 ATA box (A → G) codon 19 (A → G); -90

C → T, -88 C → A; -88 C → T, -87 C → A; -87 C → G, -87 C → T; -86 C → G, 31 A → G results in a milder disease [27].

Some β-thalassemia mutations are completely silent and have been shown to cause a milder form of the disease. The most common is the -101 (C → T) mutation which interacts with different severe β-thalassemia alleles to produce a mild form of the disease [28]. Co-inheritance of severe β-thalassemia allele ($β^0$) with hemoglobin E (HbE) allele also results in variability of the phenotype. Alternative to the splicing of HbE globin pre-mRNA, the amount of mRNA spliced may also play a role in the phenotypic variability.

5.2. Secondary modifiers

Secondary genetic modifiers affect the clinical severity of the disease by reducing the globin chain imbalance, therefore resulting in a milder form of the disease phenotype [29]. Genome-wide studies (GWAS) have shown the association of genetic polymorphisms in three major loci Xmn1-HBG2, HBS1L-MYB intergenic region (HMIP) on chromosome 6q23, and BCL11A on chromosome 2p16, accountable for a relatively large proportion of the phenotypic variation in HbF levels. The gene encoding for zinc fingers and homeobox 2 (ZHX2) transcription factor located on 8q24 has emerged as a potential candidate gene for γ-globin regulation.

- Xmn-1 (Xanthomonas maniholis-1) Restriction Site

The presence of one polymorphism Xmn-1 restriction site at -158 position of the Gγ gene has been co-related with the increased production of HbF in adults under haematopoietic stress. A specific (C → T) mutation at the -158 position in the promoter region of the Gγ gene creates a restriction site for the Xmn-1 endonuclease. Higher expression of the fetal hemoglobin (HbF) in adulthood has been indicated to ameliorate the morbidity and mortality in sickle cell disease (SCD). Nemati et al. have studied the frequency of Xmn1 polymorphic sites in β-thalassemia major patients from Western Iran. The study revealed that the presence of this polymorphic site caused a positive influence on HbF production and the G-γ percent, which could improve the clinical symptoms of β-thalassemia patients [30]. In another study carried out by Pandey et al., the phenotypes of Indian sickle cell patients were found to be greatly influenced by Xmn1polymorphism [31].

In a recent study, we have evaluated the association of Xmn1 polymorphism with mild, moderate, and severe groups of β-thalassemia as well as sickle cell anemia (SCA). A significant association of TT genotype and T allele was observed with milder disease phenotype. In addition, we also evaluated the association of Xmn1 polymorphism with HbF levels to estimate whether this variant modifies the phenotype of homozygous β-thalassemia as well as SCA by modulating the HbF levels. A significant difference in the high and low percentage of HbF in CC, CT, and TT bearing individuals ($P<0.01$) were observed. This study confirms that increased γG-globin expression, associated with the Xmn1 polymorphism ameliorates the clinical severity in β-thalassemia as well as SCA in the study population [32].

- Zinc-fingers and homeoboxes 2 (ZHX2) gene

The gene coding for ZHX2 or KIAA0854 in human is located on chromosome 8q24.13 in the position 123863082-124055936. Four exons code for 837 amino acid protein of approximately

92 kDa. The ZHX2 mRNA is expressed among various tissues. ZHX2 is a transcriptional repressor [33] and has been identified as a factor which is involved in postnatal repression of fetal expressing genes [34]. Therefore, ZHX2 is a novel candidate gene for globin regulation in erythroid cells [35]. In 2005, Perencheri et al. indicated that overexpression of a ZHX2 transgene restores H19 repression on a BALB/cj background, confirming that this gene is responsible for hereditary persistence of the α-fetoprotein (Afp) and H19 which are transcribed at high levels in the mammalian fetal liver but are rapidly repressed postnatally [36]. Down-regulation of ZHX2 was recently demonstrated in two HPFH-2 subjects by real-time PCR [35].

ZHX2 gene coincides on the quantitative trait loci (QTL) on chromosome 8q that has been reported to influence the absolute fetalhemoglobin levels [37]. Taken together, ZHX2 is a good candidate gene for regulating γ-globin gene expression. Aussara Panya et al. demonstrated the effect of ZHX2 overexpression and the down-regulation of γ-globin expression in K562 cells [38]. Further, their study supported that ZHX2 is involved in the repression of the γ-globin gene, but also provides evidence that ZHX2 has a direct effect on the γ-globin expression level and might participate in the globin gene regulation [38]. In another study, de Andrade et al. reported the marked down-regulation of ZHX2 in CD34+ cells cultured in a high fetalhemoglobin-enriched condition [39].

- B-cell lymphoma/leukemia 11A (BCL11A) Gene

The BCL11A gene is essential for normal lymphoid development [40] and has been associated with hematologic malignancies [41]. The BCL11A gene was initially identified from aberrant chromosomal translocations involving the immunoglobulin-heavy chain locus detected in B-cell non-Hodgkin lymphomas [42]. It encodes a kruppel-link zinc finger protein containing 3 C_2H_2 zinc finger motifs, a proline-rich region, and an acidic domain. BCL11A gene located on chromosome 2p16.1 is expressed predominantly in the brain, spleen, and testis.

A study has demonstrated that an intronic SNP in BCL11A, rs11886868 strongly co-relates with HbF levels in a large cohort of sickle cell patients [43], this indicates that BCL11A variants, by modulating HbF levels, act as an important ameliorating factor of the SCA and it is likely they could help ameliorate other hemoglobin disorders. Genotyping of two other SNPs rs4671393 and rs7557939 in the Brazil Sickle cell disease cohorts have shown that these SNPs were more strongly associated with HbF level variation than rs11886868 [44].

In a recent study, we evaluated the association of rs11886868 of the BCL11A gene with mild, moderate, and severe groups of β-thalassemia and SCA. A significant association of CC genotype and C allele was observed with milder disease phenotype in β-thalassemia as well as SCA [45].

- Friend of Protein (FOP)

Friend of protein arginine methyltransferase I (FOP) has been reported to be one of the targets of protein arginine methyltransferase 1 (PRMT1), which stably interacts with chromatin [46]. Initially this protein was studied for its role in estrogen-dependent gene activation and in hemoglobin switching [46]. Studies have shown that knockdown of FOP in murine fetal liver cells transgenic for the β-globin locus significantly increased expression of both the mouse embryonic and human adult peripheral blood erythroid progenitors resulting in up-regulation of γ-globe and increased production of HbF [46]. As a result of this, HbF levels were reported to increase from background levels of 6% to 7% to an average of approximately 27%. It was observed that BCL11A levels were not altered interestingly, but levels of Sex determining region Y-box 6 (SOX6) protein appeared to be reduced. Therefore, there is a possibility that FOP depletion increases globin expression via reduction of SOX6.

- Sex determining region X-box 6 (SOX6 -SRY)

SOX6 plays an important role in the silencing of the embryonic globin genes. This gene encodes a member of the D subfamily of sex determining region y-related transcription factors. It is characterized by a conserved DNA-binding domain termed the high mobility group box and has the ability to bind the minor groove of DNA. The encoded protein is a transcriptional activator which is required for normal development of the central nervous system, chondrogenesis, and maintenance of cardiac and skeletal muscle cells. This protein interacts with other family members to activate gene expression. Alternative splicing leads to multiple transcript variants. First of all, SOX6 was observed to play a role in the silencing of the mouse embryonic globin genes. It binds to the murine γ-globin promoter as observed by Chromatin immune-precipitation [47]. It was also found that SOX6 interacts with BCL11A, although SOX6 strongly binds the globin gene promoters suggesting that the SOX6-BCL11A protein-protein interaction may involve chromatin looping [48]. SOX6 binding to the γ-globin promoters requires BCL11A. Studies have shown that the knockdown of SOX6 in cultured, primary human erythroblasts led to a small up-regulation of HbF but when combined with BCL11A knock-down, further enhanced HbF production [48].

- KLF1

KLF1, known as Erythroid Kruppel-like factor, is a zinc finger protein which binds the CACCC of the adult globin gene in mice as well as humans [49–50]. This protein is important for its expression responsible for ablation in mice causing embryonic lethality due to severe anemia [51–52]. Studies have shown that both endogenous mouse embryonic and human fetal globin gene expression are not properly down-regulated in the *Eklf*$^{-/-}$ mice. The haemoglobin switching role of this protein was identified in further studies [53–54]. A GWAS scan followed by linkage analysis of a family including 27 members showed that 10 out of 27 members had Hereditary persistence of fetalhemoglobin phenotype. In this study, a nonsense mutation in KLF1 gene was identified, which ablated the DNA binding domain, resulting in haploinsufficiency in the heterozygous state [53]. The HbF levels were found to vary among individual family members, indicating the influence of other genetic and environmental factors. In addition to the binding globin gene promoter, normal KLF1 was reported to show strong binding to the BCL11A promoter, thereby activating its expression in cultured, primary adult human erythroblasts. KLF1 has been found to mediate its switching effects through a dual mechanism, acting both on the globin and BCL11A promoters. Zhou et al. also found that reduced, but not absent, KLF1 levels in genetically altered mice resulted in markedly decreased levels of BCL11A mRNA and protein [54]. The researchers found that there was a strong binding of KLF1 to the Bcl11A promoter. Further, mouse embryonic and human fetal globin transgene expressions were found to be highly increased in the setting of reduced KLF1. Similar to this, it was found that when KLF1 was knocked down in cultured adult human erythroblasts, γ-globin gene expression was up-regulated [54]. Therefore, both compelling evidence from genetic and functional data suggests that KLF1 has a significant role in the fetal to adult switch. However, a 2- to 3-fold elevated expression in adult versus fetal cells, which results in KLF1's preferential association with the β-promoter in the former and the γ-promoters in the latter, is still not clear.

- HBSL1-MYB DNA region

In a GWAS, designed to identify polymorphisms associated with the variability of HbF expression in nonanemic humans, variants in the intergenic region between the HBSL1 and MYB genes were identified [55]. Data suggests that the intergenic area is most highly associated with HbF expression and consists of properties of a regulatory element [56]. The linkage to an equilibrium block, which is most closely associated with HbF levels, is between the HBS1L and MYB genes, which are present on opposite DNA strands. Three hypersensitive sites have been found within that region. These sites have been recognized as the characteristic marks of active chromatin, including histone acetylation and RNA polymerase II binding in erythroid, but not in nonerythroid cells [56]. HBS1L is supposed to be a housekeeping gene because it is ubiquitously expressed. Whereas MYB has more of a restrictive pattern of expression and is crucial for erythroid development.

Studies have compared the expression profiles of 5 genes within this region, including MYB and HBS1L, in the erythroid cultures of 12 persons with elevated and 14 persons with normal HbF levels [57]. In this study, both MYB and HBS1L were down-regulated in persons with elevated HbF levels, whereas the other 3 genes did not change in their level of expression. Overexpression of MYB inhibited-globin gene expression in human erythroleukemia cells, whereas overexpression of HBS1L was reported with no effect. The researchers speculated that low levels of MYB result in fewer cell-cycle events early in erythropoiesis and that early maturation of erythroblasts yields red cells containing higher levels of HbF [57]. Overall, MYB has a critical role in erythropoiesis, and studies suggest that it acts, in part, by transactivation of KLF1 and LMO2 expression. 84 studies involving genotyping and resequencing have found that rare missense mutations might provide further evidence for the involvement of MYB in modulating HbF levels [50].

- TR2/TR4 DR erythroid-definitive complex

A repressor of the human embryonic ε-globin gene, the direct repeat (DR) erythroid-definitive complex consists of a heterodimer of 2 orphan nuclear receptors, TR2 and TR4 [58–59]. In vitro studies have found that this dimer, along with the nuclear factor COUP TFII binds DRs in the ε-globin gene promoter. Later, it binds to a similar repeat with the γ-globin gene promoters [60]. Endogenous murine embryonic to adult globin gene and fetal to adult human γ-globin transgene switching is delayed in mice which are null for TR2/TR4. In contrast to this, enforced expression of a dominant negative TR4 results in both loss of endogenous embryonic gene expression and human γ-globin transgene silencing. A mutation at -117 of the γ-globin promoter was indicated to be associated with HPFH, thereby affecting a DR element and influencing factor binding, adding to the evidence that this heterodimer plays a role in stage-selective repression of the human γ-globin gene [61–62].

- COUP-TFII

COUP-TFII was known as one of the 2 factors required for transcription of the chicken ovalbumin gene [63]. COUP-TFII was later found to bind to the γ-globin promoter DR in vitro as well [64]. Mutation of DR elements resulted in derepression of γ-globin transgene expression in adult mice, indicating that DR sites are involved in fetal globin gene silencing. An in vitro model of primary human erythroblast development was used to show that the cytokine stem cell factor, through activation of the Erk1/2 and/or p38 mitogen activated protein kinase pathways, suppresses COUP-TFII expression at the mRNA and protein level, resulting in a large reduction in its binding to the γ-globin promoter.

- NF-E4

NF-E4 was identified as a component of the "stage selector protein," which binds to the stage selector element in the proximal-globin promoter in human K562 erythroleukemia cells; NF-E4, in conjunction with the ubiquitous transcription factor CP2, facilitates transcription of the γ-globin gene [65–66]. The stage selector element is conserved in species having γ-globin genes and is not present in species lacking HbF. The p22 NF-E4 acts as an "activator" of γ-globin transcription via interacting with CP2 to recruit p45 NF-E2 and subsequently RNA polymerase II to the promoter. Further evidence supporting a role for NFE4 in HbF production is that, an HPFH mutation at -202 creates a new binding site for the NF-E4-CP2 complex [67]. This alternate form, p14 NF-E4, apparently generated by translational initiation from an internal methionine, has been suggested to play a role in γ-globin gene down-regulation or silencing. The smaller isoform is abundant in adult erythroid cells, and although it did not bind the-globin promoter, it appears to interact with CP2 and might function to sequester NF-E2, which prevents complexing of activating factors at the γ-globin promoter. Enforced expression of p22 NF-E4 in transgenic mice harboring the human β-globin locus delayed the switch, without elevating the expression of HbF in the adult [67].

- GATA-1

GATA-1 is a member of zinc finger transcription factor and plays a seminal role in the development and differentiation of many cell types, including mega karyocytes, erythrocytes, eosinophils, and mast cells [68–69]. β-globin locus transcriptional activation can be resolved into discrete molecular steps involving the formation of distinct GATA-1 cofactor assemblies at the promoters and the Locus control region (LCR) [70]. Data suggest that GATA-1 can act both as a repressor and activator of gene transcription. Interaction between GATA-1 and the YY1 protein is involved in the silencing of the ε-globin gene in primate and non-primate species [71]. Moreover, binding of a GATA-1–FOG-1–NuRD complex was indicated to silence hematopoietic genes in erythroid cells [69, 72].

GATA-1 has multiple partners of proteins, including Stat3, Stat5, FOG-1, TAL-1, and Gfi-1b among others [73–75]. GATA-1 was firstly identified as a transactivator [73], however, its ability to mediate gene repression can be achieved through different DNA binding sequences, e.g. palindromic GATA-1 motifs and double GATA sites [76–77]. GATA-1 repressor activity has been implicated in naturally occurring mutations in the γ-globin genes which are associated with the persistent HbF synthesis after birth. These include point mutations at base -175 (T → C) and -173 (T → C) of the γ-globin promoter, which reduces GATA-1 binding and produces elevated HbF levels in humans and transgenic mice respectively [78]. Likewise, the -567 and -566 GATA-1 sites in the Gγ- and Aγ-globin promoter, respectively, have been found to be associated with gene silencing [79–80]. Amrolia et al. defined a repressor element in the γ-globin 5′-UTR, which was bound by a complex of two proteins, identified as GATA-1 and a ubiquitous negative regulator [81]. In a study, it was suggested that Stat3 binds the γ-globin 5′UTR to silence γ-globin transcription while GATA-1 binds the same region to enhance γ-promoter activity. Collectively, these studies suggest a model whereby GATA-1 acts as either a direct repressor or interacts with factors that bind nearby canonical sites to silence gene expression as proposed by Amrolia and co-workers [81].

In support for data provided by Harju-baker et al., a T3G mutation in the 567 GATA site of the gamma-globin gene in an Iranian-American family was reported to be associated with an HPFH phenotype by David Chui [80].

5.3. Induction of γ-globin gene expression

High HbF levels modulate the phenotype of the disease and ameloriate the severity of β-thalassemia and related complications led to an idea that reactivation of γ-globin gene will be a promising approach for the treatment of the disease [82–83]. Treatment strategies can be based on the following factors: an understanding pathophysiology of the disease; perspective of HbF to alter its manifestation; and that the developmental changes in γ-globin gene can be reversed by controling cellular and molecular regulatory mechanism [21]. Different classes of HbF inducers for clinical use have been reported.

Studies have shown that there are a number of inducers of the gamma-globin gene, like epigenetic modifiers of HbF and HbF inducers from the natural world.

- Epigenetic modifiers

If the molecular events occurring during haemoglobin switching are better understood, HbF expression could be more fully reactivated in adult cells and might lead to a cure for β-thalassemia.

The expression of human β-like globin genes are tissue- and developmental stage-specific in vivo. The mechanisms involved in the regulation of globin gene expression have been the subject of consideration for many years. Studies have led to the identification of cis- and trans-acting factors that regulate the expression of the β-globin gene cluster. Such studies also led to the recognition of the important role of epigenetic modifiers of globin gene expression. DNA methylation and histone acetylation are two of the most important epigenetic modifications that are involved in the regulation of most of the eukaryotic genes, including the genes of the globin family. Thus, targeting epigenetic silencing of the fetal globin genes can be a novel therapeutic approach for patients with β-thalassemia.

Epigenetic modifiers of HbF can be grouped in several classes, with different mechanisms of action. Different epigenetic modifiers of γ-globin gene are namely: erythropoietin, short chain fatty acids and cytotoxic agents, azacytidine, and hydroxycarbamide [84] (Table 1).

Many inducers inhibit histone deacethylase (HDAC) activity [85]. While most of the inducers exhibit inhibitory effects on cell growth, very few of them trigger increased γ-globin expression without effecting cell proliferation [86]. Erythroid precursor cells from β-thalassemia patients may differ in their response to the same inducer. Combined use of HbF inducers exhibiting different mechanism of action might improve the results.

- Cytotoxic agents

Observations that the use of cytotoxic agents helps to reactivate HbF synthesis during recovery from bone marrow suppression haves given hope on the possible use of cytotoxic agents for the treatment of serious haemoglobin disorders. Several cytotoxic agents that modify the pattern of erythropoiesis, increasing the expression of fetal (γ)-globin genes, have been explored over the past two decades [87–88]. Cytotoxic compounds put an end to actively cycling progenitors and control cellular growth to trigger rapid erythroid-regeneration and the formation of F cells. Cytotoxic drugs such as vinblastine [89], busulfan [90], cytosine arabinoside [91], and hydroxyurea [92–94] are known inducers of HbF in humans through this mechanism. Rapid regeneration of erythroid cells allows progenitors with an active eHbF program to be selectively recruited for maturation.

- Short-chain fatty acids (SCFAs)

Two different studies have reported that the infants of diabetic mothers have a delayed fetal-to-adult hemoglobin switch [95–96], while the exact underlying mechanisms are not clear, it is known that hydroxybutyrate is elevated during pregnancy induced diabeties in women. Perrine and colleagues observed that butyrate or other similar short chain fatty acids may act as effective inducers of fetal hemoglobin in sheep [95].

In support to the above observation, many other studies have shown that Sodium phenylbutyrate and arginine butyrate enhance both fetal and total hemoglobin levels in patients with sickle cell disease and beta thalassemia [97–106]. However, these SCFA derivatives also inhibit histone deacetylases, which generally inhibit erythroid cell proliferation. Therefore, these are not preferred as oral therapeutics that induce fetal (γ)-globin gene expression in beta hemoglobinopathies.

Loss of response to butyrates in long term therapy is observed which may be the result of antiproliferative effects on the bone marrow [107]. Two cohort studies have examined the efficacy of the oral butyrate derivative isobutyramide to induce HbF. In some studies no change in globin chain imbalance or in markers of ineffective erythropoiesis was noted, while in other study a drop in plasma free hemoglobin was observed. It has been suggested that the loss of response to long term butyrate therapy in patients with β-thalassemia may be because of the effects of these agents on other globin chains. It was shown that butyrate increases α-globin expression in progenitor-derived erythroid cells from patients with β-thalassemia. Thus, suggesting that the complementary effects of the butyrate-induced γ-globin expression on α/

β-chain imbalance in β-thalassemia may be decreased as a result of the associated increase in α-globin expression [108].

Using insilico modeling, Perrine and associates have tested several SCFA derivatives to deduce the functional group(s) required for γ-globin reactivation [109]. Compounds such as phenoxyacetic acid, and 2, 2 dimethylbutyric acid and α-methyl hydrocinnamic acid, induce Stat-5 cell signaling and the growth-related immediate early genes c-myc and cmyb to achieve HbF induction independent of HDAC inhibition; butyrate has similar effects [101,110].

Short chain fatty acids, like Phenylbutyrate and Valproic acid, are also known to induce HbF levels in vivo [111–112]. Animal model studies have shown that propionate, phenyl acetic, and phenylalkyl acids induces HbF in baboons, transgenic mice, cultures, and in primates [103, 113–115].

- DNA methyl transferase (DNMT) inhibitors

DNA methylation is an epigenetic method of modulating gene expression carried out by enzyme DNA methyltransferases (DNMT) in both eukaryotes and prokaryotes [116]. These enzymes catalyze the addition of a methyl group from a donor S-adenosylmethionine to the 5′ position of cytosine, predominantly within the CpG dinucleotide [117–118].

CpG methylation in the promoter of adult erythroid cells is known to silence γ-globin gene expression [119]. The cytosine analogues such as, 5-azacytidine and 5-aza-2′-deoxycytidine (decitabine), are known to inhibit DNMTs and can be used to reactivate γ-gene expression [120–122].

The γ-globin genes are structurally and functionally similar in baboons and humans and are developmentally silenced by methylation of CpG residues [123]. 5-Azacytidine was shown to increase HbF levels in baboons and sickle cell patients, but concerns over the carcinogenic effect of 5-azacytidine hampered its development for human treatment [124–126].

Another DNA methylation inhibitor adenosine-2 3-dialdehyde (Adox) is known to inhibit both DNA methylation and protein methylation including histone tail methylation. It is known to inhibit adenosylhomocysteine hydrolase activity, thereby indirectly inhibiting methyltransferases that catalyze adenosylmethionine to adenosylhomocysteine [127]. In order to test the effect of Adox to induce γ-globin, He et al. performed a series of studies. Firstly, they treated K562 cells and showed a dose response effect on activation. Next, they performed a time-course analysis of γ-globin induction by Adox. They observed that from day two, γ-globin expression was readily detected, but after day six, induction stopped suggesting that Adox could induce γ-globin very quick and it could also be metabolized during cell proliferation. Adox also induced a dose-dependent inhibition of in vitro proliferation of K562 cells. They also performed bisulfite DNA sequencing experiments on globin genes. Using decitabine as a positive control, they found that Adox significantly reduced DNA methylation. Together, these results suggested that Adox was a potent inducer of γ-globin expression in K562 cells [128].

In their previous study, the levels of histone mark H4R3me2s on the γ-globin promoter triggered by PRMT5 were significantly reduced in Adox-treated and decitabine-treated cells compared to untreated cells. PRMT5 inhibition by Adox treatment followed a dose response that occurred over the same drug concentration range as γ-globin induction, indicating specificity of Adox for γ-globin gene.

However, DNA hypomethylation by Adox treatment may not be a major cause of the reactivation γ-globin expression in human β-thalassemia cells. But we can't exclude the possibility that by Adox treatment, different erythroid specific transcription factors play roles upon γ-globin induction. Alternatively, histone modification or repressor complex (e.g., NURD complex) reconstitution might also contribute to the γ-globin gene reactivation [129–131].

- Histone Deacetylase (HDAC) inhibitors

Histone deacetylases (HDACs) remove the acetyl group from histones resulting in the formation of tightly supercoiled, transcriptionally silent, "heterochromatin" structure that exerts antagonistic epigenetic controls on gene expression through chromatin re-modeling resulting in gene activation or repression [132–136]. HDACs are also known to deacetylase non-histone proteins, including many regulatory genes and transcriptional factors involved in cell signalling path and metabolism [137–138]. These observations suggest that HDACs plays an important role as co-repressors and co-activators of gene expression [139].

Till now, 18 mammalian HDAC genes have been identified that have been classified into four groups based on sequence homologies and catalytic mechanism [138, 140]. Class I includes HDACs 1-3, 8 and are expressed ubiquitously and consist mainly of a deacetylase domain. Class II includes HDACs 4-7 and 9-10, and are highly expressed in muscle, brain, and T cells [141]. Class I, II, and IV HDACs are evolutionarily related Zn^{+}-dependent hydrolases whereas, Class III HDACs have homology with yeast HDAC, silent information regulator 2, and use nicotinamide adenine dinucleotide as a co-substrate [142]. They have an extended N-terminus, which serves as a target for post-translational modifications and protein-protein interactions, such as phosphorylation, important for their function and governing nuclear-cytoplasmic shuttling [143].

A study by Forsberg et al. have shown that some specific histone acetylation patterns play a role in β-globin switch in murines, suggesting that the HDACs might participate in a complex mechanism of γ-globin repression, hence can be used for pharmacological reactivation of γ-globin expression [85, 144].

Shalini et al. (2010) screened Class II HDAC family members. They choose this class because they are highly tissue-specific in expression and have nuclear localization and import signals required for cell proliferation and differentiation [145–147]. Histone deacetylase inhibitors, including sodium butyrate (NaB) and trichostatin A (TSA) and hemin are known to significantly alter the mRNA levels of HDAC7, -9, and -10 and histone deacetylase-related protein (HDRP) at the same time activating γ-globin expression, as the result of loss in HDAC activity at the promoter or can also be because of changes in the expression of other genes [147]. This was verified by studying siHDAC9 in K562 cells, a dose-dependent decrease in γ-globin gene expression was observed, where forced expression of HDAC9 reactivated the γ-globin expression [147]. This study suggests that HDAC9 might have a positive role in regulating γ-globin expression.

A rapid and efficient method for detecting HbF inducers, based on a recombinant DNA construct was developed by Skarpidi and colleagues [148]. In this method, the coding sequences of the firefly and renilla luciferase genes were substituted for the human γ-globin and β-globin genes, respectively. Many new HDAC inhibitors were identified in this system and were further confirmed in human erythroid progenitor cultures [148]. With the help of the same reporter system, Makala and Pace found a stable reporter system in human KU812 cells [149]. The chemical analogues of HDAC inhibitor FK228 were identified as novel HbF inducers in primary erythroid progenitors. Last two decades has seen tremendous growth to identify other agents, systems with the help of high throughput screening techniques. Using this approach, selective HDAC 1/2 inhibitors (e.g., ACY-957) which induced HbF were reported [150]. Studies with ACY-957 have demonstrated elevated HbF expression in human erythroid progenitors [151].

Inducer	Mechanism of action	References (a)
Peptiole nucleic acids (PNAs)	Artificial promoters	Wang et al. (1999)
Cisplatin and analogues	DNA-binding drug	Bianchi et al. (2000)
Triple-helix oligodeoxynucleotides	Activation of γ-globin gene promote	Xu et al. (2000)
Trichostatin	HDAC inhibitors	Marianna et al. (2001)
Tallimustine and analogues	DNA-binding drug	Bianchi et al. (2001)
Angelicin	DNA-binding drug	Lampronti et al. (2003)
Mithramycin	DNA-binding drug	Fibach et al. (2003)
Citarabine	Hypomethylation of DNA	Sauthararajah et al, 2003
Hydroxyurea	Inhibition of DNA synthesis	Fibach et al. (2003)
Apicidin	HDAC inhibitors	Witt et al. (2003)
Rapamycin	FRAP-mTOR signal transduction	Mischiati et al. (2003) Fibach et al. (2006)
Scriptaid	HDAC inhibitors	Johnson et al. (2005)

Table 1. Inducers of Fetal Hemoglobin in Erythroid Precursor Cells from Human Donors

5.4. Other novel agents under development

Usually, developing a novel agent from bench to bedside takes more than 20 years on an average; thus, repurposing that FDA approved agents is a strategy encouraged by drug companies and government funding agents to expand the agents available to treat β-hemoglobinopathies. One such agent is the FDA approved Tecfidera (dimethyl fumarate), used for the treatment of multiple sclerosis. This agent acts via mediating immunemodulatory actions [152] with limited side effects. Dimethyl fumarate activates NRF2 signaling involved in drug mediated HbF induction [153–154]. Researchers have reported that dimethyl fumarate induces γ-globin expression in KU812 and primary erythroid cells generated from sickle cell patients, thereby supporting repurposing of Tecfidera for SCD [155].

Another FDA approved agent pomalidomide is under development for SCD. This agent stimulates proliferation of erythroid progenitors and HbF induction [156]. In a pre-clinical study, pomalidomide was investigated in the SCD knockout transgenic mouse produced by Townes and colleagues and was shown to induce HbF similar to hydroxylurea without myelo suppression. This study led to a Phase 1 clinical trial completion [157–159].

Preclinical studies to support the repurpose of the monoamine oxidase inhibitor tranylcypromine for SCD have been completed. The nuclear receptors TR2 and TR4 repress γ-globin expression by association with the co-repressors DNMT1 and lysine-specific demethylase 1 (LSD1) [58–59]. LSD1 removes methyl groups from mono- and dimethyl histone H3 lysine 4 producing an activating epigenetic signature [160]. The role of LSD1 in globin gene regulation in human erythroid cells was examined by Shi and colleagues [161]. They demonstrated that LSD1 was inhibited by tranylcypromine which mediated and enhanced HbF expression. Subsequent pre-clinical studies using β-YAC transgenic mice treated with tranylcypromine produced HbF induction. This served the basis for a clinical trial to test the ability of this agent in order to induce HbF in β-hemoglobinopathy patients [16].

5.5. Clinical development of HbF inducer

Till date, the most successful HbF inducer in the pharmacological armamentarium of drugs is Hydroxurea (HU). The first description of HU treatment in patients with SCD dates back to the year 1984 [162]. Since then, HU was found to elevate HbF levels and decrease the clinical complications of SCD and finally in 1998 it became the only FDA approved drug for SCD. In a Multicenter Study of Hydroxyurea (MSH), adult subjects with SCD were randomized on HU therapy or placebo and individuals in the HU group had ~50% reduction in vaso-occlusive rates [163]. Patients with maximal change in HbF levels had the highest reduction in white blood cell counts, indicating a hematologic response was associated with the clinical response [164]. The MSH data also demonstrated that treatment with HU was not associated with significant toxicities and was effective at reducing healthcare costs associated with complications due to SCD [163, 165]. Long-term follow up of MSH patients up to 17.5 years reported that there was a reduction in mortality [166]. Similar to these results, it was observed in the 17-year open label Laikon Study of HU in Sickle Cell Syndromes [167]; the probability of 10-year survival was 86% and 65% for HU and non-HU patients, respectively [167].

5.6. HU treatment in children

The efficacy and safety in adult trials was proved, and therefore the investigations of HU were undertaken in children. A pilot study of HU (HUSOFT) was conducted in 28 children with SCD where HU therapy was found to be feasible, well tolerated, and efficacious in young children. In addition, based on liver, spleen scans, HU could possibly delay functional asplenia [168]. Long-term follow-up data of patients in the HUSOFT extension study showed a reduction in acute SCD complications, improved splenic function, and improved growth rates in children taking HU therapy [169]. Based on these findings, BABY-HUG, a Phase III randomized controlled trial, was conducted in children with SCD (mean age 13.6 months) [170]. The primary endpoints of improved splenic function and renal glomerular filtration rates were not achieved. HU was effective at reducing the acute complications of SCD, such as pain episodes, dactylitis, acute chest syndrome, and red blood transfusions [170]. The researchers were interested to use HU to prevent the long-term organ damage of SCD or to avoid chronic transfusions for children with severe phenotypes. Evidence of organ protection from HU in the current literature led to investigations of HU in this setting [171–173]. The Stroke With Transfusions Changing to Hydroxyurea (SWiTCH) study was a Phase III multicentred randomized trial compared the HU or phlebotomy with transfusions and chelation for the prevention of secondary stroke and reduction of transfusion iron overload [174–175]. There were no subsequent strokes on the transfusions/chelation arm but (10%) on the HU/phlebotomy arm. No major difference in liver iron content was found between the groups; therefore, the study was closed early. The investigators confirmed that the transfusions and chelation remain the standard of management of children with SCD and stroke complicated by iron overload [174]. Moreover, the studies in children have yet to demonstrate a role of HU in the prevention or management of chronic complications.

5.7. Natural inducers

Recently, scientists have conducted many studies to identify the natural remedies that could possibly be applied for the treatment of β-thalassemia (Table 2) [176]. Several studies have found that the extracts from medicinal plants for biomedical purposes [177–186] including therapeutic strategies can be used for the treatment of a number of diseases.

In case of hemoglobinopathies, only a few examples are available. For instance, the extract of Aegle Marmelos containing bergatene was found to activate erythroid differentiation and HbF induction in human leukemic K562 cells [187–188]. Citropten and bergatene are the two active ingredients in bergamot juice. They are potent inducers of Erythroid cell differentiation, $^{G}\gamma$-globin gene expression and fetal hemoglobin synthesis in human erythroid cells. Thus, it is known as a possible therapeutic approach for both β-thalassemia and Sickle cell anemia [187].

Another example of HbF inducer from the natural world is Angelicin, which can be found in the fruit of *Angelica arcangelica.* There is evidence demonstrating that angelicin is a strong inducer of Erythroid cell differentiation, improvement of the HbF synthesis, and γ-globin mRNA accumulation of human leukemia K562 cells [84, 179]. Red wine, particularly the skin of black grapes, contains resveratrol which mimics the HbF-inducing activity of HU. Its role in increasing the γ-globin mRNA in human erythroid precursors has been confirmed [84]. Since β-thalassemia cells present a high level of oxidative stress resulting in short time survival of erythroid cells in β-thalassemia patients, resveratrol which exhibits both antioxidant activity and HbF inducing property can be a very good HbF inducer from the natural world [88].

Rapamycin, which is isolated from *Streptomyces hygroscopicus,* is a bacterial species found in soil of Easter Island has the capability of increasing HbF production in cultures of erythroid precursors from β-thalassemia patients without any cytotoxicity or growth-inhibitory effect. Apart from Rapamycin, Mithramycin is a DNA-binding drug that is easily isolated from Streptomyces has the potential to induce γ-globin mRNA accumulation and HbF production in erythroid cells from healthy subjects as well as β-thalassemia patients [189].

Inducer	Source	Biological effects	References
Bergaptene	*A. marmelos*	Erythroid differentiation of K562 cells	Lampronti et al. (2003)
Angelicin	*A. arcangelica*	HbF production	Lampronti et al. (2003)
Rapamycin	*S. hygroscopicus*	HbF production	Mischiati et al. (2004)
Resveratrol	Redwine, grape skin and darakchasava	HbF production	Rodrigue et al. (2001)
Mithramycn	*Streptomyces* species	HbF production	Bianchi et al. (1999)
YiSui ShengXue Granule		Erythroid survival, proliferation, and terminaldifferentiation of K562 cells and HbF production	Zhang and Wu (2008)
Cucurbitacn D	Ethanol extract of Fructus trichosanthis, which is the fruit of Trichosanthes kirilowii MAXIM	HbF production and Erythroid differentiation of K562cells	Liu et al. (2010); Li et al. (2011)
Terminalia catappa distilled water active fraction (TCDWF)	*Terminalia catappa leaves*	Erythropoiesis, cell proliferation, and transcription	Aimola et al. (2014)

Table 2. Inducers of HbF from natural sources

6. Discussion and conclusion

The Human Genome Project has improved efforts of developing gene-based therapy for β-hemoglobinopathies alongside chemical inducers. GWAS have found certain major genetic modifiers of γ-globin, including -158 XmnI HBG2, HBS1-MYB and BCL11A accounting for ~50% of inherited HbF variance [190–191]. Orkin and colleagues advanced the field significantly by defining mechanisms through which BCL11A repressed γ-globin expression and holds the promise for the development of gene-based therapy in the future.

The occurrence of inherited mutations in KLF1 that produce HPFH suggested that this factor is a viable target for gene therapy and might be accomplished by RNAi technology to create a haploinsufficiency state. Promising molecular targets such as KLF1 and BCL11A for therapeutic efforts aimed at HbF induction have been identified: however, additional pre-clinical data are needed before manipulation of transcription factors can be translated into therapeutic options at the bedside.

Agents which improve HbF synthesis represent a rational approach for the treatment of β-thalassemia. For more than three decades, many chemical agents have been tested in tissue culture as HbF inducers, but few have crossed the path from clinical trials and have reached to the bedside. One major roadblock is the lack of suitable pre-clinical models to test agents in vivo. Baboon studies led to the clinical development of HU, butyrate, decitabine, and

HQK-1001 in SCD and β-thalassemia [93, 120–121, 124–125, 192–197]. With the establishment of SCD mouse models, newer agents such as pomalidomide have been progressed to clinical trials, however, the limited availability of the knockout SCD mouse model has affected progress in this area [155]. Townes and colleagues had designed a second knockin SCD mouse model with γ-globin and β-globin constructs [157]. However, HbF induction has not been effectively achieved with HU therapy (Pace, unpublished data). Therefore, the knock-in mouse may not be ideal for future pre-clinical drug screens. An alternative model, the β-YAC mouse was used to confirm in vivo HbF induction by 5-azacytidine, scriptaid, and transcyclomide showing the utility of this mouse for pre-clinical drug screening [161, 198–199]. Currently, very few agents are in clinical trials targeting HbF induction and drugs aimed at other complications of SCD, such as nitric oxide deficiency, endothelium antagonist, anti-platelet agents, anti-sickle agents, and so forth are still under development (clinicaltrials.gov). These can be combined with HU or other HbF inducers to produce an additive or synergistic clinic benefit [155].

Despite the success of HU in clinical trials conducted on adults and children and its proven safety and efficacy, it remains underutilized in SCD [163–164, 166, 168–170, 173, 200–201]. Possible causes include: (1) limited access to comprehensive sickle cell medical care; 2) lack of coordination between subspecialists and community based clinicians; 3) concern over potential genotoxicity; and 4) lack of patient adherence with the medication regimen. Future studies are needed to address early initiation of HU, the role of HU therapy in prevention of chronic complications, and improved methods for HU therapy delivery to all patients with SCD. There remains a question about the optimal age to initiate HU therapy. The Baby HUG trial established safety in young children, but additional clinical safety data are needed for children <6 months at the highest risk of infection and spleen and kidney dysfunction. Whether the early HU therapy administration will prevent the γ- to β-globin switch has not been demonstrated.

Curative therapy for SCD and β-thalassemia includes hematopoietic stem cell transplantation, however, this option is limited by the availability of suitable donors in <20% of children with SCD [202–203]. Ongoing clinical trials exploring alternative approaches such as matched unrelated donors and the development of new regimens using haplo-identical donors in the future will increase the transplant option for the majority of SCD patients [204]. Another approach to cure β-hemoglobinopathies is efforts to develop gene therapy, e.g., recently there was a successful treatment of two β-thalassemia patients with a modified β-globin lentivirus based vector. This progress holds promise for SCD patients [205–206].

Landmark studies have developed an excitement that fully differentiated somatic cells can be reprogrammed to make induced pluripotent stem cells [207]. Subsequent studies demonstrated rectification of a mouse model of SCD using this innovative approach, therefore opened the way to the use of these cells to cure β-hemoglobinopathies beside few limitations [208]. One limitation was the inability to restore all hematopoietic lineages with induced pluripotent stem cells which precludes using human therapy [209]. Therefore, until transplantation and gene therapy is more widely available, chemical inducers of HbF remain the most effective way to treat β-thalassemia and SCD.

Author details

Anjana Munshi[1*], Sneha Dadeech[2], M. Sai Babu[2] and Preeti Khetarpal[1]

*Address all correspondence to: anjanadurani@yahoo.co.in

1 Centre for Human Genetics, Central University of Punjab, Bathinda, India

2 Department of Molecular Biology, Institute of Genetics and Hospital for Genetic Diseases, Osmania University, Hyderabad, India

References

[1] Galehdari H, Salehi B, Azmoun S, Keikhaei B, Zandian KM, Pedram M. Comprehensive spectrum of the β-Thalassemia mutations in Khuzestan, southwest Iran. Hemoglobin. 2010; 34(5):461-8.

[2] Kohne E. Hemoglobinopathies: clinical manifestations, diagnosis, and treatment. Dtsch Arztebl Int. 2011; 108(31-32):532-40.

[3] Trehan A, Sharma N, Das R, Bansal D, Marwaha RK. Clinicoinvestigational and demographic profile of children with thalassemia major. Indian J Hematol Blood Transfus. 2015; 31(1):121-6.

[4] Thein SL. Pathophysiology of beta thalassemia—a guide to molecular therapies. Hematology Am Soc Hematol Educ Program. 2005:31-7.

[5] Weatherall DJ. Phenotype-genotype relationships in monogenic disease: lessons from the thalassaemias. Nat Rev Genet. 2001; 2(4):245-55.

[6] Rund D, Rachmilewitz E. Beta-thalassemia. N Engl J Med. 2005; 353(11):1135-46.

[7] Cao A, Galanello R. Beta-thalassemia. Genet Med. 2010; 12(2):61-76.

[8] Thein SL. Genetic association studies in β-hemoglobinopathies. Hematology Am Soc Hematol Educ Program. 2013; 2013:354-61.

[9] Galanello R, Origa R. Beta-thalassemia. Orphanet J Rare Dis. 2010; 5:11.

[10] Cao A, Moi P, Galanello R. Recent advances in β-thalassemias. Pediatr Rep. 2011; 3(2):17.

[11] Nienhuis AW, Nathan DG. Pathophysiology and Clinical Manifestations of the β-Thalassemias. Cold Spring Harb Perspect Med. 2012; 2(12):011726.

[12] Olivieri NF, Pakbaz Z, Vichinsky E. Hb E/beta-thalassaemia: a common & clinically diverse disorder. Indian J Med Res. 2011; 134:522-31.

[13] Premawardhena A, De Silver S, Arambepola M, Olivieri NF, Vichinsky EP, Merson L, Muraco G, Allen A, Fisher C, Peto T, Weatherall DJ. Hemoglobin E-beta-thalassemia: Progress report from the International Study Group. Ann N Y Acad Sci. 2005; 1054:33-9.

[14] Joly P, Pondarre C, Badens C. Beta-thalassemias: molecular, epidemiological, diagnostical and clinical aspects. Ann Biol Clin (Paris). 2014; 72(6):639-668.

[15] Bard H, Prosmanne J. Relative rates of fetal hemoglobin and adult hemoglobin synthesis in cord blood of infants of insulin-dependent diabetic mothers. Pediatrics. 1985; 75(6): 1143-7.

[16] Bard H, Prosmanne J. Elevated levels of fetal hemoglobin synthesis in infants with bronchopulmonary dysplasia. Pediatrics. 1990; 86(2):193-6.

[17] Bard H, Lachance C, Widness JA, Gagnon C. The reactivation of fetal hemoglobin synthesis during anemia of prematurity. Pediatr Res. 1994; 36(2):253-6.

[18] Bard H, Gagnon C, Peri KG. HbF synthesis during stress erythropoiesis as determined by gamma-mRNA/non-alpha-mRNA quantification. Pediatr Res. 1999; 45(51):684-6.

[19] Bard H. The effect of placental insufficiency on fetal and adult hemoglobin synthesis. Am J Obstet Gynecol. 1974; 120(1):67-72.

[20] Blau CA. Therapy for globin-chain disorders. N Engl J Med. 1993; 329(5):364.

[21] Stamatoyannopoulos G, Nienhuis AW. Therapeutic approaches to hemoglobin switching in treatment of hemoglobinopathies. Annu Rev Med. 1992; 43:497-521.

[22] Karimi M, Haghpanah S, Taher AT, Cappellini MD. β-Thalassemia: New Therapeutic Modalities, Genetics, Complications, and Quality of Life. Anemia. 2012; 2012:902067.

[23] Breda L, Rivella S, Zuccato C, Gambari R. Combining gene therapy and fetal hemoglobin induction for treatment of β-thalassemia. Expert Rev Hematol. 2013; 6(3): 255-64.

[24] Fathallah H, Atweh GF. DNA hypomethylation therapy for hemoglobin disorders: molecular mechanisms and clinical applications. Blood Rev. 2006; 20(4):227-34.

[25] Ronzoni L, Sonzogni L, Fossati G, Modena D, Trombetta E, Porretti L, Cappellini MD. Modulation of gamma globin genes expression by histone deacetylase inhibitors: an in vitro study. Br J Haematol. 2014; 165(5):714-21.

[26] Mtatiro SN, Makani J, Mmbando B, Thein SL, Menzel S, Cox SE. Genetic variants at HbF-modifier loci moderate anemia and leukocytosis in sickle cell disease in Tanzania. Am J Hematol. 2015; 90(1):1-4.

[27] Svasti S, Paksua S, Nuchprayoon I, Winichagoon P, Fucharoen S. Characterization of a novel deletion causing (deltabeta)0-thalassemia in a Thai family. Am J Hematol. 2007; 82(2):155-61.

[28] Weatherall DJ. Phenotype-genotype relationships in monogenic disease: lessons from the thalassaemias. Nat Rev Genet. 2001; 2(4):245-55.

[29] Galanello R, Origa R. Beta-thalassemia. Orphanet J Rare Dis. 2010; 5:11.

[30] Nemati H, Rahimi Z, Bahrami G. The Xmn1 polymorphic site 5' to the (G)gamma gene and its correlation to the (G)gamma:(A)gamma ratio, age at first blood transfusion and clinical features in beta-thalassemia patients from Western Iran. Mol Biol Rep. 2010; 37(1):159-64.

[31] Pandey S, Pandey S, Mishra RM, Sharma M, Saxena R. Genotypic influence of α-deletions on the phenotype of Indian sickle cell anemia patients. Korean J Hematol. 2011; 46(3):192-5.

[32] Dadheech S, Jain S, Madhulatha D, Sharma V, Joseph J, Jyothy A, Munshi A. Association of Xmn1 -158 γG variant with severity and HbF levels in β-thalassemia major and sickle cell anaemia. Mol Biol Rep. 2014; 41(5):3331-7.

[33] Kawata H, Yamada K, Shou Z, Mizutani T, Yazawa T, Yoshino M, Sekiguchi T, Kajitani T, Miyamoto K. Zinc-fingers and homeoboxes (ZHX) 2, a novel member of the ZHX family, functions as a transcriptional repressor. Biochem J. 2003; 373(3):747-57.

[34] Spear BT, Jin L, Ramasamy S, Dobierzewska A. Transcriptional control in the mammalian liver: liver development, perinatal repression, and zonal gene regulation. Cell Mol Life Sci. 63(24):2922-38.

[35] de Andrade TG, Peterson KR, Cunha AF, Moreira LS, Fattori A, Saad ST, Costa FF. Identification of novel candidate genes for globin regulation in erythroid cells containing large deletions of the human beta-globin gene cluster. Blood Cells Mol Dis. 2006; 37(2):82-90.

[36] Perincheri S, Dingle RW, Peterson ML, Spear BT. Hereditary persistence of alpha-fetoprotein and H19 expression in liver of BALB/cJ mice is due to a retrovirus insertion in the Zhx2 gene. Proc Natl Acad Sci U S A. 2005; 102(2):396-401.

[37] Garner C, Silver N, Best S, Menzel S, Martin C, Spector TD, Thein SL. Quantitative trait locus on chromosome 8q influences the switch from fetal to adult hemoglobin. Blood. 2004; 104(7):2184-6.

[38] Aussara Panyaa, Nunghathai Sawasdeeb, Chatchawan Srisawata, Pa-thai Yenchitsomanusb, Chayanon Peerapittayamongkola. Expression of zinc finger and homeobox 2 in erythroleukaemic cells and gamma-globin expression. ScienceAsia. 2010; 36:342-345.

[39] De Andrade T, Moreira L, Duarte A, Lanaro C, De Albuquerque D, Saad S, Costa F. Expression of new red cell-related genes in erythroid differentiation. Biochem Genet. 2010; 48(1-2):164-71.

[40] Liu P, Keller JR, Ortiz M, Tessarollo L, Rachel RA, Nakamura T, Jenkins NA, Copeland NG. Bcl11a is essential for normal lymphoid development. Nat. Immunol. 2003; 4:525-532.

[41] Weniger MA, Pulford K, Gesk S, Ehrlich S, Banham AH, Lyne L, Martin-Subero JI, Siebert R, Dyer MJ, Möller P, Barth TF. Gains of the proto-oncogene BCL11A and nuclear accumulation of BCL11A(XL) protein are frequent in primary mediastinal B-cell lymphoma. Leukemia. 2006; 20(10):1880-2.

[42] Satterwhite E, Sonoki T, Willis TG, Harder L, Nowak R, Arriola EL, Liu H, Price HP, Gesk S, Steinemann D, Schlegelberger B, Oscier DG, Siebert R, Tucker PW, Dyer MJ. The BCL11 gene family: involvement of BCL11A in lymphoid malignancies. Blood. 2001; 98(12):3413-20.

[43] Uda M, Galanello R, Sanna S, Lettre G, Sankaran VG, Chen W, Usala G, Busonero F, Maschio A, Albai G, Piras MG, Sestu N, Lai S, Dei M, Mulas A, Crisponi L, Naitza S, Asunis I, Deiana M, Nagaraja R, Perseu L, Satta S, Cipollina MD, Sollaino C, Moi P, Hirschhorn JN, Orkin SH, Abecasis GR, Schlessinger D, Cao A. Genome-wide association study shows BCL11A associated with persistent fetal hemoglobin and amelioration of the phenotype of beta-thalassemia. Proc Natl Acad Sci U S A. 2008; 105(5): 1620-5.

[44] Lettre G, Sankaran VG, Bezerra MA, Araújo AS, Uda M, Sanna S, Cao A, Schlessinger D, Costa FF, Hirschhorn JN, Orkin SH. DNA polymorphisms at the BCL11A, HBS1L-MYB, and beta-globin loci associate with fetal hemoglobin levels and pain crises in sickle cell disease. Proc Natl Acad Sci U S A. 2008; 105(33):11869-74.

[45] SnehaDadheech, D. Madhulatha D, SumanJjain, James Joseph , A Jyothy, AnjanaMunshi. Association of BCL11A Genetic Variant (rs11886868) with severity in β-Thalassemia Major and Sickle Cell Anemia. Indian J Med Res (2015) (Accepted for publication in IJMR).

[46] van Dijk TB, Gillemans N, Pourfarzad F, van Lom K, von Lindern M, Grosveld F, Philipsen S. Fetal globin expression is regulated by Friend of Prmt1. Blood. 2010; 116(20):4349-52.

[47] Yi Z, Cohen-Barak O, Hagiwara N, Kingsley PD, Fuchs DA, Erickson DT, Epner EM, Palis J, Brilliant MH. Sox6 directly silences epsilon globin expression in definitive erythropoiesis. PLoS Genet. 2006; 2(2):14.

[48] Xu J, Sankaran VG, Ni M, Menne TF, Puram RV, Kim W, Orkin SH. Transcriptional silencing of gamma-globin by BCL11A involves long-range interactions and cooperation with SOX6. Genes Dev. 2010; 24(8):783-798.76.

[49] Miller IJ, Bieker JJ. A novel, erythroid cell-specific murine transcription factor that binds to the CACCC element and is related to the Kruppel family of nuclear proteins. Mol Cell Biol. 1993; 13(5):2776-2786.

[50] Donze D, Townes TM, Bieker JJ. Role of Erythroid Kruppel-like factor in huma gamma- to beta-globin gene switching. J Biol Chem. 1995; 270(4):1955-1959.

[51] Perkins AC, Sharpe AH, Orkin SH. Lethal betathalassaemia in mice lacking the Erythroid CACCC-transcription factor EKLF. Nature. 1995; 375(6529):318-322.

[52] Nuez B, Michalovich D, Bygrave A, Ploemacher R, Grosveld F. Defective haematopoiesis in fetal liver resulting from inactivation of the EKLF gene. Nature. 1995; 375(6529):316-318.

[53] Borg J, Papadopoulos P, Georgitsi M, Gutiérrez L, Grech G, Fanis P, Phylactides M, Verkerk AJ, van der Spek PJ, Scerri CA, Cassar W, Galdies R, van Ijcken W, Ozgür Z, Gillemans N, Hou J, Bugeja M, Grosveld FG, von Lindern M, Felice AE, Patrinos GP, Philipsen S. Haploinsufficiency for the erythroid transcription factor KLF1 causes hereditary persistence of fetal hemoglobin. Nat Genet. 2010; 42(9):801-805.

[54] Zhou D, Liu K, Sun CW, Pawlik KM, Townes TM. KLF1 regulates BCL11A expression and gamma- to beta-globin gene switching. Nat Genet. 2010; 42(9):742-744.

[55] Thein SL, Menzel S, Peng X, Best S, Jiang J, Close J, Silver N, Gerovasilli A, Ping C, Yamaguchi M, Wahlberg K, Ulug P, Spector TD, Garner C, Matsuda F, Farrall M, Lathrop M. Intergenic variants of HBS1L-MYB are responsible for a major quantitative trait locus on chromosome 6q23 influencing fetal hemoglobin levels in adults. Proc Natl Acad Sci U S A. 2007; 104(27):11346-11351.

[56] Wahlberg K, Jiang J, Rooks H, Jawaid K, Matsuda F, Yamaguchi M, Lathrop M, Thein SL, Best S. The HBS1LMYB intergenic interval associated with elevated HbF levels shows characteristics of a distal regulatory region in erythroid cells. Blood. 2009; 114(6):1254-1262.

[57] Jiang J, Best S, Menzel S, Silver N, Lai MI, Surdulescu GL, Spector TD, Thein SL. cMYB is involved in the regulation of fetal hemoglobin production in adults. Blood. 2006; 108(3):1077-1083.

[58] Tanabe O, Katsuoka F, Campbell AD, Song W, Yamamoto M, Tanimoto K, Engel JD. An embryonic/fetal beta-type globin gene repressor contains a nuclear receptor TR2/TR4 heterodimer. EMBO J. 2002; 21(13):3434-3442.

[59] Tanabe O, McPhee D, Kobayashi S, Shen Y, Brandt W, Jiang X, Campbell AD, Chen YT, Chang Cs, Yamamoto M, Tanimoto K, Engel JD. Embryonic and fetal beta-globin gene repression by the orphan nuclear receptors, TR2 and TR4.EMBO J. 2007; 26(9): 2295-2306.

[60] Omori A, Tanabe O, Engel JD, Fukamizu A, Tanimoto K. Adult stage gamma-globin silencing is mediated by a promoter direct repeat element. Mol Cell Biol. 2005; 25(9): 3443-3451.

[61] Berry M, Grosveld F, Dillon N. A single point mutation is the cause of the Greek form of hereditary persistence of fetal haemoglobin. Nature. 1992; 358(6386):499-502.

[62] Collins FS, Mentherall JE, Yamakawa M, Pan J, Weissman SM, Forget BG. À point mutation in the A gamma-globin gene promoter in Greek hereditary persistence of fetal haemoglobin. Nature. 1985; 313(6000):325-326.

[63] Sagami I, Tsai SY, Wang H, Tsai MJ, O'Malley BW. Identification of two factors required for transcription of the ovalbumin gene. Mol Cell Biol. 1986; 6(12):4259-4267.

[64] Filipe A, Li Q, Deveaux S, Godin I, Roméo PH, Stamatoyannopoulos G, Mignotte V. Regulation of embryonic/fetal globin genes by nuclear hormone receptors: A novel perspective on hemoglobin switching. EMBO J. 1999; 18(3):687-697.

[65] Jane SM, Nienhuis AW, Cunningham JM. Hemoglobin switching in man and chicken is mediated by a heteromeric complex between the ubiquitous transcription factor CP2 and a developmentally specific protein. EMBO J. 1995;14(1):97-105.

[66] Zhou W, Zhao Q, Sutton R, Cumming H, Wang X, Cerruti L, Hall M, Wu R, Cunningham JM, Jane SM. The role of p22 NF-E4 in human globin gene switching. J Biol Chem. 2004; 279(25):26227-32.

[67] Jane SM, Gumucio DL, Ney PA, Cunningham JM, Nienhuis AW. Methylation-enhanced binding of Sp1 to the stage selector element of the human gamma-globin gene promoter may regulate development specificity of expression. Mol Cell Biol. 1993; 13(6):3272-3281.

[68] Wilson NK, Foster SD, Wang X, Knezevic K, Schütte J, Kaimakis P, Chilarska PM, Kinston S, Ouwehand WH, Dzierzak E, Pimanda JE, de Bruijn MF, Göttgens B. Combinatorial transcriptional control in blood stem/progenitor cells: genome-wide analysis of ten major transcriptional regulators. Cell Stem Cell. 2010; 7(4):532-44.

[69] Chakalova L, Fraser P. Organization of transcription. Cold Spring Harb Perspect Biol. 2010; 2(9):000729.

[70] Kollias G, Wrighton N, Hurst J, Grosveld F. Regulated expression of human A gamma-, beta-, and hybrid gamma beta-globin genes in transgenic mice: manipulation of the developmental expression patterns. Cell. 1986; 46(1):89-94.

[71] Dzierzak E. Opening act in a hematopoietic program. Blood. 2009; 114(2):229-230.

[72] Magram J, Chada K, Costantini F. Developmental regulation of a cloned adult beta-globin gene in transgenic mice. Nature. 1985; 315(6017):338-340.

[73] Cantor AB1, Orkin SH. Transcriptional regulation of erythropoiesis: an affair involving multiple partners. Oncogene. 2002; 21(21):3368-76.

[74] Ezoe S, Matsumura I, Gale K, Satoh Y, Ishikawa J, Mizuki M, Takahashi S, Minegishi N, Nakajima K, Yamamoto M, Enver T, Kanakura Y. GATA transcription factors inhibit cytokine-dependent growth and survival of a hematopoietic cell line through the inhibition of STAT3 activity. J Biol Chem. 2005; 280(13):13163-70.

[75] Grosveld F1, Rodriguez P, Meier N, Krpic S, Pourfarzad F, Papadopoulos P, Kolodziej K, Patrinos GP, Hostert A, Strouboulis J. Isolation and characterization of hema-

topoietic transcription factor complexes by in vivo biotinylation tagging and mass spectrometry. Ann N Y Acad Sci. 2005; 1054:55-67.

[76] Trainor CD, Omichinski JG, Vandergon TL, Gronenborn AM, Clore GM, Felsenfeld G. A palindromic regulatory site within vertebrate GATA-1 promoters requires both zinc fingers of the GATA-1 DNA-binding domain for high-affinity interaction. Mol Cell Biol. 1996; 16:2238-2247.

[77] Trainor CD, Ghirlando R, Simpson MA. GATA zinc finger interactions modulate DNA binding and transactivation. J Biol Chem. 2000; 275:28157-28166.

[78] Magis W, Martin DI. HMG-I binds to GATA motifs: implications for an HPFH syndrome. Biochem Biophys Res Commun. 1995; 214:927-933.

[79] Chen Z, Luo HY, Basran RK, Hsu TH, Mang DW, Nuntakarn L, Rosenfield CG, Patrinos GP, Hardison RC, Steinberg MH, Chui DH. A T-to-G transversion at nucleotide -567 upstream of HBG2 in a GATA-1 binding motif is associated with elevated hemoglobin F. Mol Cell Biol. 2008; 28(13):4386-93.

[80] Harju-Baker S, Costa FC, Fedosyuk H, Neades R, Peterson KR. Silencing of Agamma-globin gene expression during adult definitive erythropoiesis mediated by GATA-1-FOG-1-Mi2 complex binding at the -566 GATA site. Mol Cell Biol. 2008; 28(10): 3101-13.

[81] Amrolia PJ, Cunningham JM, Ney P, Nienhuis AW, Jane SM. Identification of two novel regulatory elements within the 5'-untranslated region of the human A gamma-globin gene. J Biol Chem. 1995; 270(21):12892-8.

[82] Haley JD, Smith DE, Schwedes J, Brennan R, Pearce C, Moore C, Wang F, Petti F, Grosveld F, Jane SM, Noguchi CT, Schechter AN. Identification and characterization of mechanistically distinct inducers of gamma-globin transcription. Biochem Pharmacol. 2003; 66(9):1755-68.

[83] Mabaera R, Greene MR, Richardson CA, Conine SJ, Kozul CD, Lowrey CH. Neither DNA hypomethylation nor changes in the kinetics of erythroid differentiation explain 5-azacytidine's ability to induce human fetal hemoglobin. Blood. 2008; 111(1): 411-20.

[84] El-Beshlawy A, Hamdy M, El Ghamrawy M. Fetal globin induction in beta-thalassemia. Hemoglobin. 2009; 33(1):197-203.

[85] Cao H. Pharmacological induction of fetal hemoglobin synthesis using histone deacetylase inhibitors. Hematology. 2004; 9:223-233.

[86] Gambari R, Fibach E. Medicinal chemistry of fetal hemoglobin inducers for treatment of beta-thalassemia. Curr Med Chem. 2007; 14(2):199-212.

[87] Fathallah H, Atweh GF. Induction of fetal hemoglobin in the treatment of sickle cell disease. Hematology Am Soc Hematol Educ Program. 2006:58-62.

[88] Gambari R, Fibach E. Medicinal chemistry of fetal hemoglobin inducers for treatment of beta-thalassemia. Curr Med Chem. 2007; 14(2):199-212.

[89] Veith R, Galanello R, Papayannopoulou T, Stamatoyannopoulos G. Stimulation of f-cell production in patients with sickle-cell anemia treated with cytarabine or hydroxyurea. N Engl J Med. 1985; 313(25):1571-5.

[90] Liu DP, Liang CC, Ao ZH, Jia PC, Chen SS, Wang RX, et al. Treatment of severe beta-thalassemia (patients) with myleran. Am J Hematol. 1990; 33:50-55.

[91] Papayannopoulou T, Torrealba de Ron A, Veith R, Knitter G, Stamatoyannopoulos G. Arabinosylcytosine induces fetal hemoglobin in baboons by perturbing erythroid cell differentiation kinetics. Science. 1984; 224:617-619.

[92] Galanello R, Stamatoyannopoulos G, Papayannopoulou T. Mechanism of Hb F stimulation by S-stage compounds. In vitro studies with bone marrow cells exposed to 5-azacytidine, are-C, or hydroxyurea. J Clin Invest. 1988; 81:1209-1216.

[93] Musallam KM, Taher AT, Cappellini MD, Sankaran VG. Clinical experience with fetal hemoglobin induction therapy in patients with β-thalassemia. Blood. 2013; 121(12):2199-212; quiz 2372.

[94] Bayanzay K, Khan R. Meta-analysis on effectiveness of hydroxyurea to treat transfusion-dependent beta-thalassemia. Hematology. 2014 Dec 23. [Epub ahead of print].

[95] Perrine SP, Greene MF, Faller DV. Delay in the fetal globin switch in infants of diabetic mothers. N Engl J Med. 1985; 312(6):334-8.

[96] Bard H, Prosmanne J. Relative rates of fetal hemoglobin and adult hemoglobin synthesis in cord blood of infants of insulin-dependent diabetic mothers. Pediatrics. 1985; 75(6):1143-7.

[97] Perrine SP, Ginder GD, Faller DV, Dover GH, Ikuta T, Witkowska HE, Cai SP, Vichinsky EP, Olivieri NF. A short-term trial of butyrate to stimulate fetal-globin-gene expression in the beta-globin disorders. N Engl J Med. 1993; 328(2):81-6.

[98] Little JA, Dempsey NJ, Tuchman M, Ginder GD. Metabolic persistence of fetal hemoglobin. Blood. 1995; 85:1712-8.

[99] Atweh GF, Sutton M, Nassif I, Boosalis V, Dover GJ, Wallenstein S, Wright E, McMahon L, Stamatoyannopoulos G, Faller DV, Perrine SP. Sustained induction of fetal hemoglobin by pulse butyrate therapy in sickle cell disease. Blood. 1999; 93(6):1790-7.

[100] Steinberg MH, Rodgers GP. Pathophysiology of sickle cell disease: role of cellular and genetic modifiers. Semin Hematol. 2001; 38(4):299-306.

[101] Boosalis MS, Bandyopadhyay R, Bresnick EH, Pace BS, Van DeMark K, Zhang B, Faller DV, Perrine SP. Short-chain fatty acid derivatives stimulate cell proliferation and induce STAT-5 activation. Blood. 2001; 97(10):3259-67.

[102] Pace BS, White GL, Dover GJ, Boosalis MS, Faller DV, Perrine SP. Short-chain fatty acid derivatives induce fetal globin expression and erythropoiesis in vivo. Blood. 2002; 100:4640-4648.

[103] Perrine SP. Fetal globin induction—can it cure beta thalassemia? Hematology Am Soc Hematol Educ Program. 2005:38-44.

[104] Perrine SP, Castaneda SA, Boosalis MS, White GL, Jones BM, Bohacek R. Induction of fetal globin in beta-thalassemia: Cellular obstacles and molecular progress. Ann N Y Acad Sci. 2005; 1054:257-65.

[105] Castaneda S, Boosalis MS, Emery D, Thies A, Faller DV, Perrine SP. Enhancement of growth and survival and alterations in Bcl-family proteins in beta-thalassemic erythroid progenitors by novel short-chain fatty acid derivatives. Blood Cells Mol Dis. 2005; 35(2):217-26.

[106] Perrine SP. Fetal globin stimulant therapies in the beta-hemoglobinopathies: principles and current potential. Pediatr Ann. 2008; 37(5):339-46.

[107] Atweh GF, Sutton M, Nassif I, Boosalis V, Dover GJ, Wallenstein S, Wright E, McMahon L, Stamatoyannopoulos G, Faller DV, Perrine SP. Sustained induction of fetal hemoglobin by pulse butyrate therapy in sickle cell disease. Blood. 1999; 93(6):1790-7.

[108] Fathallah H, Taher A, Bazarbachi A, Atweh GF. Differences in response to fetal hemoglobin induction therapy in beta-thalassemia and sickle cell disease. Blood Cells Mol Dis. 2009; 43(1):58-62.

[109] Boosalis MS, Ikuta T, Pace BS, da Fonseca S, White GL, Faller DV, Perrine SP. Abrogation of IL-3 requirements and stimulation of hematopoietic cell proliferation in vitro and in vivo by carboxylic acids. Blood Cells Mol Dis. 1997; 23(3):434-42.

[110] Kutlar A, Meiler S, Swerdlow P, Knight R. Thalidomide and its analogs for hemoglobinopathies: two birds with one stone? Expert Rev Hematol. 2012; 5(1):9-11.

[111] Collins AF, Dover GJ, Luban NL. Increased fetal hemoglobin production in patients receiving valproic acid for epilepsy. Blood. 1994; 84:1690-1691.

[112] Dover GJ, Brusilow S, Charache S. Induction of fetal hemoglobin production in subjects with sickle cell anemia by oral sodium phenylbutyrate. Blood. 1994; 84(1): 339-43.

[113] Liakopoulou E, Blau CA, Li Q, Josephson B, Wolf JA, Fournarakis B, Raisys V, Dover G, Papayannopoulou T, Stamatoyannopoulos G. Stimulation of fetal hemoglobin production by short chain fatty acids. Blood. 1995; 86(8):3227-35.

[114] Torkelson S, White B, Faller DV, Phipps K, Pantazis C, Perrine SP. Erythroid progenitor proliferation is stimulated by phenoxyacetic and phenylalkyl acids. Blood Cells Mol Dis. 1996; 22 (2):150-8.

[115] Mankidy R, Faller DV, Mabaera R, Lowrey CH, Boosalis MS, White GL, Castaneda SA, Perrine SP. Short-chain fatty acids induce gamma-globin gene expression by displacement of a HDAC3-NCoR repressor complex. Blood. 2006; 108(9):3179-86.

[116] Noyer-Weidner M, Trautner TA. Methylation of DNA in prokaryotes. EXS. 1993; 64:39-108.

[117] Momparler RL, Eliopoulos N, Ayoub J. Evaluation of an inhibitor of DNA methylation, 5-aza-2'-deoxycytidine, for the treatment of lung cancer and the future role of gene therapy. Adv Exp Med Biol. 2000; 465:433-46.

[118] Robertson KD. DNA methylation, methyltransferases, and cancer. Oncogene. 2001; 20(24):3139-55.

[119] van der Ploeg LH, Flavell RA. DNA methylation in the human gamma delta beta-globin locus in erythroid and nonerythroid tissues. Cell. 1980; 19(4):947-58.

[120] Torrealba de Ron A, Papayannopoulou T, Stamatoyannopoulos G. Studies of Hb F in adult nonanemic baboons: Hb F expression in erythroid colonies decreases as the level of maturation of Erythroid progenitors advances. Exp Hematol. 1985; 13:919-925.

[121] DeSimone J, Koshy M, Dorn L, Lavelle D, Bressler L, Molokie R, Talischy N. Maintenance of elevated fetal hemoglobin levels by decitabine during dose interval treatment of sickle cell anemia. Blood. 2002; 99(11):3905-8.

[122] Saunthararajah Y, DeSimone J. Clinical studies with fetal hemoglobin-enhancing agents in sickle cell disease. Semin Hematol. 2004; 41(46):11-6.

[123] Lavelle DE. The molecular mechanism of fetal hemoglobin reactivation. Semin Hematol. 2004; 41:3-10.

[124] DeSimone J, Heller P, Hall L, Zwiers D. 5-Azacytidine stimulates fetal hemoglobin synthesis in anemic baboons. Proc Natl Acad Sci U S A. 1982; 79:4428-4431.

[125] Ley TJ, DeSimone J, Anagnou NP, Keller GH, Humphries RK, Turner PH, Young NS, Keller P, Nienhuis AW. 5-azacytidine selectively increases gamma-globin synthesis in a patient with beta$^+$ thalassemia. N Engl J Med. 1982; 307(24):1469-75.

[126] Carr BI, Reilly JG, Smith SS, Winberg C, Riggs A. The tumorigenicity of 5-azacytidine in the male Fischer rat. Carcinogenesis. 1984; 5:1583-1590.

[127] Hermes M, Osswald H, Kloor D. Role of S-adenosylhomocysteine hydrolase in adenosine-induced apoptosis in HepG2 cells. Exp Cell Res. 2007; 313(2):264-83.

[128] He M, Fan J, Jiang R, Tang WX, Wang ZW. Expression of DNMTs and genomic DNA methylation in gastric signet ring cell carcinoma. Mol Med Rep. 2013; 8(3):942-8.

[129] Rupon JW, Wang SZ, Gaensler K, Lloyd J, Ginder GD. Methyl binding domain protein 2 mediates gamma-globin gene silencing in adult human betaYAC transgenic mice. Proc Natl Acad Sci U S A. 2006; 103(17):6617-22.

[130] Chin MH, Mason MJ, Xie W, Volinia S, Singer M, Peterson C, Ambartsumyan G, Aimiuwu O, Richter L, Zhang J, Khvorostov I, Ott V, Grunstein M, Lavon N, Benvenisty N, Croce CM, Clark AT, Baxter T, Pyle AD, Teitell MA, Pelegrini M, Plath K, Lowry WE. Induced pluripotent stem cells and embryonic stem cells are distinguished by gene expression signatures. Cell Stem Cell. 2009; 5(1):111-23.

[131] Bauer S, Robinson PN, Gagneur J. Model-based gene set analysis for Bioconductor. Bioinformatics. 2011; 27: 1882-1883.

[132] Turner B.M. Histone acetylation and control of gene expression. J. Cell Science. 1991; 99:13-20.

[133] Hassig CA, Schreiber SL. Nuclear histone acetylases and deacetylases and transcriptional regulation: HATs off to HDACs. Curr Opin Chem Biol. 1997; 1(3):300-8.

[134] Mizzen CA, Allis CD. Linking histone acetylation to transcriptional regulation. Cell Mol Life Sci. 1998; 54(1):6-20.

[135] Kuo MH, Allis CD. Roles of histone acetyltransferases and deacetylases in gene regulation. Bioessays. 1998; 20(8):615-26.

[136] Felsenfeld G, Groudine M. Controlling the double helix. Nature. 2003; 421(6921): 448-53.

[137] Glozak MA, Sengupta N, Zhang X, Seto E. Acetylation and deacetylation of non-histone proteins. Gene. 2005; 363:15-23.

[138] Yang XJ, Seto E. HATs and HDACs: from structure, function and regulation to novel strategies for therapy and prevention. Oncogene. 2007; 26(37):5310-8.

[139] Smith CL. A shifting paradigm: histone deacetylases and transcriptional activation. Bioessays. 2008; 30(1):15-24.

[140] Dokmanovic M, Clarke C, Marks PA. Histone deacetylase inhibitors: overview and perspectives. Mol Cancer Res. 2007; 5(10):981-9.

[141] Seto E, Yoshida M. Erasers of histone acetylation: the histone deacetylase enzymes. Cold Spring Harb Perspect Biol. 2014; 6(4):018713.

[142] Imai S, Armstrong CM, Kaeberlein M, Guarente L-Transcriptional silencing and longevity protein Sir2 is an NAD-dependent histone deacetylase. Nature. 2000; 403:795-800.

[143] Verdin E, Dequiedt F, Kasler HG. Class II histone deacetylases: versatile regulators. Trends Genet. 2003; 19(5):286-93.

[144] Forsberg EC, Downs KM, Christensen HM, Im H, Nuzzi PA, Bresnick EH. Developmentally dynamic histone acetylation pattern of a tissue-specific chromatin domain. Proc Natl Acad Sci U S A. 2000; 97(26):14494-9.

[145] Mai A, Massa S, Rotili D, Cerbara I, Valente S, Pezzi R, Simeoni S, Ragno R. Histone deacetylation in epigenetics: an attractive target for anticancer therapy. Med Res Rev. 2005; 25(3):261-309.

[146] Martin DG, Grimes DE, Baetz K, Howe L. Methylation of histone H3 mediates the association of the NuA3 histone acetyltransferase with chromatin. Mol Cell Biol. 2006; 26:3018-3028.

[147] Shalini A. Muralidhar, Valya Ramakrishnan, Inderdeep S. Kalra, Wei Li, Betty S. Pace. Histone Deacetylase 9 Activates γ-Globin Gene Expression in Primary ErythroidCells. J Biol Chem. 2011; 286(3):2343-2353.

[148] Skarpidi E, Vassilopoulos G, Li Q, Stamatoyannopoulos G. Novel in vitro assay for the detection of pharmacologic inducers of fetal hemoglobin. Blood. 2000; 96:321-326.

[149] Makala L, Di Maro S, Lou TF, Sivanand S, Ahn JM, Pace BS. FK228 Analogues Induce Fetal Hemoglobin in Human Erythroid Progenitors. Anemia. 2012; 2012:428137.

[150] Bradner JE, Mak R, Tanguturi SK, Mazitschek R, Haggarty SJ, Ross K, Chang CY, Bosco J, West N, Morse E, Lin K, Shen JP, Kwiatkowski NP, Gheldof N, Dekker J, DeAngelo DJ, Carr SA, Schreiber SL, Golub TR, Ebert BL. Chemical genetic strategy identifies histone deacetylase 1 (HDAC1) and HDAC2 as therapeutic targets in sickle cell disease. Proc Natl Acad Sci U S A. 2010; 107(28):12617-22.

[151] Shearstone JR vDJ, Bradner JE, Mazitschek R, Jones SS, Jarpe M. Induction of Human Fetal Hemoglobin Expression by Selective Inhibitors of Hilstone Deacetylase 1 and 2 (HDAC 1/2). Blood. 2012; 120:3259.

[152] Kappos L, Gold R, Arnold DL, Bar-Or A, Giovannoni G, Selmaj K, Sarda SP, Agarwal S, Zhang A, Sheikh SI, Seidman E, Dawson KT. Quality of life outcomes with BG-12 (dimethyl fumarate) in patients with relapsing-remitting multiple sclerosis: the DEFINE study. Mult Scler. 2014; 20(2):243-52.

[153] Macari ER, Schaeffer EK, West RJ, Lowrey CH. Simvastatin and t-butylhydroquinone suppress KLF1 and BCL11A gene expression and additively increase fetal hemoglobin in primary human erythroid cells. Blood. 2013; 121:830-839.

[154] Fox RJ, Kita M, Cohan SL, Henson LJ, Zambrano J, Scannevin RH, O'Gorman J, Novas M, Dawson KT, Phillips JT. BG-12 (dimethyl fumarate): a review of mechanism of action, efficacy, and safety. Curr Med Res Opin. 2014; 30(2):251-62.

[155] Makala L, Promsote W, Li B, Ganapathy V, Pamela M, Pace BS. Monomethylfumarate (MMF), a Novel Inducer of Fetal Hemoglobin in Human Erythroid Progenitors and Retinal Pigment Epithelial Cells.. Blood. 2013; 122:317.

[156] Menzel S, Garner C, Gut I, Matsuda F, Yamaguchi M, Heath S, Foglio M, Zelenika D, Boland A, Rooks H, Best S, Spector TD, Farrall M, Lathrop M, Thein SL. A QTL influencing F cell production maps to a gene encoding a zinc-finger protein on chromosome 2p15. Nat Genet. 2007; 39(10):1197-9.

[157] Townes TM, Behringer RR. Human globin locus activation region (LAR): role in temporal control. Trends Genet. 1990; 6:219-223.

[158] Ryan TM, Ciavatta DJ, Townes TM. Knockout-transgenic mouse model of sickle cell disease. Science. 1997; 278:873-876.

[159] Meiler SE, Wade M, Kutlar F, Yerigenahally SD, Xue Y, Moutouh-de Parseval LA, Corral LG, Swerdlow PS, Kutlar A. Pomalidomide augments fetal hemoglobin production without the myelosuppressive effects of hydroxyurea in transgenic sickle cell mice. Blood. 2011; 118(4):1109-12.

[160] Shi Y, Lan F, Matson C, Mulligan P, Whetstine JR, Cole PA, Casero RA, Shi Y. Histone demethylation mediated by the nuclear amine oxidase homolog LSD1. Cell. 2004; 119(7):941-53.

[161] Shi L, Cui S, Engel JD, Tanabe O. Lysine-specific demethylase 1 is a therapeutic target for fetal hemoglobin induction. Nat Med. 2013; 19:291-294.

[162] Platt OS, Orkin SH, Dover G, Beardsley GP, Miller B, Nathan DG. Hydroxyurea enhances fetal hemoglobin production in sickle cell anemia. J Clin Invest. 1984; 74:652-656.

[163] Charache S, Terrin ML, Moore RD, Dover GJ, Barton FB, Eckert SV, McMahon RP, Bonds DR. Effect of hydroxyurea on the frequency of painful crises in sickle cell anemia. Investigators of the Multicenter Study of Hydroxyurea in Sickle Cell Anemia. N Engl J Med. 1995; 332(20):1317-22.

[164] Steinberg MH, Lu ZH, Barton FB, Terrin ML, Charache S, Dover GJ. Fetal hemoglobin in sickle cell anemia: determinants of response to hydroxyurea. Multicenter Study of Hydroxyurea. Blood. 1997; 89:1078-1088.

[165] Moore RD, Charache S, Terrin ML, Barton FB, Ballas SK. Cost effectiveness of hydroxyurea in sickle cell anemia. Investigators of the Multicenter Study of Hydroxyurea in Sickle Cell Anemia. Am J Hematol. 2000; 64:26-31.

[166] Steinberg MH, McCarthy WF, Castro O, Ballas SK, Armstrong FD, Smith W, Ataga K, Swerdlow P, Kutlar A, DeCastro L, Waclawiw MA. Investigators of the Multicenter Study of Hydroxyurea in Sickle Cell Anemia and MSH Patients' Follow-Up. The risks and benefits of long-term use of hydroxyurea in sickle cell anemia: A 17.5 year follow-up. Am J Hematol. 2010; 85(6):403-8.

[167] Voskaridou E, Christoulas D, Bilalis A, Plata E, Varvagiannis K, Stamatopoulos G, Sinopoulou K, Balassopoulou A, Loukopoulos D, Terpos E. The effect of prolonged administration of hydroxyurea on morbidity and mortality in adult patients with sickle cell syndromes: results of a 17-year, single-center trial (LaSHS). Blood. 2010; 115(12): 2354-63.

[168] Wang WC, Wynn LW, Rogers ZR, Scott JP, Lane PA, Ware RE. A two year pilot trial of hydroxyurea in very young children with sickle cell anemia. J Pediatr. 2001; 139:790-796.

[169] Hankins JS, Ware RE, Rogers ZR, Wynn LW, Lane PA, Scott JP, Wang WC. Long-term hydroxyurea therapy for infants with sickle cell anemia: the HUSOFT extension study. Blood. 2005; 106(7):2269-75.

[170] Wang WC1, Ware RE, Miller ST, Iyer RV, Casella JF, Minniti CP, Rana S, Thornburg CD, Rogers ZR, Kalpatthi RV, Barredo JC, Brown RC, Sarnaik SA, Howard TH, Wynn LW, Kutlar A, Armstrong FD, Files BA, Goldsmith JC, Waclawiw MA, Huang X, Thompson BW; BABY HUG investigators. Hydroxycarbamide in very young children with sickle cell anaemia: a multicentre, randomised, controlled trial (BABY HUG). Lancet. 2011; 377(9778):1663-72.

[171] Zimmerman SA, Schultz WH, Burgett S, Mortier NA, Ware RE. Hydroxyurea therapy lowers transcranial Doppler flow velocities in children with sickle cell anemia. Blood. 2007; 110:1043-1047.

[172] Hankins JS, Helton KJ, McCarville MB, Li CS, Wang WC, Ware RE. Preservation of spleen and brain function in children with sickle cell anemia treated with hydroxyurea. Pediatr Blood Cancer. 2008; 50:293-297.

[173] Thornburg CD, Dixon N, Burgett S, Mortier NA, Schultz WH, Zimmerman SA, Bonner M, Hardy KK, Calatroni A, Ware RE. A pilot study of hydroxyurea to prevent chronic organ damage in young children with sickle cell anemia. Pediatr Blood Cancer. 2009; 52(5):609-15.

[174] Ware RE, Schultz WH, Yovetich N, Mortier NA, Alvarez O, Hilliard L, Iyer RV, Miller ST, Rogers ZR, Scott JP, Waclawiw M, Helms RW. Stroke With Transfusions Changing to Hydroxyurea (SWiTCH): a phase III randomized clinical trial for treatment of children with sickle cell anemia, stroke, and iron overload. Pediatr Blood Cancer. 2011; 57(6):1011-7.

[175] Ware RE, Helms RW, SWiTCH Investigators. Stroke With Transfusions Changing to Hydroxyurea (SWiTCH). Blood. 2012; 119:3925-3932.

[176] Noel N, Ko C. Natural Remedies for the Treatment of Beta-Thalassemia and Sickle Cell Anemia—Current Status and Perspectives in Fetal Hemoglobin Reactivation. Hindawi Publishing Corporation International Scholarly Research Notices. Volume 2014, (123257): 11.

[177] Heinrich M, Gibbons S. Ethnopharmacology in drug discovery: an analysis of its role and potential contribution. J Pharm Pharmacol. 2001; 53:425-32.

[178] Khan MT, Lampronti I, Martello D, Bianchi N, Jabbar S, Choudhuri MS, et al. Identification of pyrogallol as an antiproliferative compound present in extracts from the

medicinal plant Emblica officinalis: effects on in vitro cell growth of human tumor cell lines.Int J Oncol. 2002; 21:187-92.

[179] Lampronti I, Martello D, Bianchi N, Borgatti M, Lambertini E, Piva R, Jabbar S, Choudhuri MS, Khan MT, Gambari R. In vitro antiproliferative effects on human tumor cell lines of extracts from the Bangladeshi medicinal plant Aegle marmelos Correa. Phytomedicine. 2003; 10(4):300-8.

[180] Lambertini E, Piva R, Khan MT, Lampronti I, Bianchi N, Borgatti M, Gambari R. Effects of extracts from Bangladeshi medicinal plants on in vitro proliferation of human breast cancer cell lines and expression of estrogen receptor alpha gene. Int J Oncol. 2004; 24(2):419-23.

[181] Xie F, Wu CF, Lai WP, Yang XJ, Cheung PY, Yao XS, Leung PC, Wong MS. The osteoprotective effect of Herba epimedii (HEP) extract in vivo and in vitro. Evid Based Complement Alternat Med. 2005; 2(3):353-61.

[182] Saad B, Azaizeh H, Said O. Tradition and perspectives of arab herbal medicine: a review. Evid Based Complement Alternat Med. 2005;2:475-9.

[183] Lampronti I, Khan MT, Bianchi N, Ather A, Borgatti M, Vizziello L, Fabbri E, Gambari R. Bangladeshi medicinal plant extracts inhibiting molecular interactions between nuclear factors and target DNA sequences mimicking NF-kappaB binding sites. Med Chem. 2005; 1(4):327-33.

[184] Adams LS, Seeram NP, Hardy ML, Carpenter C, Heber D. Analysis of the interactions of botanical extract combinations against the viability of prostate cancer cell lines. Evid Based Complement Alternat Med. 2006; 3:117-24.

[185] Luo JZ, Luo L. American ginseng stimulates insulin production and prevents apoptosis through regulation of uncoupling Protein-2 in cultured beta cells. Evid Based Complement Alternat Med 2006; 3:365-72.

[186] Jagetia GC, Rao SK. Evaluation of cytotoxic effects of dichloromethane extract of guduchi (Tinospora cordifoliaMiers ex Hook F & THOMS) on cultured HeLa cells. Evid Based Complement Alternat Med. 2006; 3:267-72.

[187] Guerrini A, Lampronti I, Bianchi N, Zuccato C, Breveglieri G, Salvatori F, Mancini I, Rossi D, Potenza R, Chiavilli F, Sacchetti G, Gambari R, Borgatti M. Bergamot (Citrus bergamia Risso) fruit extracts as γ-globin gene expression inducers: phytochemical and functional perspectives. J Agric Food Chem. 2009; 57(10):4103-11.

[188] H. Li , C. H. Ko, S. Y. Tsang, P. C. Leung, M. C. Fung, and K. P. Fung., The ethanol extract of Fructus trichosanthis promotes fetal hemoglobin production via p38 MAPK activation and Erk inactivation in K562 cells. Evidence-Based Complementary and Alternative Medicine, vol. 2011, Article ID 657056, 8.

[189] Fibach E, Bianchi N, Borgatti M, Prus E, Gambari R. Mithramycin induces fetal hemoglobin production in normal and thalassemic human erythroid precursor cells. Blood. 2003; 102(4):1276-81.

[190] Menzel S1, Garner C, Gut I, Matsuda F, Yamaguchi M, Heath S, Foglio M, Zelenika D, Boland A, Rooks H, Best S, Spector TD, Farrall M, Lathrop M, Thein SL. A QTL influencing F cell production maps to a gene encoding a zinc-finger protein on chromosome 2p15. Nat Genet. 2007; 39(10):1197-9.

[191] Thein SL, Menzel S. Discovering the genetics underlying foetal haemoglobin production in adults. Br J Haematol. 2009; 145:455-467.

[192] van der Ploeg LH, Flavell RA. DNA methylation in the human gamma delta beta-globin locus in erythroid and nonerythroid tissues. Cell. 1980; 19:947-958.

[193] Letvin NL, Linch DC, Beardsley GP, McIntyre KW, Nathan DG. Augmentation of fetal-hemoglobin production in anemic monkeys by hydroxyurea. N Engl J Med. 1984; 310:869-873.

[194] DeSimone J, Heller P, Molokie RE, Hall L, Zwiers D. Tetrahydrouridine, cytidine analogues, and hemoglobin F. Am J Hematol. 1985; 18:283-288.

[195] Saunthararajah Y, Hillery CA, Lavelle D, Molokie R, Dorn L, Bressler L, Gavazova S, Chen YH, Hoffman R, DeSimone J. Effects of 5-aza-2'-deoxycytidine on fetal hemoglobin levels, red cell adhesion, and hematopoietic differentiation in patients with sickle cell disease. Blood. 2003; 102(12):3865-70.

[196] Lavelle D, Chin J, Vaitkus K, Redkar S, Phiasivongsa P, Tang C, Will R, Hankewych M, Roxas B, Singh M, Saunthararajah Y, Desimone J. Oral decitabine reactivates expression of the methylated gamma-globin gene in Papio anubis. Am J Hematol. 2007; 82(11):981-5.

[197] Inati A, Kahale M, Perrine SP, Chui DH, Taher AT, Koussa S, Abi Nasr T, Abbas HA, Ghalie RG. A phase 2 study of HQK-1001, an oral fetal haemoglobin inducer, in β-thalassaemia intermedia. Br J Haematol. 2014; 164(3):456-8.

[198] Peterson KR, Navas PA, Stamatoyannopoulos G. beta-YAC transgenic mice for studying LCR function. Ann N Y Acad Sci. 1998; 850:28-37.

[199] Johnson J, Hunter R, McElveen R, Qian XH, Baliga BS, Pace BS. Fetal hemoglobin induction by the histone deacetylase inhibitor, scriptaid. Cell Mol Biol (Noisy-le-grand). 2005; 51:229-238.

[200] Moore RD, Charache S, Terrin ML, Barton FB, Ballas SK. Costeffectiveness of hydroxyurea in sickle cell anemia. Investigators of the Multicenter Study of Hydroxyurea in Sickle Cell Anemia. Am J Hematol. 2000; 64:26-31.

[201] Lanzkron S, Haywood C Jr, Segal JB, Dover GJ. Hospitalization rates and costs of care of patients with sickle cell anemia in the state of Maryland in the era of hydroxyurea. Am J Hematol. 2006; 81:927-932.

[202] Walters MC1, Storb R, Patience M, Leisenring W, Taylor T, Sanders JE, Buchanan GE, Rogers ZR, Dinndorf P, Davies SC, Roberts IA, Dickerhoff R, Yeager AM, Hsu L, Kurtzberg J, Ohene-Frempong K, Bunin N, Bernaudin F, Wong WY, Scott JP, Margolis D, Vichinsky E, Wall DA, Wayne AS, Pegelow C, Redding-Lallinger R, Wiley J, Klemperer M, Mentzer WC, Smith FO, Sullivan KM. Impact of bone marrow transplantation for symptomatic sickle cell disease: An interim report. Multicenter investigation of bone marrow transplantation for sickle cell disease. Blood. 2000 Mar; 95(6): 1918-24.

[203] Locatelli F, Rocha V, Reed W, Bernaudin F, Ertem M, Grafakos S, Brichard B, Li X, Nagler A, Giorgiani G, Haut PR, Brochstein JA, Nugent DJ, Blatt J, Woodard P, Kurtzberg J, Rubin CM, Miniero R, Lutz P, Raja T, Roberts I, Will AM, Yaniv I, Vermylen C, Tannoia N, Garnier F, Ionescu I, Walters MC, Lubin BH, Gluckman E; Eurocord Transplant Group. Related umbilical cord blood transplantation in patients with thalassemia and sickle cell disease. Blood. 2003; 101(6):2137-43.

[204] Kharbanda S, Smith AR, Hutchinson SK, McKenna DH, Ball JB, Lamb LS Jr, Agarwal R, Weinberg KI, Wagner JE Jr. Unrelated donor allogeneic hematopoietic stem cell transplantation for patients with hemoglobinopathies using a reduced-intensity conditioning regimen and third-party mesenchymal stromal cells. Biol Blood Marrow Transplant. 2014; 20(4):581-6.

[205] Cavazzana-Calvo M, Payen E, Negre O, Wang G, Hehir K, Fusil F, Down J, Denaro M, Brady T, Westerman K, Cavallesco R, Gillet-Legrand B, Caccavelli L, Sgarra R, Maouche-Chrétien L, Bernaudin F, Girot R, Dorazio R, Mulder GJ, Polack A, Bank A, Soulier J, Larghero J, Kabbara N, Dalle B, Gourmel B, Socie G, Chrétien S, Cartier N, Aubourg P, Fischer A, Cornetta K, Galacteros F, Beuzard Y, Gluckman E, Bushman F, Hacein-Bey-Abina S, Leboulch P. Transfusion independence and HMGA2 activation after gene therapy of human β-thalassaemia. Nature. 2010; 467(7313):318-22.

[206] Leboulch P. Gene therapy: primed for take-off. Nature. 2013; 500:280-282.

[207] Takahashi K, Yamanaka S. Induction of pluripotent stem cells from mouse embryonic and adult fibroblast cultures by defined factors. Cell. 2006; 126:663-676.

[208] Hanna J, Wernig M, Markoulaki S, Sun CW, Meissner A, Cassady JP, Beard C, Brambrink T, Wu LC, Townes TM, Jaenisch R. Treatment of sickle cell anemia mouse model with iPS cells generated from autologous skin. Science. 2007; 318(5858):1920-3.

[209] Yu J, Vodyanik MA, Smuga-Otto K, Antosiewicz-Bourget J, Frane JL, Tian S, Nie J, Jonsdottir GA, Ruotti V, Stewart R, Slukvin II, Thomson JA. Induced pluripotent stem cell lines derived from human somatic cells. Science. 2007; 318(5858):1917-20.

2

Cancer Gene Therapy

Hakan Akbulut, Muge Ocal and Gizem Sonugur

Abstract

Cancer treatment has been the major goal of the gene therapy studies over the decades. Although there is no cancer gene therapy drug in the market yet, substantial progress has been made in defining potential targets and in developing viral and nonviral gene delivery systems recently. Numerous genes have been studied as the targets for cancer gene therapy so far. Various gene therapy strategies, including suicide gene therapy, oncolytic viral therapies, antiangiogenesis, and gene therapy vaccines have been developed. The combination of gene therapy with conventional methods, such as chemotherapy, radiotherapy, and immunotherapy, has further improved the therapeutic efficacy. Although the preclinical and experimental studies have yielded highly encouraging results, there are still few gene therapy agents at phase III trials. In the current chapter, we will review gene transfer systems, targets, gene targeting strategies, and cancer gene therapy in the clinic.

Keywords: Cancer gene therapy, viral vectors, nonviral vectors, gene targeting

1. Introduction

The improvements in the past 20 years in the molecular biology have evoked optimism in the treatment of cancer and yielded a number of targeted drugs in the market. However, the curative treatment of the cancer has still been possible with only the early diagnosis and early intervention in the vast majority of the solid tumors. Almost half of the cancer patients diagnosed each year have been dying of the disease throughout the world. In particular, the patients with distant metastasis have no hope of cure with the current treatment modalities.

2. Cancer is a complex genetic disease

It has long been suggested that the cancer has evolved from a single cell transformed by the influence of the environmental factors such as physical, chemical factors, and viruses. Changes in hundreds of genes, so-called mutations, are required to transform a normal cell into a cancer cell. The major functional changes that transform a cell are mainly the activation of oncogenes or inactivation of tumor suppressor genes.

The overexpression of oncogenes and loss of function of tumor suppressor genes usually induce malignant transformation. Those changes are also required for further growth of tumor cells.

A transformed cell usually gains some important biological properties to establish a malignant disease. Those properties, including uncontrolled proliferation, evasion of growth suppressors, inhibition of apoptosis, replicative immortality, angiogenesis, proliferative signals, invasion, and metastasis, are discussed in detail in a recent review of Hanahan and Weinberg [1]. Although the conventional chemotherapy has mainly focused on direct tumor cell killing, a vast majority of current targeted therapies have aimed to eliminate one or more of the above-mentioned properties of cancer cells.

The targeting of angiogenesis, proliferation pathways, and immune system has yielded a number of drugs that are already in the market. Nodules of cancer cells cannot grow beyond 1–2 mm without expanding their blood supply to access every increasing need for oxygen and nutrients. In order to generate the additional blood supply, the tumor tissue stimulates the elaboration of its own vessel network, through a process called angiogenesis [2]. If one could cut the blood supply of the tumor, it cannot grow beyond 1–2 mm, which means that they cannot grow enough to be diagnosed by the current diagnostic technology and cannot cause a clinical disease. The tumor vascular targeting therapy or antiangiogenetic therapies like bevacizumab and aflibercept targeting ligands of angiogenesis or small tyrosine kinase inhibitors of angiogenesis pathway receptors or signaling molecules have already emerged as standard therapeutic drugs in various tumors [3].

The overexpression of oncogenes and the loss of function of tumor suppressor genes are usually involved in both malignant conversion of the cells and further growth of tumor cells. A new generation of small molecules targeting proliferation pathways, like gefitinib, erlotinib, and imatinib, has been developed to block the cancer-causing signals within cancer cells and become standard treatments in those patients with mutations of EGFR or c-KIT [4]. Antibody molecules, targeting the EGFR family of receptors like trastuzumab, cetuximab, and panitumumab also block the growth-promoting signals that push cancer cells into an unregulated pattern of growth [5]. In contrast to standard chemotherapy, which is quite damaging to the normal tissues of the body as well as the cancer tissue, the targeted drugs are quite specific for the cancer cells and therefore relatively free of side effects.

Although majority of the cancer patients has a fairly intact immune system, the cells of the immune system do not usually respond to tumor cells because the immune system cannot differentiate the normal and cancer cells and therefore cannot fight against them. Immunotherapy or cancer vaccine therapy aims to activate immune system against tumors. Recently, ipilumumab/tremelimumab and pembrolizumab/nivolumumab targeting checkpoints of immune response such as CTLA-4 or PD1 have also been approved [6]. Likewise, a dendritic cell-based vaccine, sipuleucel T, for the treatment of metastatic prostate cancer has been approved 2 years ago [7].

Hundreds of genes have been involved in the action and regulation of those pathways. The generation of cancer through a series of changes in the normal cellular genes makes the disease a genetic disease at the cellular base. The involvement of genes in the development of the disease also makes the disease a good candidate for gene therapy. Therefore, gene therapy has emerged as the hope of curative treatment modality in cancer.

3. What is gene therapy?

Gene therapy can be defined as the delivery of genetic elements to the cancer cell or to the cells of the immune response in order to correct the abnormalities in the cancer tissue or to induce an immune response against the cancer cells. The corrective strategies can involve replacing missing or defective genes, i.e., tumor suppressor genes [8], suppressing the action of cancer promoting oncogenes [9], or programming normal or cancer cells to release into the systemic circulation molecules which suppress the growth of cancer cells or their vasculature [10].

There are some prerequisites for a successful gene therapy program in cancer, such as a suitable target to be replaced or modified, a carrier to reach the interest of gene to the cell, a successful targeting of the vector, and a sufficient expression of the therapeutic genes in the target cells. Besides a strong therapeutic efficacy, safety is also mandatory for the success of the treatment.

Unraveling the mystery of the genetic changes in the development of cancer has been proposed many genes as targets for gene therapy studies. The second step in gene therapy following the identification of a suitable gene is to introduce it into the target cell. Different vehicles (vectors) have been used to introduce the genes into the cells, such as viral vectors, nonviral vectors, and cell-based carriers. The mainly used viral vectors in cancer gene therapy are retroviruses, adenoviruses, and adeno-associated viruses. The gene therapist uses the capability of the virus to enter and reprogram the action of cells for purposes of therapy. The therapeutic genetic element is first placed into a viral backbone to produce a complete therapeutic viral vector. Alternatively, the therapeutic genetic elements can be delivered into the cancer cells through droplets of fat called liposomes or nanoparticles. The genes themselves, in the form of naked DNA or DNA packed into particles can be administered locally or systemically.

A third way of delivering genes to the target tissues is accomplished by using living cells such as irradiated tumor cells, blood cells, and mesenchymal or neuronal stem cells. All of these cells have the capability to home to particular types of target tissue through the blood stream. In this way, the therapeutic genes can be placed into the brain or other target tissues because of the homing properties of those cells.

For the safety of the procedure and the increased therapeutic efficacy, the genes of interest should be expressed in only target cells or tissues. Sparing of the normal cells and tissues is one of the keystones in their clinical use. The target specificity of the vectors could be achieved by the targeting of those specific to the tumor cells or tissues.

4. Gene transfer systems of cancer gene therapy

There are three main ways of transferring genes into the tumor cells: nonviral vectors, viral vectors, and cell-based vehicles. For most of the tumors, a relatively short-term expression of therapeutic genes may be sufficient to kill the tumor cells. Rapid clearance of viral vectors from the blood stream has enabled the development of synthetic gene delivery vectors. However, an important drawback for these approaches is to carry the DNA of interest to the distant metastatic deposits. The nonviral gene delivery vectors have usually been injected locally to the tumors. Although local injection is reasonable for tumors as melanoma, head and neck cancers, or peritoneal carcinomatosis; it is not suitable in patients with hematogenous metastases. The limitations of the viral vectors are also valid for the nonviral vectors for gene therapy. They have to survive through the blood stream to be arrested in the target tumor tissue, to extravasate, and to bind to specific cells and to enter the cells and then to reach the nucleus.

4.1. Nonviral vectors

Plasmid DNA, which is mostly used as nonviral gene therapy modality, is easily degraded by nucleases [11]. Therefore, some strategies to reduce the size and prevent the degradation have been developed. The most commonly used agents for gene delivery are *cationic lipids* [12]. The cationic head group of the lipids binds to DNA and the lipid tail enables the collapse of the DNA lipid complex [13]. Cationic lipid DNA complexes (lipoplexes) (LPD/DNA) enter the target cell through an endosomal pathway. However, the transgene expression efficiency is very low with lipoplexes. It has been shown that only a very small portion of the systemically injected DNA could be reached to tumor tissue [14].

Lipid-based formulations of gene delivery have been predominantly limited to the intratumoral or local applications. The systemic administration carries the potential risk of adverse inflammatory and immune reactions. The development of systemic lipid delivery systems with the modifications to reduce the systemic toxicity could have the potential for clinical use in cancer gene therapy. In an animal model of breast cancer, folate-targeted lipid–protamine DNA complexes (LPD-PEG-folate) have been shown to reduce the tumor volume and increase the survival when administered systemically [14].

Neutral liposomes composed of DOPC (1,2-dioleyl-sn-phosphatidyl choline) and DOPE (1,2-dioleyl-sn-phosphatidyl ethanol amine) and polycationic carrier proteins as protamine, polylysine, polyarginine, polyhistidine, or polyethynilemine (PEI) are also suitable to carry the DNA [15–18]. The *hydrophobic polymers*, such as polyethylene glycol (PEG), polyhydroxy propylmethacrylamide (pHPMA), and polyvinyl pyrrolidine (pVPyrr), have also been used to mask the positive charge of DNA to extend its half-life in the blood [19,20]. Both the neutral liposomes and hydrophobic polymers yield less toxicity when administered systemically. The leaky nature of the blood vessels of the tumors allows the influx of macromolecules as polymer shielded DNA into the tumor. The PEGylation of plasmid DNA has been reported to circulate in the blood several hours and passively accumulate in the subcutaneous tumors in animals [21].

4.2. Viral vectors

Viruses have the natural ability to deliver the nucleic acids within its own genome to specific cell types, including cancer cells. This ability makes those attractive and popular gene-delivery vehicles. Retroviruses, adenoviruses, adeno-associated viruses, herpes simplex virus, poxviruses, and baculoviruses are commonly modified and used as gene therapy vectors in cancer. Additionally, chimeric viral-vector systems combining the properties of two or more virus type are also developed.

Retroviral vectors derived from retroviruses contain a linear single-stranded RNA of around 7–10 kb and have a lipid envelope. The viral particles enter the mammalian cells expressing appropriate receptors for retroviruses [22]. After entering the cell, the viral reverse transcriptase transcribes the virus RNA into double-stranded DNA (dsDNS). The dsDNA transcribed in the cytoplasm forms a nucleoprotein preintegration complex (PIC) by binding cellular proteins [23]. The PIC migrates to the nucleus and thereby integrates the host genome. The ability of transgene expression in only dividing cells is an advantage of retroviral vectors for cancer gene therapy to avoid undesired expression in nondividing cells of surrounding tissues. The incorporation of retroviral genes into the host genome provides long-term expression of transgenes. Although this is advantageous, a nonspecific incorporation of viral DNA could impair the function of host gene or induce aberrant expression of a cellular oncogene [24]. Although retroviral vectors have been the most widely used gene transfer vehicles in the clinic, the risk of insertional oncogenesis seen in the trial of X-SCID infants in 2003 has limited the use of retroviral gene transfer systems in humans [25]. The possibility of generating replication-competent retroviruses is another safety issue regarding the clinical use of those vectors [26].

Lentiviral vectors derived from retroviruses can cause stable integration of the transgene into the host genome with long-term gene expression. The ability of transducing both dividing and nondividing cells make those vectors more suitable and efficient gene transfer vehicle over retroviruses. Targeting strategies of vectors at the level of cell entry and transgene transcription improved the use of lentiviral vectors in gene therapy trials [27]. However, the biosafety concerns of random integration to the host genome as in retroviruses are the limitations of those vectors.

Adenoviral vectors are widely used to introduce the therapeutic genes into the tumor cells. They can infect a broad range of cell types, transfer the genes being not dependent on cell division, and have high titers and high level of gene expression [28]. The most widely used serotypes of adenoviruses to develop vectors in human cancer gene therapy studies are type 5 (Ad5) and type 2 (Ad2). They have the capacity of approximately 8–10 kb of therapeutic genes with first-generation vectors and up to 36 kbp with gutless third generation adenoviral vectors [29]. However, along with the immunogenic potential, the broad range of host cells by adenovirus limits its systemic use in human cancer gene therapy trials [30]. Targeting strategies have enabled the use of adenoviral vectors in human gene therapy trials. Adenoviral vectors cannot integrate to cellular genome and express the transgene episomally. They cannot induce random mutations. However, the transgene expression is limited to 7–10 days postinfection [31]. Therefore, repeated administrations of the vector are needed to achieve sustainable responses in cancer treatment. Adenoviruses could be engineered either as replication deficient by deleting the immediate early genes of E1 or replication-competent keeping the E1 region. Replication-competent adenoviral vectors will be further discussed in the section of oncolytic viruses.

Adeno-associated viruses (AAV) are simple viruses with approximately single-stranded DNA of 4.7 kb in size [32]. They belong to parvovirus family and require a helper virus such as adenovirus or herpes virus for lytic replication and release from the cell [33]. They can infect a wide variety of cells independent of cell cycle. This property makes AAV as suitable vectors for cancer gene therapy. Furthermore, unlike adenoviruses, they elicit little immune response when infect the normal host cells. Another advantage of AAV over adenoviruses is their ability to integrate the transgene into a particular spot on the 19th chromosome of human cells [34]. Unlike retroviruses, AAV cannot induce mutations. However, the major drawback of AAV is its limited cargo capacity of approximately 4 kbp of therapeutic genes. AAV could transduce certain cell types. Therefore, targeting strategies such as modification of viral capsid proteins, binding monoclonal antibodies, or bispecific proteins have been developed to improve the efficiency of AAV systems in cancer gene therapy [35,36].

Baculoviruses are enveloped viral particles with a large dsDNA of approximately 80–180 kb. They naturally infect insect cells. There have been no diseases related to baculoviruses in humans. Along with their highly safety profile in humans, they seem very useful gene therapy vehicles with their highly large cargo capacity of approximately 40 kb with possible multiple inserts, easy manipulation, and production [37]. *Autographa californica* multiple nucleopolyhedrovirus (*Ac*MNPV) is the most widely used types of baculovirus in gene therapy studies. It has a circular dsDNA genome of 135 kb [38]. They can easily transduce mammalian cells, including many types of cancer cells, and cause high transgene expression in the host cell [39]. They are already approved for the production of human vaccine components such as Cervarix (GlaxoSmithKline) in cervical cancer and Provenge (Dendreon) in prostatic cancer [40].

Herpes simplex virus (HSV) is a large DNA virus with approximately 152 kb of dsDNA genome. It has a natural tropism to nerve tissues and cannot integrate into the host genome [41]. The HSV vectors can be designed in three different types as amplicons, replication-defective, and replication-competent vectors [42]. In general, the replication-competent HSV vectors are used as oncolytic agents in cancer gene therapy studies [43].

Poxviruses were the first viruses to be used as gene therapy vectors. They have been used in the in vitro production of proteins and as live vaccines. The attenuated forms of poxviruses have been developed and used in the development of genetic cancer vaccine trials [44]. The immunostimulatory properties of poxviruses make them preferable agents to induce immunity against tumors. In particular, the attenuated MVA virus derived from chorioallantoid vaccinia Ankara (CVA), a Turkish smallpox vaccine strain, has been widely used in cancer vaccine development strategies [45].

5. Cells as the carriers of cancer gene therapy vectors

The systemic administration of the gene therapy vectors usually failed because of low titer achieved in the target tissue and insufficient transgene expression. The clearance of the vector by the immune system, sequestration, and nonspecific binding to nontarget tissues are the major drawbacks of viral and nonviral vectors [46,47]. In general, in vivo targeting has relied mainly upon the enhanced leakiness of the tumor vessels, allowing the extravasation and access to tumor cells. Besides, the target tropism, extravasations in tumor site, and poor penetration of the vectors into the tumor tissue are the major problems for the vectors to eradicate the metastatic tumor deposits.

Cell carriers have the potential of eliminating those problems. They are stable and most of them have tumor homing properties and can be administered locally, such as intraperitoneal or intratumoral injections or systemically. In case of the use of autologous cells, they will not be cleared by the immune system. Macrophages, bone marrow mesenchymal stem cells (MSC), T cells, NK cells, and eosinophils are the known cells infiltrating the tumor tissues. Also, the tumor cells themselves naturally have the potential of homing to the tumor deposits throughout the body.

Macrophages have been used to deliver therapeutic genes because of their naturally trafficking ability to sites of neoplastic diseases [48]. Further refinement of the targeting of these cells by using transcriptional promoters could avoid the transgene expression in other parts of the body where the macrophages naturally traveled [49].

T cells can be used to transfer the therapeutic genes to target tissues because of their ability to circulate through the body and arrest in tumor tissues [50]. T cells have the advantage of the release of vectors that they carry in an antigen-binding-specific manner. The T cells could also provide further antitumoral activity by their cytotoxic effects. Tumor infiltrating lymphocytes (TIL) are the first example of cell-based carriers in cancer therapy in which they were transfected with cytokine genes [51].

Mesenchymal progenitor cells from either bone marrow (MSC) or adipose tissue (PLA) have the potential to expand in culture and the differentiation along the adipogenic, osteogenic, chondrogenic, and myogenic lineages [52,53]. It has been shown that lentivirally transfected mesenchymal progenitors from the adipose tissue have sustained transgene expression, even after the differentiation into adipogenic and osteogenic lineages [54]. Further modifications of PLA cells transfected ex vivo in order to target tumor tissues of their natural potential differentiation would provide an efficient gene delivery vehicle.

Some other cells such as fibroblasts and allogeneic cells have also been used as cell carriers for gene therapy vectors [55,56]. Because of their homing properties to the tumor cell deposits, tumor cells could be good candidates to target the established metastases. An animal model of MDA-MB-231 cells, transduced ex vivo by a CD carrying Ad vector, has been shown to reduce the tumor volumes in the established metastases of the tumor [57].

6. Gene targeting in cancer gene therapy

In order to maximize the therapeutic index of cancer gene therapy, the expression of therapeutic genes could be restricted to the target tissues. Therefore, the targeting of gene therapy vectors is the major key for the success of those treatments. There are two main targeting strategies: physical targeting and biological targeting.

6.1. Physical targeting

The first one is physical targeting by means of some physical methods such as local injections, catheters, gene guns, and electroporation. This strategy is usually used for local delivery of gene therapy vectors and is therefore not suitable for most of the cancer patients who may have cancer spread throughout the body. Supercoiled DNA molecules and oligonucleotides are also successfully delivered to the cells of the skin following intradermal injection to the tumor deposits accessible by local injections. However, intratumoral injection might have only the transducing capacity of the cells neighboring the needle. The tumor deposits in the body cavities such as peritoneum, pleura, and meninges and in subcutaneous tissues are the potential targets for the physical targeting of the gene therapy vectors in the clinic [58,59].

6.2. Biological targeting

In a second strategy, the viral or nonviral carriers of the genes are modified in such a way that they can only bind to tumor cells but not the normal cells. Because of the low transduction efficiency of the currently used gene therapy vectors in distant tissues when administered systemically, the specific transgene expression or viral replication in target tissues could provide an opportunity to achieve sufficient antitumor activity. To achieve this goal, *transcriptionally* and *transductionally* targeted vectors have been developed. For safety reasons, mostly the replication defective vectors have been used to transfer the therapeutic genes into tumor cells. However, because of limitations of vector delivery and relatively low levels of gene transfer capacity, replication-deficient vector systems are usually inefficient for the treatment of large solid tumors. Therefore, replicating vectors could efficiently transfer genes and also increase the therapeutic efficiency by means of its oncolytic effect. Such vectors could be targeted in such a way that they can replicate within the tumor cells but not in normal cells and cause no local or systemic toxicity.

6.3. Transcriptional targeting

The clinical utility of a cancer gene therapy program will be dependent on its therapeutic index. In order to maximize the therapeutic index, the expression of therapeutic genes could be restricted to the target tissues. The selective targeting of gene therapy vectors to specific cells enables the delivery of therapeutic genes to the target cancer cells while sparing the normal tissues. This has the potential of the reducing the dose of vectors and toxicity.

Transcriptional targeting, which utilizes DNA regulatory (promoter/enhancer) elements that enable the expression of transgenes within specific cells, would probably decrease the toxicity of the treatment while increasing the specificity. The promoters used to drive the transgenes in viral or nonviral vectors targeted in cancer therapy could be tumor-selective, inducible, or cell cycle regulated. Certain genes have been expressed specifically in tumors such as L-plastin, survivin, telomerase, and midkine [60]. The vector constructs carrying tumor-specific promoters such as L-plastin, survivin, and midkine have been shown to efficiently eradicate tumor cells while sparing normal cells [61–63].

Likewise, the tumor-type-specific group of selective promoters shows a pattern of tumor tissue specificity. The promoters of oncofetal antigens such as carcinoembryonic antigen (CEA) and alpha-feto protein (AFP), mucin 1 (muc1), and oncogenes such as c-erbB2 and MYC have been used widely in the transcriptional targeting of gene therapy vectors to achieve specific transgene expression in tumor tissue [64–68].

The phenotypically heterogeneous expression of certain genes in certain tissues constitutes the basis of tissue-specific promoters in cancer gene therapy. The tissue specificity of those genes is largely regulated at the transcriptional level. Therefore, the promoters of those genes have been used to target cancer gene therapy vectors to specific tumor types in a specific manner of their origin of tissues. The tissue-specific promoters such as PSA in prostatic cancer [69], tyrosinase in melanoma [70], albumin in hepatocellular carcinoma [71], thyroglobulin (TG) in thyroid cancers [72], glial fibrillary acidic protein (GFAP) in glioblastoma [73], and osteocalcin (OC) in osteosarcoma [74] have been used to specifically target those tumors.

The inherent problems of tissue or tumor-specific promoters such as relative weakness and lack of true restriction of gene expression to the tumor tissues have led to the use of new promoters whose activity can be controlled exogenously. These systems also provide temporal control of gene expression. Various stress genes of the body are usually silent under normal conditions, but they are activated during the stress to protect the tissues. The stress genes up-regulated during stress such as heat, hypoxia, glucose deprivation, irradiation, and chemotherapy have opened a new avenue to the development of the tumor-specific targeting of gene therapy. The use of human heat shock protein (HSP)-driven HSV-TK or CD suicide gene therapy vectors has been a significant activity when combined with hyperthermia [75]. The promoter region of the hypoxia-inducible factor (HIF-1), a key regulator of the transcriptional response to oxygen, has been successfully used to target tumor cells [76]. MDR-1 gene encodes a 170-kDa P-glycoprotein and belongs to the ATP-binding cassette (ABC) family of transporters, which mediates the transport of some chemo drugs out of the cells thereby decreasing the efficacy of the treatment [77]. Therefore, the use of vector constructs carrying therapeutic genes under the control of MDR-1 promoter could efficiently target chemo-resistant tumor cells [78].

Uncontrolled cell proliferation is the prominent feature of cancer cells. The retinoblastoma family of proteins and their upstream regulators such as cyclin D, CDK4, and p16/INK4 regulate the G1 checkpoint in the cell cycle. Tumor suppression by Rb has been linked to its ability to repress E2F-responsive promoters such as E2F-1 promoter. It has been shown that Ad vectors that contain transgenes driven by E2F-1 promoter can mediate tumor-selective gene expression in vivo in glioma cells [79]. The promoters of cell cycle genes such as cyclin D, cyclin A, cdc25c, cyclin-dependent kinase inhibitors, p16/INK4, p27, and p14 could be expected to exert cell cycle arrest, thereby increasing the apoptosis when used in vector targeting strategies in proliferating tumor or endothelial cells [80–83]. Additionally, drug-inducible systems such as tat-on/tat-off regulated by tetracycline or rapamycin could provide a wide-dose response range in the treatment [84].

6.4. Transductional targeting

The second strategy of biologic targeting is to engineer the either viral or nonviral vectors in such a way that they can be captured only in tumor tissues, and therapeutic genes are produced only in the environment of the tumor tissue. There have been numerous attempts to modify the vectors with tumor cell-specific ligands that would increase the specific binding to tumor cells and reduce the toxicity. Therefore, targeting DNA complexes to the tumor cell-specific receptors is an attractive strategy. One of the well-known strategies is coating the surface of the complexes with transferrin, an iron-binding plasma protein that is mainly an up-regulated expression on rapidly proliferating cells as tumors [85]. Likewise, coating with EGF has also been reported to cause a 50-fold increase in the transgene expression in hepatocellular carcinoma cells [86]. The suicide gene HSV-TK/PEI complex mixed with a single chain antibody (scFv) against EGFR with a negatively charged oligopeptide tail has exhibited EGFR-specific gene transfer in vitro and in vivo [87].

The nonviral systems usually fail in promoting the delivery of DNA to the nucleus. Almost 99% of the internalized DNA from a nonviral vector is degraded in the cytoplasm [88]. Trafficking of exogenous DNA from cytosol to the nucleus may be improved by using the nuclear localization signal (NLS) found in some nuclear proteins [89]. Dermaseptins, a family of antimicrobial peptides that destabilize the membrane, have been successfully linked to NLS of SV40-T antigen and HIV-1 Rev protein [90]. Likewise, mellitin, which is a membrane-active protein, and viral protein r (vpr) of HIV-1, which binds directly to nucleoporins of the nuclear pore complex, have been successfully bound to PEI/DNA complexes to improve nuclear transport [91].

The selective targeting of viral vectors to specific cells permits the cell-specific expression of transgenes and enables the systemic administration of the vectors. Avoiding the targeting of the native receptor found on immune and inflammatory cell surfaces also reduces the immunity and inflammation to those vectors. Replication-competent retroviral vectors (RCR) based on murine leukemia virus (MLV) represent an attractive system for gene delivery through their ability to replicate and provide long term transgene expression in rapidly proliferating cells [92]. However, the uncontrolled spread of the RCR might cause the infection of nontarget cells. In order to develop tumor-selective RCR vectors, several modifications have been made such as a modification of the envelope protein by inserting single chain antibodies (scFv) [93] and peptide ligands [94]. Also, the specifically targeted entry of replication-deficient retroviral vectors has been accomplished by combining cell-specific monoclonal antibodies [95,96].

The capability of an Ad vector to infect a cell is mainly based on CAR and integrin expression. Following the attachment of an adenoviral vector to the target cell via C-terminal part of the fiber protein (knob) and CAR (Coxsackie's B adenovirus receptor), the alphaV beta3 and alphaV beta5 integrins mediate the internalization of the vector [97]. The CAR deficiency of the primary tumor cells limits the success of the gene therapy protocols using Ad vectors [98]. Redirecting the Ad vectors to bind other cellular receptors would allow CAR independent virus entry into the tumor cells. There are mainly two strategies to redirect the viral vectors to the cells: conjugate-based and genetically modified viral membranes. Adenoviral vectors have been targeted to different cells by genetic modification of the capsid or by using adapter molecules. In the conjugate-based strategy, it is aimed to complex the vector with the targeting molecule that redirects the vector to the cell-specific receptors. Bispecific molecules containing a first specificity for the fiber knob to block binding to CAR and the second specificity for a cell-specific receptor, such as bispecific fusion proteins (antibodies), bispecific peptides, polymer mediated ligand coupling, and chemical modifications (biotin–avidin bridges), have been utilized to target adenoviral vectors [99–101].

Adeno-associated vectors (AAV) possess a highly favorable safety profile and have the unique potential in certain cancer models. However, they have a restricted range of cells to transduce transgenes to the target tissues. In order to augment the transduction efficiency of AAV in various tissues retargeting strategies such as engineering of viral capsid, monoclonal antibodies and specific peptides have been used to successfully retarget the AAV vectors [102,103].

7. Targets for gene therapy of cancer

Current gene therapy studies have mainly focused on introducing the genes into the tumor cells to block the action of oncogene expression and the development of tumor vasculature, or to induce the development of an immune response against the cancer tissue. The major targets of gene therapy are shown on Table 1.

Tumor suppressor genes (p53, RB, APC, BRCA1)
Oncogenes (RAS, BCL-2, MET, MYC, ERBB2, HPV E6E7, etc.)
Drug-metabolizing enzymes (cytosine deaminase, HSV-thymidine kinase, cytochrom p450, purine nucleoside phosphorylase, carboxypeptidase A)
Direct cell killing (oncolytic vectors)
Angiogenesis (endostatin, angiostatin, VEGF, tissue factor, Tie2, etc.)
Cytokines (IL-2, IL-12, GM-CSF vb)
Immune system (T-cell receptor)/cancer vaccines (tumor-specific antigens, polynucleotide vaccines, genetically modified dendritic cell-based vaccines, and adoptive immunotherapies)

Table 1. The major targets of gene therapy of cancer

7.1. Tumor suppressor genes

Loss of functions of tumor suppressor genes have crucial role in the development and spread of cancer. Therefore, those genes were among the first targets of gene therapy studies. *P53* is mutated in almost 60 percent of solid tumors. Reintroducing wild-type p53 has been one of the common gene therapy approaches within the last two decades. The introduction of wild-type p53 by retroviruses or replication-deficient adenoviral vectors into the cancer cells inhibits tumor growth both in vitro and in vivo [104]. The use of adenoviral vectors carrying p53 has yielded some clinical activities, particularly in patients with head and neck cancers and lung cancers used either as a single agent or in combination with chemotherapy or radiotherapy [105,106]. Likewise, strategies aiming at the activation of p53 pathway in patients with p53-mutated tumors have also been tried. The introduction of small synthetic peptides like CDB3 derived from p53-binding protein 2 or p53 C terminal peptide have been shown to reactivate the mutant p53 functions in vitro [107]. Furthermore, transductions of other family members of p53 like p63 and p73, which are known to transactivate the downstream genes of p53 pathway, have been shown to induce apoptosis of tumor cells [108,109].

RB1 is a tumor suppressor gene involved in cell cycle regulation. Constitutively active RB1 potently inhibits cellular proliferation and induce persistent cell cycle arrest [110]. Since the first cloning of the RB gene at the beginning of the nineties, researchers have tried to activate the tumor suppressor function of the RB pathway. Gene transfer of truncated RB protein, such as RB94, has been shown to restore the RB pathway and to induce potent tumor growth inhibition both in vitro and in vivo [111]. However, these strategies have not been tested in the clinical setting yet.

The restoration of functions of other tumor suppressor genes such as adenomatosis polyposis coli (APC) in colorectal cancer cells [112] and BRCA1 in breast and ovarian cancers [113] has been shown to slow the growth of tumor cells.

7.2. Oncogenes

The targeting of oncogenes has long been at the focus of drug development studies in cancer. Small molecules of inhibitors of oncogene functions such as tyrosine kinase inhibitors have already been used in the routine treatment of various cancers. Gene therapeutic strategies to suppress oncogene functions are usually focused on the inhibition of those genes at mRNA level. Usually small oligonucleotides or RNA inhibitors such as short-interfering RNA (siRNA), short-hairpin RNA (shRNA), or micro-RNA (miRNA) have been used to interfere the actions of oncogenes [114].

Chemically modified or unmodified small single-stranded DNA molecules, antisense oligonucleotides inhibit protein translation through the disruption of ribosome assembly or utilization of RNase H enzymes to destroy mRNA. Numerous oligonucleotides and RNA inhibitors have been designed to inhibit oncogenes, including RAS, MYC, BCL-2, or cell signaling molecules survivin, IGF, VEGF, and PKCalphfa, have been tested. Although the efficacy of these oligonucleotides has shown a great diversity, some of them have been tested in phase II/III clinical trials in various cancer types [115]. Oblimersen, an antisense oligonucleotide targeting Bcl-2, is one of the oldest agents that have already tested in phase III studies of Chronic Lymphocytic Leukemia CLL and multiple myeloma [116,117]. The members of the RAS family of oncogenes have been found mutated in various solid tumors. Therefore, the targeting of RAS would have been a hot topic in the development of recent therapeutics.

Targeting RAS with an anti-RAS mRNA plasmid yielded significant tumor inhibition when used alone or in combination with chemotherapy in hepatoma cells [118]. Antisense oligonucleotides targeting survivin, which are highly expressed in various cancer types, including liver, lung, breast, and prostate, have been employed successfully to inhibit the expression of the gene [119]. The phase I/II clinical trials have also shown some responses in cancers [120].

7.3. Gene-Directed Enzyme/Prodrug Therapy (GDEPT)

Conventional chemotherapeutic drugs are mainly directed to nonspecific direct cell killing. However, dose-limiting toxicities avoid the use of higher doses of those drugs to eradicate the disseminated cancer. However, if the drug was synthesized within the tumor tissue, then the toxicity level would only increase in tumor cells but not other parts of the body. The tumor-specific targeting of drug-metabolizing genes and the systemic use of a prodrug that is converted to a cytotoxic agent by the action of transduced enzyme called gene-directed enzyme/prodrug therapy (GDEPT) enable the achievement of that aim. GDEPT is also known as suicide gene therapy. A lot of drug-metabolizing genes have been used to develop suicide gene therapy/prodrug systems. Cytosine deaminase (CD) and herpes simplex virus 1 thymidine kinase (HSV1-TK) are the most widely studied ones in cancer gene therapy [121,122]. CD, an enzyme found in fungi and bacteria, converts the nontoxic 5-fluorocyotsine into a toxic chemotherapy drug of 5-fluorouracil. The lack of this enzyme in mammalian cells makes it a convenient gene therapy tool to achieve intaratumoral chemotherapy. Others and we have designed suicide gene therapy vectors to avoid systemic toxicity of 5-FU. We have shown that Lp-driven CD carrying adenoviral vectors (AdLpCD) specifically target the epithelial cancers, including breast, ovary, prostate, and lung [123]. It is possible to achieve a 5-FU dose in tumor tissue as much as 200-fold of the dose when the drug is used intravenously at the standard dose [123]. The 5-FU produced in the infected tumor cells can diffuse into the neighboring tumor cells and kill them even not infected by the vector, which is called bystander effect [124]. Likewise, the combination of CD carrying vectors with conventional chemotherapy or radiotherapy yields synergistic efficacy [125–127].

TK, one of the immediate early (IE) genes of HSV, converts ganciclovir (GCV) into a triphosphated form of GCV, which is an analogue of purine and inhibits DNA polymerase [128]. HSV1-TK suicide gene therapy loaded onto either adenoviral vectors or retroviral vectors has been used to treat various tumors, including pancreatic cancer, hepatocellular carcinoma, lung cancer, glioma, and leukemia [129–133]. Although the exact mechanism of HSV-TK carrying vectors to kill tumor cells is not completely understood, they can induce apoptosis sensitizing the TNF-related ligands or the sensitization of CD95-L, TNF-related apoptosis inducing ligands may contribute to cell death [134]. The transcriptional targeting of HSV1-TK vectors using tumor-specific promoters has decreased the potential side effects [130]. HSV-TK/GCV prodrug systems have also been modified with other genes such as addition of E-cadherin to increase the bystander effect of the vector [129].

Other prodrug-activating enzymes such as purine nucleoside phosphorylase to convert 6-methylpurine-2-deoxyriboside to 6-methyl purine, cytochrome p450 cyclophosphamide and ifosfamide to active metabolites of phosphoramide mustard and acrolein cyanide, and carboxypeptidase methotrexate-alpha peptides to methotrexate have also been reported to decrease tumor burden in various preclinical models [135–137].

Dying tumor cells during suicide gene therapy could induce a tumor-specific immune response. Therefore, combining prodrug/enzyme systems with an immnuomodulating cytokine would further improve the efficacy. The addition of an IL-2 gene to the HSV-TK has yielded more potent antitumoral activity when compared the each strategy alone [138]. Similarly, GM-CSF, IL-12, and IL-18 have also been used to increase the antitumoral activity of suicide gene therapy [139,140]. Suicide gene therapy also successfully combines with other strategies such as targeting tumor angiogenesis or adoptive transfer [141,142].

7.4. Oncolytic viral vectors

Viruses have long been recognized tumor cell lytic agents and tried to treat cancer patients. However, the use of unmodified oncolytic viruses usually failed in the clinic. The engineering of those viruses to increase their therapeutic index have been possible in the last two decades. Herpes simplex virus (HSV), adenoviruses, parvoviruses, Newcastle disease virus, and retroviruses have been modified as oncolytic viral vectors.

HSV with its high infective capacity of a large number of cell types has been one of the popular oncolytic agents in the treatment of cancers. By deleting the genes thymidine kinase (TK), ribonucleotide reductase (RR), or ICP34.5 alone or in combination, HSV vectors could be selectively targeted many cancer types [143,144]. In order to further increase the cancer cell specificity of the replicating vector, engineering of the expression of surface glycoproteins, attachment of a novel receptor, or other macromolecules such as bispecific antibodies have been tested [145]. Likewise, tumor cell-specific promoters to drive the immediate–early gene expression, which is essential for viral replication, has been another effective strategy to obtain tumor-selective HSV [146].

Adenoviruses can infect a wide variety of dividing and nondividing normal and tumor cells. They can be engineered to have tumor-selective oncotropic properties or to be conditionally replicative (CRAds) for selective cancer gene therapy.

In type I CRAds, usually a mutant Ad vector that replicates specifically in tumor cells with aberrant cell cycle regulation has been developed. A deletion in the E1B 55-kDa region abrogates the p53 binding of the vector, and therefore, the vector cannot replicate in cells with intact p53 [147]. Therefore, this mutant Ad vector (dl1520) could replicate in only p53-deficient tumor cells. However, further studies revealed that E1B 55-kDa mutant CRAds could also replicate in p53 intact tumor cells [148,149]. The CRAds are already tested in phase II/III clinical trials with some success in patients with p53-deficient tumors [150]. Accordingly, the combination of CRAds with conventional treatment modalities provided better tumor control [151]. Although the combination of E1B-55kD mutant Ad vector with chemotherapy has yielded a promising result of 63% partial response in patients with head and neck cancer administered intratumorally [151], no objective responses were seen when the vector used alone [152,153].

Another way to achieve tumor-specific adenoviral replication is to take the advantage of altered cell cycle regulation at G1-S phase checkpoint in which the retinoblastoma 1 (RB1] gene functions. In most of the cancer cells, there is a mutation in RB1 gene. Therefore, an Ad vector having a mutation in the RB-binding site of E1A cannot induce the quiescent cells to pass the checkpoint. A mutant CRAd carrying an E1A deletion, Ad5-Δ24, is unable to replicate in normal cells with the wild-type RB1 gene [154]. It has been shown that this E1A mutant Ad vector has strong oncolytic activity in in vitro experiments of glioblastoma cells. Also, a similar vector with E1A mutations at RB-binding sites (dl922-947) has also been shown to have strong antitumor activity in other tumor models such as breast and colon cancer [155]. An additional promising strategy to achieve specific oncolytic activity to the CRAds is the use of tumor-specific promoters that drive the genes of the vector responsible for the replication, referred to as type II CRAds. There have been many replication-competent vectors carrying tumor- or tissue-specific promoters such as prostate-specific antigen (PSA), alphafeto protein (AFP), Tcf4, MUC1, and CEA that have been developed [156–160]. We have designed replication-competent adenoviral vectors carrying Lp-driven E1A, which are specifically replicated in various tumor cell lines but not in normal cells [161]. We have also constructed a bicistronic CRAd vector carrying both cytosine deaminase (CD) gene and E1A linked by an IRES component driven by the Lp promoter (AdLpCDIRESE1A) [162]. The new bicistronic construct also has been shown to have significant oncolytic activity in the colon (HTB-38), breast (MCF-7), ovary (Ovcar 5], and prostate (LNCaP) cancer cell lines but not in normal human mammary epithelial cells [162]. Also, the combination of the construct, AdLpCDIRESE1A/ 5flourocytosine system, and chemotherapy has shown synergistic activity [163].

Different replication-competent viruses are currently being studied for their potential use in cancer gene therapy. The naturally occurring tumor-selective viruses in their replication and cytolysis might have the potential in cancer treatment. Autonomous parvoviruses (APV) have been shown to replicate more efficiently in transformed cells than normal cells [164]. The members of the rodent group of APVs such as LuIII, MVM (minute virus of mice), and H1, which can infect human cells, are currently being studied as vectors for cancer gene therapy. The replication of APV depends on cellular functions expressed during the S phase of the cell cycle. The oncogenic transformation of cells favor the replication of APVs and therefore makes them as oncolytic viruses [165]. The overexpression of the RAS signaling pathway [166] and the defects in the interferon pathway of the transformed cells [167] could possibly enhance the oncolytic activity of the APVs. Further manipulation of the specific targeting of those vectors to achieve tumor-specific transgene expression such as inserting binding sites for the hetero-dimer beta-catenin/Tcf transcription factor to the MVM P4 promoter to make it responsive to wnt signaling would make those attractive vectors for cancer gene therapy [168].

Newcastle disease virus (NDV) is an animal virus showing oncolytic activity in transformed cells. In murine tumor xenograft models, the intratumoral administration of NDV has caused significant tumor reduction [169]. Also, the intraperitoneal injection of the virus has resulted in complete regressions of tumor xenografts. A replication-competent strain of NDV, PV701, has been shown to replicate in tumor tissues of patients with solid tumors when administered intravenously [170]. In that phase, trial objective responses have also been achieved at higher and repeated doses of the virus.

The murine hepatitis coronavirus (MHV), an oncolytic virus, is a positive-strand RNA virus displaying strong species specificity with a replication cycle of 10–15 h and efficiently kills cells by fusion of the infected cells with their neighboring cells [171]. Substituting its spike protein by the other species such as porcine amino peptidase could change the host cell tropism of the MHV. The resulting recombinant corona virus pMHV thus only infects porcine cells via the porcine amino peptide N (pAPN) receptor. In vitro studies have shown that the tumor cells could be more susceptible to that recombinant corona virus [172]. It is also likely to further manipulate those vectors by using specific antibodies.

7.5. Tumor vascular targeting therapy

Unraveling the mechanisms of tumor-induced angiogenesis, which is a key event in tumor growth and metastasis, has opened a new therapeutic era in cancer treatment. The antiangiogenic gene therapy approaches have been reported to inhibit the tumor-induced angiogenesis and therefore tumor growth. The main strategies in antiangiogenic gene therapy are targeting specifically the endothelial cells (direct antiangiogenic gene therapy) and interfering with a tumor-derived angiogenic factor or the receptor for it or delivery of genes that encode angiogenesis inhibitors (indirect antiangiogenic therapy).

Proangiogenic cytokines such as vascular endothelial growth factor (VEGF) and basic fibroblast growth factor (bFGF) mainly secreted from tumor cells are required for the new vessel formation. The indirect strategies were mainly focused on the inhibition of proangiogenic cytokines or receptors involved in VEGF pathway or basic fibroblast growth factor (bFGF). VEGF binds two high affinity receptors (VEGFR1/FLT-1 and VEGFR-2/KDR) that are expressed on endothelial cells. An adenovirus-mediated transfer of a secreted form of the extracellular domain of the FLT-1 (AdsFLT) has been shown to inhibit the growth of metastatic tumor deposits when administered intravenously to preestablished splenic and liver metastases from a murine colon carcinoma cell line in syngeneic mice [173].

Likewise, the delivery of genes encoding antiangiogenic proteins such as endostatin, angiostatin, platelet factor 4, interferon alpha, and thrombospondins have also been tested [174]. The intratumoral administration of a plasmid encoding murine endostatin under the control of a CMV promoter has provided elevated concentrations of endostatin high enough to obtain growth arrest of murine renal carcinoma cells and breast cancer model [175]. Likewise, an adenoviral vector carrying human endostatin gene markedly reduced the blood vessel density of the tumor in an orthotopic liver tumor model [176].

The viral vector constructs of other angiogenesis inhibitors such as angiostatitn, thrombospondin, platelet factor 4, and hepatocyte growth factor antagonists have also been shown to successfully inhibit endothelial cell proliferation and tumor growth [177–180]. However, there are conflicting results regarding the tumor inhibiting activity of antiangiogenic gene therapy modality in experimental models. The combination of antiangiogenic gene therapy with chemotherapy or radiation could be an efficient way of the inhibition of tumor growth [181].

Many vector constructs carrying therapeutic or reporter genes driven by endothelium-specific promoters such as preproendothelin-1 (PPE-1), VEGFR kinase insert domain receptor

(KDR), VEGF, E-selectin, and endoglin/CD105 have been reported to specifically target endothelial cells [182,183]. The replication-competent adenoviral vectors driven by the regulatory elements of FLK-1 and endoglin have successfully been targeted to the dividing endothelial cells, and therefore, this strategy could be used as an antiangiogenic treatment for cancer [184]. The activation of proapoptotic caspases such as caspase 9, driven by endothelium-specific promoters such as VEGF and FGF, could be another strategy to destroy endothelial cells [185].

Antisense approaches also are being tested for the inhibition of VEGF. A recombinant adeno-associated virus (rAAV) vector encoding an antisense mRNA against VEGF has been shown to inhibit the production of endogenous tumor cell VEGF [186]. The adenovirus-mediated delivery of an uPA uPAR antagonist, which inhibits FGF, has been shown to inhibit angiogenesis-dependent tumor growth and metastasis in mice [187].

7.6. Immune system as the target of cancer gene therapy

The immune system is the most important defense mechanism of the body against cancer. Recent developments in gene therapy have suggested to many cancer therapists that cytokine–chemokine-based gene therapies, tumor antigen-specific vaccination strategies, and gene-modified cellular therapies have great potential for future use either in the treatment of an established disease or in the prevention of cancer in people having high risk of developing cancer.

Cytokine/chemokine-based gene therapy has been widely used to induce immune system against tumors. The delivery of immunomodulatory cytokines by gene therapy vectors has opened a new avenue both to decrease the toxicity of these cytokines when used systemically and to augment antitumor immunity. A wide variety of cytokines such as GM-CSF, IFN-a, IFN-g, IL-2, IL-4, IL-12, IL-18, and IL-24 have been tested so far [188–191]. Also, the vector constructs, including the combination of these cytokines, have also been tested in cancer. The coexpression of IL-12 and GM-CSF has been reported to yield significantly more immune response than the either cytokines alone [192]. In particular, implementing the cytokine genes into oncolytic viruses has great potential for use in clinical trials [193]. Chemokines recruit the immune effector cells to the tumor microenvironment. The delivery of chemokines such as CCL-5 using viral vectors has also resulted in significant tumor reduction through increasing tumor infiltration of DCs, macrophages, and CTLs [194].

Tumor-associated antigens (TAA) loaded on to gene therapy vectors have been tested in cancer treatment (DNA vaccines) [195,196]. However, the efficacy of using TAA alone is not enough to get a sufficient immune response to decrease tumor size. Therefore, researchers have focused on the augmentation of the immune response by combining immune cytokines or costimulatory molecules and TAA. This strategy seems much better than using either gene alone. We have previously shown an increased efficacy of an adenoviral vector encoding a fusion protein of CD40L and MUC1 in preclinical models [197]. The addition of prodrug/enzyme system to DNA vaccination further increased the efficacy [198]. This strategy has also been tested in early clinical trials with some success. Vector vaccinations using cytokines or costimulatory molecules and tumor-associated antigens (TAA) have increased the immune responses and caused antitumor responses in preclinical models and even some responses in earlier clinical trials. In a small clinical trial, an attenuated vaccinia vector carrying IL-2 and MUC1 has been found effective in a small group of patients with advanced prostatic cancer [199]. Likewise, a vector vaccine of canary poxvirus encoding B7.1 and CEA has been tested in a group of patients with epithelial tumors [200]. Hundreds of different DNA vaccines have been tested in clinical trials so far [202]. However, no DNA vaccine is available in the market.

Gene therapy vectors have also been used to transduce either autologous tumor cells or dendritic cells. In the earlier studies, irradiated autologous tumor cells transduced to express immunostimulatory molecules have been tested. In a syngeneic colon cancer model, the subcutaneous injection of CT26 colon cancer cells transduced with an adenoviral vector carrying GM-CSF gene has eliminated both the established tumors and prevented the growth of new tumor nodules when rechallenged with tumor cells [201]. Later on, this strategy has also been tested in human tumors. Autologous tumors transduced with GVAX, an adenovirus carrying GM-CSF, have induced tumor-specific immunity in a variety of tumors, including melanoma, prostate, and lung cancers [203]. Although a slight increase in overall survival has been reported in those trials, no significant tumor responses observed [203,204].

The ex vivo transduction of dendritic cells with gene therapy vectors carrying either immunostimulatory genes or TAAs is another promising strategy. When injected subcutaneously, the dendritic cells exposed to vectors migrate to the lymph nodes where they prime cytotoxic T cells and induce a strong immune response. A number of vectors have been designed to activate dendritic cells for the past two decades. We have tested the use of ex vivo transduced dendritic cells with an adenoviral vector carrying a fusion protein of CD40L and MUC1 in a syngeneic mouse tumor model [205]. The intratumoral injection of activated dendritic cells induced a potent tumor-specific T-cell response. Furthermore, the combination of suicide gene therapy of a CD/5FU system and activated dendritic cells caused a more potent immune response and increased tumor response [205]. Likewise, retroviral vectors and lentiviral vectors are both used to transduce dendritic cells [206]. A dendritic cell vaccine based on the ex vivo activation of mononuclear antigen presenting cells by a fusion protein consisting prostatic acid phosphatase and GM-CSF has extended the progression-free survival of patients with advanced prostatic cancer and approved by FDA in 2010 (Provenge®, Dendreon, USA) [207].

Recently, an adoptive therapy of cancer using genetically modified T cells armed with chimeric antigen receptors (CAR) has gained great popularity with the announcement of success in advanced malignancies [208]. CAR is a fusion receptor of an antibody-derived targeting domain and T-cell signaling domain and expressed on T cells by a retroviral vector [209]. CARs target antigens, including proteins, carbohydrates, and glycolipids without antigen processing or HLA recognition. They can be generated in significant quantities ex vivo and used with the minimal risk of autoimmunity or graft versus host disease [210,211]. However, because of the severe side effects, the most troublesome being cytokine-release syndrome, researchers try to obtain better CAR T cells with further refinement of receptor and better targets [212].

8. Cancer gene therapy in the clinic—Future prospects

The vast majority of the clinical trials of gene therapy have been devoted to the treatment of cancer so far. The gene therapy agents have been tested in many types of cancer in the clinic. Almost 1200 clinical trials (approximately 64% of all gene therapy trials) in cancer have been started, conducted, or completed [202]. Less than 4% of those are phase II or III and only few of them are phase IV trials [202]. Although the preclinical and experimental studies have yielded highly encouraging results, the progress in the clinic is not so remarkable. There is no gene therapy agent available in the market yet.

The most important factor that has limited the success of clinical gene therapy trials in human subjects is the delivery of the vector genetic elements or their products to the target cancer cells and their vasculature. A second problem has been toxicity. Recent advances on improving the delivery and specificity of gene therapy vectors have suggested these trials may be more successful in the coming years. This is especially true of the attempts to use vectors to activate the immune response against the tumor tissue. Continued testing of these strategies in the context of clinical trials may lead to new opportunities for individuals engaged in a personal struggle with cancer to control their disease.

Indeed, the nature of the distant spread of the disease, which causes the failure of conventional treatment modalities, is also one of the main drawbacks of gene therapy of cancer.

Author details

Hakan Akbulut*, Muge Ocal and Gizem Sonugur

*Address all correspondence to: akbulut@medicine.ankara.edu.tr

Gene Therapy Research Unit, Department of Medical Oncology, Ankara University School of Medicine, Ankara, Turkey

References

[1] Hanahan D, Weinberg RA. Hallmarks of cancer: the next generation. Cell 2011;144:646–74.

[2] Fidler IJ. Seed and soil revisited: contribution of the organ microenvironment to cancer metastasis. Surg Oncol Clin N Am 2001;10:257–69.

[3] Gacche RN, Meshram RJ. Angiogenic factors as potential drug target: efficacy and limitations of anti-angiogenic therapy. Biochim Biophys Acta 2014;1846:161–79.

[4] Zhang J, Hochwald SN. Targeting receptor tyrosine kinases in solid tumors. Surg Oncol Clin N Am 2013;22:685–703.

[5] Cheng L, Ren W, Xie L, Li M, Liu J, Hu J, Liu BR, Qian XP. Anti-EGFR MoAb treatment in colorectal cancer: limitations, controversies, and contradictories. Cancer Chemother Pharmacol 2014;74:1–13.

[6] Naidoo J, Page DB, Wolchok JD. Immune checkpoint blockade. Hematol Oncol Clin North Am 2014;28:585–600.

[7] Frohlich MW. Sipuleucel-T for the treatment of advanced prostate cancer. Semin Oncol 2012;39:245–52.

[8] Hong B, van den Heuvel AP, Prabhu VV, Zhang S, El-Deiry WS. Targeting tumor suppressor p53 for cancer therapy: strategies, challenges and opportunities. Curr Drug Targets 2014;15:80–9.

[9] Pagliarini R, Shao W, Sellers WR. Oncogene addiction: pathways of therapeutic response, resistance, and road maps toward a cure. EMBO Rep 2015;16:280–296.

[10] Katoh M. Therapeutics targeting angiogenesis: genetics and epigenetics, extracellular miRNAs and signaling networks (Review). Int J Mol Med 2013;32:763–7.

[11] Low D, Parker SE, Latimer T, Abai AM, Kuwahara-Rundell A, Doh SG, Yang ZY, Laface D, Gromkowski SH, Nabel GJ, Manthorpe M, Norman J. Cancer gene therapy using plasmid DNA: pharmacokinetic study of DNA following injection in mice. Hum Gene Ther 1995;6:53–564.

[12] Legendre JY, Szoka F Jr. Delivery of plasmid DNA into mammalian cell lines using pH-sensitive liposomes: comparison with cationic liposomes. Pharm Res 1992;9:1235–1242.

[13] Paul FW, Dutzar B, Stayton PS, Hoffman A, Anklesiaria P, Harvie P. Poly propylacrylic acid (PPAA) functions as an endosomal escape agent synergistically enhancing the transfection potency of folate targeted cationic–lipid–protamine–DNA (LPD) complexes. Mol Ther 2003;7:208.

[14] Bruckheimer EM, Harvie P, Orthel J, Dutzar B, Furstoss K, Mebel E, Anklesaria P, Paul R. In vivo efficacy of folate-targeted lipid–protamine–DNA (LPD-PEG-Folate) complexes in an immunocompetent sybgeneic model for breast adenocarcinoma. Mol Ther 2003;7:129.

[15] Bailey AL, Sullivan SM. Efficient encapsulation of DNA plasmids in small neutral liposomes induced by ethanol and calcium. Biochim Biophys 2000;1468:239–252.

[16] De Smedt Sc, Demeester J, Hennink WE. Cationic polymer based gene delivery systems. Pharm Res 2000;17:113–126.

[17] Kircheis R, Schuller S, Brunner S, Ogris M, Heider KH, Zauner W, Wagner E. Polycation-based DNA complexes for tumor-targeted gene delivery in vivo. J Gene Med 1999;1:111–120.

[18] Zou SM, Erbacher P, Remy JS, Behr JP. Systemic linear polyethynilemine (L-PEI)-mediated gene delivery in the mouse. J Gene Med 2000;2:128.

[19] Oupicky D, Ogris M, Howard KA, Dash PR, Ulbrich K, Seymour LW. Importance of lateral and steric stabilization of polyelectrolyte gene delivery vectors for extended systemic circulation. Mol Ther 2002;5:463–472

[20] Ogris M, Wagner E. Targeting tumors with non-viral gene delivery systems. Drug Discov Today 2002;15:479–485.

[21] Kircheis R, Wightman L, Schreiber A, Robitza B, Rouslar V, Kursa M, Wanger E. Polyethylenimine/DNA complexes shielded by transferring target gene expression to tumors after systemic application. Gene Ther 2001;8:28–40.

[22] Overbaugh J, Miller AD, Eiden MV. Receptors and entry cofactors for retroviruses include single and multiple transmembrane-spanning proteins as well as newly described glycophosphatidylinositol-anchored and secreted proteins. Microbiol Mol Biol Rev 2001;65:371–89.

[23] Yi Y, Jong Noh M, Hee Lee K. Current advances in retroviral gene therapy. Curr Gene Ther 2011;11:218–228.

[24] Ismail SI, Kingsman SM, Kingsman AJ, Uden M. Split-intron retroviral vectors: enhanced expression with improved safety. J Virol 2000;74:2365–71.

[25] Hacein-Bey-Abina S, von Kalle C, Schmidt M, Le Deist F, Wulffraat N, Mclntyre E, Radford I, Villeval JL, Fraser CC, Cavazzana-Calvo M, Fischer A. A serious adverse event after successful gene therapy for X-linked severe combined immunodeficiency. N Engl J Med 2003;348:255–6.

[26] Baum C, Dullmann J, Li Z, Fehse B, Meyer J, Williams DA, von Kalle C. Side effects of retroviral gene transfer into hematopoietic stem cells. Blood 2003;101:2099–114.

[27] Wold WS, Toth K. Adenovirus vectors for gene therapy, vaccination and cancer gene therapy. Curr Gene Ther 2013;1:421–33.

[28] Lopez-Gordo E, Podgorski II, Downes N, Alemany R. Circumventing antivector immunity: potential use of nonhuman adenoviral vectors. Hum Gene Ther. 2014;25:285–300.

[29] Yao XL, Nakagawa S, Gao JQ. Current targeting strategies for adenovirus vectors in cancer gene therapy. Curr Cancer Drug Targets 2011;11:810–25.

[30] Khare R, Chen CY, Weaver EA, Barry MA. Advances and future challenges in adenoviral vector pharmacology and targeting. Curr Gene Ther 2011;11:241–58.

[31] Kasala D, Choi JW, Kim SW, Yun CO. Utilizing adenovirus vectors for gene delivery in cancer. Expert Opin Drug Deliv 2014;11:379–92.

[32] Lerch TF, Xie Q, Chapman MS. The structure of adeno-associated virus serotype 3B (AAV-3B): insights into receptor binding and immune evasion. Virology 2010;403[1]: 26–36.

[33] Luo J, Luo Y, Sun J, Zhou Y, Zhang Y, Yang X. Adeno-associated virus-mediated cancer gene therapy: current status. Cancer Lett 2015;356:347–56.

[34] Dunbar CE, Emmons RV. Gene transfer into hematopoietic progenitor and stem cells: progress and problems. Stem Cells 1994;12:563–76.

[35] Carruthers KH, Metzger G, During MJ, Muravlev A, Wang C, Kocak E. Gene-directed enzyme prodrug therapy for localized chemotherapeutics in allograft and xenograft tumor models. Cancer Gene Ther 2014;21:434–40.

[36] Kotterman MA, Schaffer DV. Engineering adeno-associated viruses for clinical gene therapy. Nat Rev Genet 2014;15:445–451.

[37] Airenne KJ, Hu Y-C, Kost TA, Smith RH, Kotin RM, Ono C, Matsuura Y, Wang S, Yla-Herttsala S. Baculovirus: an insect-derived vector for diverse gene transfer applications. Mol Ther 2013;21:739–749.

[38] Hu Y-C. Baculovirus vectors for gene therapy. Adv Virus Res 2006;68:287–320.

[39] Luo WY, Shih YS, Hung CL, Lo KW, Chiang CS, Lo WH, Huang SF, Wang SC, Yu CF, Chien CH, Hu YC. Development of the hybrid sleeping beauty: baculovirus vector for sustained gene expression and cancer therapy. Gene Ther 2012;19: 844–851.

[40] van Oers MM, Pijlman GP, Vlak JM. Thirty years of baculovirus–insect cell protein expression: from dark horse to mainstream technology. J Gen Virol 2015;96:6–23.

[41] Baldo A, van den Akker E, Bergmans HE, Lim F, Pauwels K. General considerations on the biosafety of virus-derived vectors used in gene therapy and vaccination. Curr Gene Ther 2013;13:385–394.

[42] Manservigi R, Argnani R, Marconi P. HSV recombinant vectors for gene therapy. Open Virol J 2010;4:123–156.

[43] Zhang G, Jin G, Nie X, Mi R, Zhu G, Jia W, Liu F. Enhanced antitumor efficacy of an oncolytic herpes simplex virus expressing an endostatin–angiostatin fusion gene in human glioblastoma stem cell xenografts. PLoS One 2014;9:e95872.

[44] Moss B. Genetically engineered poxviruses for recombinant gene expression, vaccination, and safety. Proc Natl Acad Sci U S A 1996; 93:11341–11348.

[45] Gómez CE, Nájera JL, Krupa M, Esteban M. The Poxvirus vectors MVA and NYVAC as gene delivery systems for vaccination against infectious diseases and cancer. Curr Gene Ther 2008;8:97–120.

[46] Vile RG, Russel S, Lemoine N. Cancer gene therapy: hard lessons and new courses. Gene Ther 2000;7:2–8.

[47] Zhang L, Dailey PJ, Gettie A, Blanchard J, Ho DD. The liver is a major organ clearing simian immunodeficiency virus in rhesus monkeys. J Virol 2002;76:5271–5273.

[48] Mantovani A, Bototazzi B, Colotta F, Sozzani S, Ruco L. The origin and function of tumor-associated macrophages. Immunol Today 1992;10:265–270.

[49] Pastorino S, Massaza S, Cilli M, Varesio L, Bosco MC. Generation of high titer retroviral vector-producing macrophages as vehicles for in vivo gene transfer. Gene Ther 2001;8:431–441.

[50] Griffith KD, Read Ej, Carrasquilly JA, Carter CS, Yang JC, Fisher B, Aebersold P, Packard BS, Yu MY, Rosenberg SA. In vivo distribution of adoptively transferred indium-111 labeled tumor infiltrating lymphocytes and peripheral blood lymphocytes in patients with metastatic melanoma. J Natl Cancer Inst 1989;81:1709–1717.

[51] Chang AE, Li Q, Bishop DK, Normolle Dp, Redman BD, Nickoloff BJ. Immunogenetic therapy of human melanoma utilizing autologous tumor cells transduced to secrete granulocyte-macrophage colony stimulating factor. Hum Gene Ther 2000;11:839–850.

[52] Porada CD, Almeida-Porada G. Mesenchymal Stem Cells as Therapeutics and Vehicles for Gene and Drug Delivery. Adv Drug Deliv Rev 2010;62:1156–1166.

[53] Zuk PA, Zhu M, Mizuno H, Huang J, Futrell JW, Katz AJ, Benhaim P, Lorenz HP, Hedrick MH. Multilineage cells from human adipose tissue: implications for cell-based therapies. Tisue Eng 2001;7:211–228.

[54] Morizono K, De Ugarte DA, Zhu M, Zuk P, Elbarbary A, Ashjian P, Benhaim P, Chen ISY, Hedrick MH. Multilineage cells from adipose tissue as gene delivery vehicles. Hum Gene Ther 2003;14:59–66.

[55] Kang WK, Park C, Yoon HL, Kim WS, Yoon SS, Lee MH, Park K, Kim K, Jeong HS, Kim JA, Nam SJ, Yang JH, Son YI, Baek CH, Han J, Ree HJ, Lee ES, Kim SH, Kim DW, Ahn YC, Huh SJ, Choe YH, Lee JH, Park MH, Kong GS, Park EY, Kang YK, Bang YJ, Paik NS, Lee SN, Kim SH, Kim S, Robbins PD, Tahara H, Lotze MT, Park CH. Interleukin 12 gene therapy of cancer by peritumoral injection of transduced autologous fibrobloasts: outcome of a phase I study. Hum Gene Ther 2001;12:671–684.

[56] Löhr M, Hoffmeyer A, Kröger J, Freund M, Hain J, Holle A, Karle P, Knöfel WT, Liebe S, Müller P, Nizze H, Renner M, Saller RM, Wagner T, Hauenstein K, Günzburg WH, Salmons B. Microencapsulated cell-mediated treatment of inoperable pancreatic carcinoma. Lancet 2001;357:1591–1593.

[57] Moret-Tatay I, Díaz J, Marco FM, Crespo A, Aliño SF. Complete tumor prevention by engineered tumor cell vaccines employing nonviral vectors. Cancer Gene Ther 2003;10:887–897.

[58] Vasey PA, Shulman LN, Campos S, Davis J, Gore M, Johnston S, Kirn DH, O'Neill V, Siddiqui N, Seiden MV, Kaye SB. Phase I trial of intraperitoneal injection of the E1B-55-kd-gene-deleted adenovirus ONYX-015 (dl1520) given on days 1 through 5every 3 weeks in patients with recurrent/refractory epithelial ovarian cancer. J Clin Oncol 2002;20:1562–9.

[59] Li L, Liu RY, Huang JL, Liu QC, Li Y, Wu PH, Zeng YX, Huang W. Adenovirus-mediated intra tumoral delivery of the human endostatin gene inhibits tumor growth in nasopharyngeal carcinoma. Int J Cancer 2006;118:2064–71.

[60] Markert JM, Medlock MD, Rabkin SD, Gillespie GY, Todo T, Hunter WD, Palmer CA, Feigenbaum F, Tornatore C, Tufaro F, Martuza RL. Conditionally replicating herpes simplex virus mutant, G207 for the treatment of malignant glioma: results of a phase I trial. Gene Ther 2000;7:1–4.

[61] Rampling R, Cruickshank G, Papanastassiou V, Nicoll J, Hadley D, Brennan D,Petty R, MacLean A, Harland J, McKie E, Mabbs R, Brown M. Toxicity evaluation of replication-competent herpes simplex virus (ICP34.5 null mutant 1716] in patients with recurrent malignant glioma. Gene Ther 2000;7:859–866.

[62] Das SK, Sarkar S, Dash R, Dent P, Wang XY, Sarkar D, Fisher PB. Cancer terminator viruses and approaches for enhancing therapeutic outcomes. Adv Cancer Res 2012;115:1–38.

[63] Dorer DE, Nettelbeck DM. Targeting cancer by transcriptional control in cancer gene therapy and viral oncolysis. Adv Drug Deliv Rev 2009;61:554–71.

[64] Osaki T, Tanio Y, Tachibana I, Hosoe S, Kumagal T, Kawase I, Oikawa S, Kishimoto T. Gene therapy for carcinoembryonic antigen-producing human lung cancer cels by cell type-specific expression of herpes simplex virus thymidine kinase gene. Cancer Res 1994;54:5258–5261.

[65] Takahashi M, Sato T, Sagawa T, Lu Y, Sato Y, Iyama S, Yamada Y, Fukaura J, Takahashi S, Miyanishi K, Yamashita T, Sasaki K, Kogawa K, Hamada H, Kato J, Niitsu Y. E1B-55K-deleted adenovirus expressing E1A-13S by AFP-enhancer/promoter is capable of highly specific replication in AFP-producing hepatocellular carcinoma and eradication of established tumor. Mol Ther 2002;5:627–34.

[66] Gupta VK, Park JO, Kurihara T, Koons A, Mauceri HJ, Jaskowiak NT, Kufe DW, Weichselbaum RR, Posner MC. Selective gene expression using a DF3/MUC1 promoter in a human esophageal adenocarcinoma model. Gene Ther 2003;10:206–12.

[67] Pandha HS, Martin L-A, Rigg A, Hurst HC, Stamp GWH, Sikora K, Lemoine NR. Genetic prodrug activation therapy for breast cancer: a phase I clinical trial of c-erbB2 directed suicide gene expression. J Clin Oncol 1999;17:2180–2189.

[68] Nishino K, Osaki T, Kumagai T, Kijima T, Tachibana I, Goto H, Arai T, Kimura H, Funakoshi T, Takeda Y, Tanio Y, Hayashi S. Adenovirus-mediated gene therapy spe-

cific for small cell lung cancer cells using a Myc-Max binding motif. Int J Cancer 2001;91:851–6.

[69] Latham JP, Searle PF, Mautner V, James ND. Prostate specificantigen promoter/ enhancer driven gene therapy for prostate cancer: construction and testing of a tissue specific adenovirus vector. Cancer Res 2000;60:334–341.

[70] Vile RG, Nelson JA, Castleden S, Chong H, Hart IR. Systemic gene therapy of immune melanoma using tissue specific expression of the HSVtk gene involves an immune component. Cancer Res 1994;54:228–234.

[71] Miyatake SI, Tani S, Feigenbaum F, Sundaresan P, Toda H,Narumi O, Kikuchi H, Hashimoto N, Hangai M, Martuza RL, Rabkin SD. Hepatoma-specific anti-tumor activity of an albumin enhancer/promoter regulated herpes simplex virus in vivo. Gene Ther 1999;6:564–572.

[72] Kitazono M, Chuman Y, Aikou T, Fojo T. Adenovirus HSV-TK construct with thyroid-specific promoter: enhancement of activity and specificity with histone deacetylase inhibitors and agents modulating the camp pathway. Int J Cancer 2002;99:453–9.

[73] McKie EA, Graham DI, Brown SM. Selective astrocytic transgene expression in vitro and in vivo from the GFAP promoter in a HSV RL1 null mutant vector-potential glioblastoma targeting. Gene Ther 1998;5:440–450.

[74] Kubo H, Gardner TA, Wada Y, Koeneman KS, Gotoh A, Yang L, Kao C, Lim SD, Amin MB, Yang H, Black ME, Matsubara S, Nakagawa M, Gillenwater JY, Zhau HE, Chung LW. Phase I dose escalation clinical trial of adenovirus vector carrying osteocalcin promoter-driven herpes simplex virus thymidine kinase in localized and metastatic hormone-refractory prostate cancer. Hum Gene Ther 2003;14:227–241.

[75] Li GC, He F, Shao X, Urano M, Shen L, Kim D, Borrelli M, Leibel SA, Gutin PH, Ling CC. Adenovirus-mediated heat-activated antisense Ku70 expression radiosensitizes tumor cells in vitro and in vivo. Cancer Res 2003; 63:3268–74.

[76] Ruan H, Su H, Hu L, Lamborn KR, Kan YW, Deen DF. A hypoxia-regulated adeno-associated virus vector for cancer-specific gene therapy. Neoplasia 2001;3:255–63.

[77] Walther W, Wendt J, Stein U. Employment of the mdr1 promoter for the chemotherapy-inducible expression of therapeutic genes in cancer gene therapy. Gene Ther 1997; 4:544–52.

[78] Walther W, Stein U, Fichtner I, Alexander M, Shoemaker RH, Schlag PM. Mdr1 promoter-driven tumor necrosis factor-alpha expression for a chemotherapy-controllable combined in vivo gene therapy and chemotherapy of tumors. Cancer Gene Ther 2000 7:893–900.

[79] Parr MJ, Manome Y, Tanaka T, Wen P, Kufe DW, Kaelin WG Jr, Fine HA. Tumor-selective transgene expression in vivo mediated by an E2F-responsive adenoviral vector. Nat Med 1997;3:1145–1149.

[80] Tsihlias J, Kapusta L, Slingerland J. The prognostic significance of altered cyclin-dependent kinase inhibitors in human cancer. Annu Rev Med 1999;50:401–423.

[81] Naruse I, Hashiro H, Doboushi K, Minato K, Saito R, Mori M. Over-expression of p27 (kip1] induces growth arrest and apoptosis mediated by changes of Rb expression in lung cancer cell lines. Int J Cancer 2000;88:377–83.

[82] Yang CT, You L, Yeh CC, Chang JWC, Zhang F, McCormick F, Jablons DM. Adenovirus-mediated p14 (ARF) gene transfer in human mesothelioma cells. J Natl Cancer Inst 2000;92:636–641.

[83] Nettelbeck DM, Zwicker J, Lucibello FC, Gross C, Liu N, Brusselbach S, Muller R. Cell cycle regulated promoters for the targeting of tumor endothelium. Adv Exp Med Biol 1998;451:437–40.

[84] Kimchi-Sarfaty C, Gottesman MM. SV40 pseudovirions as highly efficient vectors for gene transfer and their potential application in cancer therapy. Curr Pharm Biotechnol 2004;5:451–8.

[85] Kursa M, Walker GF, Roessler V, Ogris M, Roedl W, Kircheis R, Wagner E. Novel shielded transferrin-polyethylene glycol-polyethynilemine/DNA complexes for systemic tumor-targeted gene transfer. Bioconjug Chem 2003;14 :222–231.

[86] Liu X, Tian P, Yu Y, Yao M, Cao X, Gu J. Enhanced antitumor effect of EGF R targeted p21WAF-1 and GM-CSF gene transfer in the established murine hepatoma by peritumoral injection. Cancer Gene Ther 2002;9:100–108.

[87] Suzuki M, Takayanagi A, Shimizu N. Recombinant single-chain antibodies with various oligopeptide tails for targeted gene delivery. Gene Ther 2003;10:781–88.

[88] Davis ME. Non-viral gene delivery systems. Curr Opin Biotechnol 2002;13:128–131.

[89] Neves C, Escriov V, Byk G, Schermann P, Wils P. Intracellular fate and nuclear targeting of plasmid DNA. Cell Biol Toxicol 1999;15:193–202.

[90] Harriton-Gazal E, Feder R, Mor A, Graessmann A, Brack-Werner R, Jons D, Gilon C, Loyter A. Targeting of non-karyophilic cell-permeable peptides into the nuclei of intact cells by covalently attached nuclear localization signals. Biochemistry 2002;41:9208–9214.

[91] Ogris M, Carlisle RC, Bettinger T, Seymour LW. Mellitin enables efficient vesicular escape and enhanced nuclear access of non-viral gene delivery vectors. J Biol Chem 2001;276:47550–47555.

[92] Logg R, Tai CK, Logg A, Anderson WF, Kasahara N. A uniquely stable replication-competent retrovirus vector achieves efficient gene delivery in vitro and in solid tumors. Hum Gene Ther 2001;12:921–932.

[93] Martin F, Chowdrhury S, Neil SJ, Chester KA, Gosset F-L, Collins MK. Targeted retroviral infection of tumor celss by receptor cooperation. J Virol 2003;77:2753–2756.

[94] Kasahara N, Dozy AM, Kan YW. Tissue specific targeting of retroviral vectors through ligand-receptor interactions. Science 1994;266:1373–1376.

[95] Khare PD, Liao S, Hirose Y, Kuroki M, Fujimura S, Yamauchi Y. Tumor growth suppression by a retroviral vector displaying scFv antibody to CEA and carrying the iNOS gene. Anticancer Res 2002;22:2443–2446.

[96] Tai C-K, Logg CR, Park JH, Anderson WF, Press MF, Kasahara N. Antibody-mediated targeting of replication competent retroviral vectors. Hum Gene Ther 2003;14:789–802.

[97] Bergelson JM, Cunningham JA, Droguett G, Kurt-Jones EA, Krithivas A, Hong JS, Horwitz MS, Crowell RL, Finberg RW. Isolation of a common receptor for coxsackie B viruses and adenoviruses 2 and 5. Science 1997;275:1320–1323.

[98] Wickham TJ, Tzeng E, Shears LL, Roelvink PW, Li Y, Lee GM, Brough DE, Lizonova A, Kovesdi I. Increased in vitro and in vivo gene transfer by adenovirus vectors containing chimeric fiber proteins. J Virol 1997;71:8221–8229.

[99] Haisma HJ, Grill J, Curiel DT, Hoogeland S, van Beusechem VW, Pinedo HM, Gerritsen WR. Targeting of adenoviral vectors through a bispecific single-chain antibody. Cancer Gene Ther 2000;7:901–904.

[100] Grill J, van Beusechem VW, Van Der Valk P, Dirven CM, Leonhart A, Pherai DS, Haisma HJ, Pinedo HM, Curiel DT, Gerritsen WR. Combined targeting of adenoviruses to integrins and epidermal growth factor receptors increases gene transfer into primary glioma cells and spheroids. Clin Cancer Res 2001;7:641–650.

[101] Hong SS, Galaup A, Peytavi N, Chazal N, Boulanger P. Enhancement of adenovirus-mediated gene delivery by use of an oligopeptide with dual binding specificity. Hum Gene Ther 1999;10:2577–2586.

[102] Bartlet JS, Kleinschmidt J, Boucher RC, Samulski RJ. Targeted adenoassociated virus vector transduction of non-permissive cells mediated by a bispecific (ab-g) antibody. Nat Biotechnol 1999;17:181–186.

[103] Perabo L, Büning H, Kofler DM, Ried MU, Girod A, Wendtner CM, Enssle J, Hallek M. In vitro selection of viral vectors with modified tropism: the adenoassociated virus display. Mol Ther 2003;8:151–157.

[104] Lane DP, Cheok CF, Lain S. p53-based cancer therapy. Cold Spring Harb Perspect Biol 2010;2:a001222.

[105] Tassone P, Old M, Teknos TN, Pan Q. p53-based therapeutics for head and neck squamous cell carcinoma. Oral Oncol 2013;49:733–7.

[106] Beckta JM, Ahmad SF, Yang H, Valerie K. Revisiting p53 for cancer-specific chemo- and radiotherapy: ten years after. Cell Cycle 2014;13:710–3.

[107] Issaeva N, Friedler A, Bozko P, Wiman KG, Fersht AR, Selivanova G. Rescue of mutants of the tumor suppressor p53 in cancer cells by a designed peptide. Proc Natl Acad Sci U S A 2003;100:13303–7.

[108] Oshima Y, Sasaki Y, Negishi H, Idogawa M, Toyota M, Yamashita T, Wada T, Nagoya S, Kawaguchi S, Yamashita T, Tokino T. Antitumor effect of adenovirus-mediated p53 family gene transfer on osteosarcoma cell lines. Cancer Biol Ther 2007;6:1058–66.

[109] Das S, Nama S, Antony S, Somasundaram K. p73 β-expressing recombinant adenovirus: a potential anticancer agent. Cancer Gene Ther 2005;12:417–426.

[110] Knudsen KE, Weber E, Arden KC, Cavenee WK, Feramisco JR, Knudsen ES. The retinoblastoma tumor suppressor inhibits cellular proliferation through two distinct mechanisms: inhibition of cell cycle progression and induction of cell death. Oncogene 1999;18: 5239–45.

[111] Liu F, Li Q, Zhang P, Chen F, Cheng Y. Role of adenovirus-mediated retinoblastoma 94 in the treatment of human non-small cell lung cancer. Mol Med Rep 2015;11:3349–3353.

[112] Macnab SA, Turrell SJ, Carr IM, Markham AF, Coletta PL, Whitehouse A. Herpesvirus saimiri-mediated delivery of the adenomatous polyposis coli tumour suppressor gene reduces proliferation of colorectal cancer cells. Int J Oncol 2011; 39:1173–1181.

[113] Tait DL, Jensen RA, Holt JT, Johnson DH, Gralow J, King MC. Gene therapy for breast and ovarian cancer with BRCA1. Breast Dis 1998;10:89–98.

[114] Farooqi AA, Rehman ZU, Muntane J. Antisense therapeutics in oncology: current status. Onco Targets Ther 2014;3:2035–42.

[115] Bedikian AY, Garbe C, Conry R, Lebbe C, Grob JJ; Genasense Melanoma Study Group. Dacarbazine with or without oblimersen (a Bcl-2 antisense oligonucleotide) in chemotherapy-naive patients with advanced melanoma and low-normal serum lactate dehydrogenase: 'The AGENDA trial'. Melanoma Res 2014;24:237–243.

[116] O'Brien S, Moore JO, Boyd TE, Larratt LM, Skotnicki A, Koziner B, Chanan-Khan AA, Seymour JF, Bociek RG, Pavletic S, Rai KR. Randomized phase III trial of fludarabine plus cyclophosphamide with or without oblimersen sodium (Bcl-2 antisense) in patients with relapsed or refractory chronic lymphocytic leukemia. J Clin Oncol 2008;26:820.

[117] Chanan-Khan AA, Niesvizky R, Hohl RJ, Zimmerman TM, Christiansen NP, Schiller GJ, Callander N, Lister J, Oken M, Jagannath S. Phase III randomised study of dexamethasone with or without oblimersen sodium for patients with advanced multiple myeloma. Leuk Lymphoma 2009;50:559–65.

[118] Sun HX, He HW, Zhang SH, Liu TG, Ren KH, He QY, Shao RG. Suppression of N-Ras by shRNA-expressing plasmid increases sensitivity of HepG2 cells to vincristine-induced growth inhibition. Cancer Gene Ther 209;16:693- 702.

[119] Altieri DC. 2008. Survivin, cancer networks and pathway-directed drug discovery. Nat Rev Cancer 2008;8:61–70.

[120] Talbot DC, Ranson M, Davies J, Lahn M, Callies S, André V, Kadam S, Burgess M, Slapak C, Olsen AL, McHugh PJ, de Bono JS, Matthews J, Saleem A, Price P. Tumor survivin is downregulated by the antisense oligonucleotide LY2181308: a proof-of-concept, first-in-human dose study. Clin Cancer Res 2010;16:6150–8.

[121] Vassaux G, Martin-Duque P. Use of suicide genes for cancer gene therapy: study of the different approaches. Expert Opin Biol Ther 2004;4:519–530.

[122] Tomicic MT, Thust R, Kaina B. Ganciclovir-induced apoptosis in HSV-1 thymidine kinase expressing cells: critical role of DNA breaks, Bcl-2 decline and caspase-9 activation. Oncogene 2002;21:2141–2153.

[123] Liu Y, Ye T, Maynard J, Akbulut H, Deisseroth A. Engineering conditionally replication-competent adenoviral vectors carrying the cytosine deaminase gene increases the infectivity and therapeutic effect for breast cancer gene therapy. Cancer Gene Ther 2006;13:346–56.

[124] Zhang L, Akbulut H, Tang Y, Peng X, Pizzorno G, Sapi E, Manegold S, Deisseroth A. Adenoviral vectors with E1A regulated by tumor-specific promoters are selectively cytolytic for breast cancer and melanoma. Mol Ther 2002;6:386–93.

[125] Akbulut H, Tang Y, Maynard J, Zhang L, Pizzorno G, Deisseroth A. Vector targeting makes 5-fluorouracil chemotherapy less toxic and more effective in animal models of epithelial neoplasms. Clin Cancer Res 2004;10:7738–7746.

[126] Prados J, Melguizo C, Rama A, Ortiz R, Boulaiz H, Rodriguez-Serrano F,Caba O, Rodriguez-Herza JJ, Ramos JL, Aranega A. Combined therapy using suicide gef gene and paclitaxel enhances growth inhibition of multicellular tumour spheroids of A-549 human lung cancer cells. Int J Oncol 2008;33:121–127.

[127] Liao Z, Huang C, Zhou F, Xiong J, Bao J, Zhang H, Sun W, Xie C, Zhou Y. Radiation enhances suicide gene therapy in radioresistant laryngeal squamous cell carcinoma via activation of a tumor-specific promoter. Cancer Lett 2009;283:20–8.

[128] Matthews T, Boehme R. Antiviral activity and mechanism of action of ganciclovir. Rev Infect Dis 1998;10:490–4.

[129] Garcia-Rodríguez L, Abate-Daga D, Rojas A, González JR, Fillat C. E-cadherin contributes to the bystander effect of TK/GCV suicide therapy and enhances its antitumoral activity in pancreatic cancer models. Gene Ther 2011;18:73–8.

[130] Sangro B, Mazzolini G, Ruiz M, Ruiz J, Quiroga J, Herrero I, Qian C, Benito A, Larrache J, Olagüe C, Boan J, Peñuelas I, Sádaba B, Prieto J. A phase I clinical trial of thy-

midine kinase-based gene therapy in advanced hepatocellular carcinoma. Cancer Gene Ther 2010;17:837–43.

[131] Zhang J, Wei F, Wang H, Li H, Qiu M, Ren P, Chen X, Huang Q. Potent anti-tumor activity of telomerase-dependent and HSVTK armed oncolytic adenovirus for non-small cell lung cancer in vitro and in vivo. J Exp Clin Cancer Res 2010;29:52.

[132] Miletic H, Fischer YH, Giroglou T, Rueger MA, Winkeler A, Li H, Himmelreich U, Stenzel W, Jacobs AH, von Laer D. Normal brain cells contribute to the bystander effect in suicide gene therapy of malignant glioma. Clin Cancer Res 2007;13:6761–6768.

[133] Blumenthal M, Skelton D, Pepper KA, Jahn T, Methangkool E, Kohn DB. Effective suicide gene therapy for leukemia in a model of insertional oncogenesis in mice. Mol Ther 2007;15:183–192.

[134] Beltinger C, Fulda S, Kammertoens T, Meyer E, Uckert W, Debatin KM. Herpes simplex virus thymidine kinase/ganciclovir induced apoptosis involves ligand independent death receptor aggregation and activation of cas- pases. Proc Natl Acad Sci U S A 1999;96:8699–704.

[135] Gadi VK, Alexander SD, Kudlow JE, Allan P, Parker WB, Sorscher EJ. In vivo sensitization of ovarian tumors to chemotherapy by expression of E. coli purine nucleoside phosphorylase in a small fraction of cells. Gene Ther 2000;20:1738–1743.

[136] Karle P, Renner M, Salmons B, Günzburg WH. Necrotic, rather than apoptotic, cell death caused by cytochrome P450-activated ifosfamide. Cancer Gene Ther 2001;8: 220–30.

[137] Hamstra DA, Pagé M, Maybaum J, Rehemtulla A. Expression of endogenously activated secreted or cell surface carboxypeptidase A sensitizes tumor cells to methotrexate-alpha-peptide prodrugs. Cancer Res 2000;60:657–665.

[138] Ambade AV, Joshi GV, Mulherkar R. Effect of suicide gene therapy in combination with immunotherapy on antitumour immune response & tumour regression in a xenograft mouse model for head & neck squamous cell carcinoma. Indian J Med Res 2010;312:415–422.

[139] Cao X, Huang X, Ju DW, Zhang W, Hamada H, Wang J. Enhanced antitumoral effect of adenovirus-mediated cytosine deaminase gene therapy by induction of antigen-presenting cells through stem cell factor/granulocyte-macrophage colony-stimulating factor gene transfer. Cancer Gene Ther 2000;7:177–186.

[140] Khatri A, Husaini Y, Ow K, Chapman J, Russell PJ.Cytosine deaminase-uracil phosphoribosyltransferase and interleukin (IL)-12 and IL-18: a multimodal anticancer interface marked by specific modulation in serum cytokines. Clin Cancer Res 2009;15:2323–2334.

[141] Chen CT, Yamaguchi H, Lee HJ, Du Y, Lee HH, Xia W, Yu WH, Hsu JL, Yen CJ, Sun HL, Wang Y, Yeh ET, Hortobagyi GN, Hung MC. Dual targeting of tumor angiogen-

esis and chemotherapy by endostatin–cytosine deaminase– uracil phosphoribosyltransferase. Mol Cancer Ther 2011;10:1327–1336.

[142] Restifo NP, Dudley ME, Rosenberg SA. Adoptive immunotherapy for cancer: harnessing the T cell response. Nat Rev Immunol 2012;12:269–281.

[143] Kaufman HL, Bines SD. OPTIM trial: a Phase III trial of an oncolytic herpes virus encoding GM-CSF for unresectable stage III or IV melanoma. Future Oncol 2010;6:941–9.

[144] Goshima F, Esaki S, Luo C, Kamakura M, Kimura H, Nishiyama Y. Oncolytic viral therapy with a combination of HF10, a herpes simplex virus type 1 variant and granulocyte-macrophage colony-stimulating factor for murine ovarian cancer. Int J Cancer 2014;134:2865–77.

[145] Goins WF, Huang S, Cohen JB, Glorioso JC. Engineering HSV-1 vectors for gene therapy. Methods Mol Biol 2014;1144:63–79.

[146] Lim F, Khalique H, Ventosa M, Baldo A. Biosafety of gene therapy vectors derived from herpes simplex virus type 1. Curr Gene Ther 2013;13:478–91.

[147] Bischoff JR, Kirn DH, Williams A, Heise C, Horn S, Muna M, Ng L, Nye JA, Sampson-Johannes A, FattaeKammertoens Ty A, McCormick F. An adenovirus mutant that replicates selectively in p53-deficient human tumor cells. Science 1996;274:373–376.

[148] Hay JG, Shapiro N, Sauthoff H, Heitner S, Phupakdi W, Rom WN. Targeting the replication of adenoviral gene therapy vectors to lung cancer cells: the importance of the adenoviral E1b-55kD gene. Hum Gene Ther 1999;10:579–590.

[149] Rothman T, Hungstermann A, Whitaker NJ, Scheffner M, zur Hausen H. Replication of ONYX-015 a potential anticancer adenovirus, is independent of p53 status in tumor cells. J Virol 1998;72:9470–9478.

[150] Liu S, Chen P, Hu M, Tao Y, Chen L, Liu H, Wang J, Luo J, Gao G. Randomized, controlled phase II study of post-surgery radiotherapy combined with recombinant adenoviral human p53 gene therapy in treatment of oral cancer. Cancer Gene Ther 2013;20:375–8.

[151] Khuri FR, Nemunaitis J, Ganly I, Arseneau J, Tannock IF, Romel L, Gore M, Ironside J, MacDougall RH, Heise C, Randlev B, Gillenwater AM, Bruso P, Kaye SB, Hong WK, Kirn DH. A controlled trial of intratumoral ONYX-015, a selectively replicating adenovirus in combination with cisplatin and 5-fluorouracil in patients with recurrent head and neck cancer. Nat Med 2000;6:879–885.

[152] Ganly I, Kirn D, Eckhardt G, Rodriguez GI, Soutar DS, Otto R, Robertson AG, Park O, Gulley ML, Heise C, Von Hoff DD, Kaye SB. A phase I study of ONYX-015, an E1B attenuated adenovirus, administered intratumorally to patient with recurrent head and neck cancer. Clin Cancer Res 2000;6:798–806.

[153] Vasey PA, Schulman LN, Campos S, Davis J, Gore M, Johnston S, Kirn DH, O'Neill V, Siddiqui N, Seiden MV, Kaye SB. Phase I trial of intraperitoneal injection of the E1B-55kd-gene deleted adenovirus ONYX-015 (dl1520) given on days 1 through 5 every 3 weeks in patients with recurrent/refractory epithelial ovarian cancer. J Clin Oncol 2002;20:1562–1569.

[154] Fueyo J, Gomez-Manzano C, Alemany R, Lee P, McDonnel T, Mitliangel P, Shi YX, Levin VA, Yung WK, Kyritsis AP. A mutant oncolytic adenovirus targeting the Rb pathway produces anti-glioma effect in vivo. Oncogene 1999;19:1–11.

[155] Heise C, Hermiston T, Johnson L, Brooks G, Sampson-Johannes A, Williams A, Hawkins L, Kirn D. An adenovirus E1A mutant that demonstrates potent and selective systemic anti-tumoral efficacy. Nat Med 2000;6:1134–1139.

[156] Rodriguez R, Schuer ER, Yeong L, Henderson GA, Simons JW, Henderson DR. Prostate attenuated replication competent adenovirus (ARCA) CN706 a selective cytotoxic for prostate specific antigen postive prostate cancer cells. Cancer Res 1997;57:2559–2563.

[157] Hallenbeck PL, Chang YN, Hay C, Golightly D, Stewart D, Lin J, Phipps S, Chiang YL. A novel tumor-specific replication restricted adenoviral vector for gene therapy of hepatocellular carcinoma. Hum Gene Ther 1999;10:1721–1733.

[158] Brunori M, Malerba M, Kashiwasaki H, Iggo R. Replicating adenoviruses that target tumors with constitutive activation of the wnt signallig pathway. J Virol 2001;75:2857–2865.

[159] Kurihara T, Brough DE, Komesdi I, Kufe DW. Selectivity of a replication-competent adenovirus for human breast carcinoma cells expressing the MUC1 antigen. J Clin Invest 2000;106:763–771.

[160] Wildner O, Moris JC. Therapy of peritoneal carcinomatosis from colon cancer with oncolytic adenoviruses. J Gene Med 2000;2:353–360.

[161] Chung I, Deisseroth AB. Recombinant adenoviral vector containing tumor-specific L-plastin promoter fused to cytosine deaminase gene as atranscription unit: generation and functional test. Arch Pharm Res. 2004;27:633–639.

[162] Akbulut H, Zhang L, Tang Y, Deisseroth A. The cytotoxic effect of replication competent adenoviral vectors carrying L-plastin promoter regulated E1A and cytosine deaminase genes in cancers of the breast, ovary and colon. Cancer Gene Ther 2003;10:388–395.

[163] Akbulut H, Tang Y, Deisseroth A. Vector vaccination and vector targeted chemotherapy in solid tumors. J BUON 2009;14:141–146.

[164] Hashiro G, Loh PC, Jav ST. The preferential cytotoxicity of reovirus for cetain transformed cell lines. Arch Virol 1977;75:3335–3342.

[165] Maxwell IH, Terrel KL, Maxwell F. Autonomous parvovirus vectors. Methods 2002;28:168–181.

[166] Strong JE, Coffey MC, Tang D, Sabinin P, Lee PWK. The molecular basis of viral oncolysis: usurpation of tha RAS signaling pathway by rheovirus. EMBO J 1998;12:3351–3362.

[167] Stojdl DF, Lichty B, Knowles S, Marius R, Atkins H, Sonenberg N, Bell JC. Exploiting tumor-specific defects in the interferon pathway with a previously unknown oncolytic virus. Nat Med 2000;6:821–825.

[168] Malerba M, Daeffler L, Rommelaere J, Iggo D. Replicating parvoviruses that target colon cancer cells. J Virol 2003;77:6683–6691.

[169] Phangsdo A, Lorence RM, Reichard KW, Peoples ME, Walter RJ. New castle disease virus therapy of human tumor xenografts: anti-tumor effects of local or systemic administration. Cancer Lett 2001;172:27–36.

[170] Pecora AL, Rizvi N, Cohen GI, Menopol NJ, Sterman D, Marshal JL, Goldberg S, Gross P, O'Neil JD, Groene WS, Roberts MS, Rabin H, Bamat MK, Lorence RM. Phase I trial of intravenous administration of PV701, an oncolytic virus, in patients with solid tumors. J Clin Oncol 2002;20:2251–2266.

[171] Kuo L, Godeke GJ, Ramsanman MJB, Masters PS, Rottier PJM. Retargeting of coronavirus by substitution of the spike glycoprotein ectodomain: crossing the host cell species barrier. J Virol 2000;74:1393–1406.

[172] Ortego J, Escors D, Laude H, Enjuanes L. Generation of a replication competent, propagation-deficient virus vector based on the transmissible gastroenteritis coronavirus genome. J Virol 2002;76:11518–11529.

[173] Kong HL, Hecht D, Song W, Kovesdi I, Hackett NR, Yayon A, Crystal RG. Regional suppression of tumor growth by in vivo transfer of a cDNA encoding a secreted form of the extracellular domain of the flt-1 vascular endothelial growth factor receptor. Hum Gene Ther 1998;10:823–833.

[174] Takayama K, Ueno H, Nakanishi Y, Sakamato T, Inoue K, Shimizu K, Oohashi H, Hara N. Suppression of tumor angiogenesis and growth by gene transfer of a soluble form of vascular endothelial growth factor receptor into a remote organ. Cancer Res 2000;60:2169–2177.

[175] Szary J, Szala S. Intra-tumoral administration of naked plasmid DNA encoding mouse endostatin inhibits renal carcinoma growth. Int J Cancer 2001; 91:835–839.

[176] Tai KF, Chen PJ, Chen DS, Hwang LH. Concurrent delivery of GM-CSF and endostatin genes by a single adenoviral vector provides a synergistic effect on the treatment of orthotopic liver tumors. J Gene Med 2003;5:386–398.

[177] Ma HI, Lin SZ, Chiang YH, Li J, Chen SL, Tsao YP, Xiao X. Intratumoral gene therapy of malignant brain tumor in a rat model with angiostatin delivered by adeno-associated viral (AAV) vector. Gene Ther 2002; 9:2–11.

[178] Jin RJ, Kwak C, Lee SG, Lee CH, Soo CG, Park MS, Lee E, Lee SE.. The application of an anti-angiogenic gene (thrombospondin-1] in the treatment of human prostate cancer xenografts. Cancer Gene Ther 2000;7:1537–1542.

[179] Tanaka T, Manome Y, Wen P, Kufe DW, Fine HA. Viral vector-mediated transduction of a modified platelet factor 4 cDNA inhibits angiogenesis and tumor growth. Nat Med 1997;3:437–442.

[180] Maemondo M, Narumi K, Saijo Y, Usui K, Tahara M, Tazawa R, K, Matsumoto K, Nakamura T, Nukiwa T. Targeting angiogenesis and HGF function using an adenoviral vector expressing the HGF antagonist NK4 for cancer therapy. Mol Ther 2002;5:177–185.

[181] Griscelli F, Li H, Cheong C, Opolon P, Bennaceur-Griscelli A, Vassal G, Soria J, Soria C, Lu H, Perricaudet M, Yeh P. Combined effects of radiotherapy and angiostatin gene therapy in glioma tumor model. Proc Natl Acad Sci U S A 2000; 97:6698–6703.

[182] Varda-Bloom N, Shaish A, Gonen A, Levanon K, Greenbereger S, Ferber S, Levkovitz H, Castel D, Goldberg I, Afek A, Kopolovitc Y, Harats D. Tissue specific gene therapy directed to tumor angiogenesis. Gene Ther 2001;8:819–827.

[183] Kaliberov SA, Buchsbaum DJ, Gillespie GY, Curiel DT, Arafat WO, Carpenter M, Stackhouse MA. Adenovirus-mediated transfer of BAX driven by the vascular endothelial growth factor promoter induces apoptosis in lung cancer cells. Mol Ther 2002;6:190–198.

[184] Savontaus MJ, Sauter BV, Huang TG, Woo SL. Transcriptional targeting of conditionally replicating adenovirus to dividing endothelial cells. Gene Ther 2002;9:972–979.

[185] Nör JE, Hu Y, Song W, Spencer DM, Núñez G. Ablation of microvessels in vivo upon dimerization of Caspase-9. Gene Ther 2002; 9:444–451.

[186] Nguyen JT, Wu P, Clouse ME, Hlatky L, Terwilliger EF. Adeno-associated virus-mediated delivery of antiangiogenic factors as an antitumor strategy. Cancer Res 1998;58:5673–5677.

[187] Li H, Lu H, Griscelli F, Opolon P, Sun LQ, Ragot T, Y, Belin D, Soria J, Soria C, Perricaudet M, Yeh P. Adenovirus-mediated delivery of a uPA/uPAR antagonist suppresses angiogenesis dependent tumor growth and dissemination in mice. Gene Ther 1998;5:1105–1113.

[188] Dranoff G. GM-CSF-based cancer vaccines. Immunol Rev 2002; 188: 147–154.

[189] Shashkova EV, Spencer JF, Wold WS, Doronin K. Targeting interferon-alpha increases antitumor efficacy and reduces hepatotoxicity of E1A-mutated spread- enhanced oncolytic adenovirus. Mol Ther 2007; 15: 598–607.

[190] Choi IK, Lee JS, Zhang SN, Park J, Sonn CH, Lee KM, Yun CO. Oncolytic adenovirus co-expressing IL-12 and IL-18 improves tumor-specific immunity via differ- entiation of T cells expressing IL-12Rbeta2 or IL-18Ralpha. Gene Ther 2011; 18: 898–909.

[191] Jinushi M, Tahara H. Cytokine gene-mediated immunotherapy: current status and future perspectives. Cancer Sci 2009; 100: 1389–1396.

[192] Choi KJ, Zhang SN, Choi IK, Kim JS, Yun CO. Strengthening of antitumor immune memory and prevention of thymic atrophy mediated by adenovirus expressing IL-12 and GM-CSF. Gene Ther 2012; 19: 711–723.

[193] Pesonen S, Diaconu I, Cerullo V, Escutenaire S, Raki M, Kangasniemi L, Nokisalmi P, Dotti G, Guse K, Laasonen L, Partanen K, Karli E, Haavisto E, Oksanen M, Karioja-Kallio A, Hannuksela P, Holm SL, Kauppinen S, Joensuu T, Kanerva A, Hemminki A. Integrin targeted oncolytic adenoviruses Ad5-D24-RGD and Ad5-RGD-D24-GMCSF for treatment of patients with advanced chemotherapy refractory solid tumors. Int J Cancer. 2012;130:1937–1947.

[194] Lapteva N, Aldrich M, Weksberg D, Rollins L, Goltsova T, Chen SY, Huang XF. Targeting the intratumoral dendritic cells by the oncolytic adenoviral vaccine expressing RANTES elicits potent antitumor immunity. J Immunother 2009; 32:145–156.

[195] Charles LG, Xie YC, Restifo NP, Roessler B, Sanda MG. Antitumor efficacy of tumor-antigen-encoding recombinant poxvirus immunization in Dunning rat prostate cancer: implications for clinical genetic vaccine development. World J Urol. 2000;18:136–142.

[196] Deisseroth A, Tang Y, Zhang L, Akbulut H, Habib N. TAA/ecdCD40L adenoviral prime-protein boost vaccine for cancer and infectious diseases. Cancer Gene Ther. 2013;20[2]:65–69.

[197] Tang Y, Akbulut H, Maynard J, Petersen L, Fang X, Zhang WW, Xia X, Koziol J, Linton PJ, Deisseroth A. Vector prime/protein boost vaccine that overcomes defects acquired during aging and cancer. J Immunol 2006;177: 5697–56707.

[198] Akbulut H, Tang Y, Akbulut KG, Maynard J, Deisseroth A. Addition of adenoviral vector targeting of chemotherapy to the MUC-1/ecdCD40L VPPP vector prime protein boost vaccine prolongs survival of mice carrying growing subcutaneous deposits ofLewis lung cancer cells. Gene Ther. 2010;17[11]:1333–1340.

[199] Rochlitz C, Figlin R, Squiban P, Salzberg M, Pless M, Herrmann R. Phase I immunotherapy with a modified vaccinia virus (MVA) expressing human MUC1 as antigen-specific immunotherapy in patients with MUC1-positive advanced cancer. J Gene Med 2003;5:690–699.

[200] Von Mehren M, Arlen P, Tsang KY, Rogatko A, Meropol N, Cooper HS. Pilot study of a dual gene recombinant avipox vaccine containing both carcinoembryonic antigen (CEA) and B7.1 transgenes in patients with recurrent CEA-expressing adenocarcinomas. Clin Cancer Res 2000;6:2219–2228.

[201] Nagai E, Ogawa T, Kielian T, Ikubo A, Suzuki T. Irradiated tumor cells adenovirally engineered to secrete granulocyte/macrophage-colony-stimulating factor establish antitumor immunity and eliminate pre-existing tumors in syngeneic mice. Cancer Immunol Immunother 1998;47:72–80.

[202] Ginn SL, Alexander IE, Edelstein ML, Abedi MR, Wixon J. Gene therapy clinical trials worldwide to 2012—an update. J Gene Med 2013;15:65–77.

[203] Nemunaitis J. Vaccines in cancer: GVAX, a GM-CSF gene vaccine. Expert Rev Vaccines 2005;4:259–274.

[204] Nemunaitis J, Jahan T, Ross H, Sterman D, Richards D, Fox B. Phase 1/2 trial of autologous tumor mixed with an allogeneic GVAX vaccine in advanced-stage non-small-cell lung cancer. Cancer Gene Ther 2006;13:555–562.

[205] Akbulut H, Tang Y, Akbulut KG, Maynard J, Zhang L, Deisseroth A. Antitumor immune response induced by i.t. injection of vector-activated dendritic cells and chemotherapy suppresses metastatic breast cancer. Mol Cancer Ther. 2006;5:1975–1985.

[206] Breckpot K, Dullaers M, Bonehill A, van Meirvenne S, Heirman C, de Greef C. Lentivirally transduced dendritic cells as a tool for cancer immunotherapy. J Gene Med 2003;5:654–667.

[207] Di Lorenzo G, Buonerba C and Kantoff PW. Immunotherapy for the treatment of prostate cancer. Nat Rev Clin Oncol 2011;8: 551–561.

[208] Barrett DM, Singh N, David L. Porter DL, Grupp SA, Carl H. Chimeric antigen receptor therapy for cancer. Annu Rev Med 2014;65: 333–347.

[209] Sun M, Shi H, Liu C, Liu J, LiuX, Sun Y. Construction and evaluation of a novel humanized HER2-specific chimeric receptor. Breast Cancer Res 2014;16:R61.

[210] Jensen MC, Riddel SR. Design and implementation of adoptive therapy with chimeric antigen receptor-modified T cellsImmunol Rev. Immunol Rev 2014 J;257:127–144.

[211] Shi H, Sun M, Liu L, Wang Z. Chimeric antigen receptor for adoptive immunotherapy of cancer: latest research and future prospects. Mol Cancer 2014;13:219.

3

Methods of Transfection with Messenger RNA Gene Vectors

Oleg E. Tolmachov and Tanya Tolmachova

Abstract

Non-viral gene delivery vectors with messenger RNA (mRNA) as a carrier of genetic information are among the staple gene transfer vectors for research in gene therapy, gene vaccination and cell fate reprogramming. As no passage of genetic cargo in and out of the nucleus is required, mRNA-based vectors typically offer the following five advantages: 1) fast start of transgene expression; 2) ability to express genes in non-dividing cells with an intact nuclear envelope; 3) insensitivity to the major gene silencing mechanisms, which operate in the nucleus; 4) absence of potentially mutagenic genomic insertions; 5) high cell survival rate after transfection procedures, which do not need to disturb nuclear envelope. In addition, mRNA-based vectors offer a simple combination of various transgenes through mixing of several mRNAs in a single multi-gene cocktail or expression of a number of proteins from a single mRNA molecule using internal ribosome entry sites (IRESes), ribosome skipping sequences and proteolytic signals. However, on the downside, uncontrolled extracellular and intracellular decay of mRNA can be a substantial hurdle for mRNA-mediated gene transfer. Procedures for mRNA delivery are analogous to DNA transfer methods, which are well-established. In general, there are three actors in the gene delivery play, namely, the vector, the cell and the transfer environment. The desired outcome, that is, the efficient delivery of a gene to a target cell population, depends on the efficient interaction of all three parties. Thus, the vector should be customised for the target cell population and presented in a form that is resistant to the aggressive factors in the delivery *milieu*. At the same time, the delivery environment should be adjusted to be more vector-friendly and more cell-friendly. The recipient cells should be subjected to a specific regimen or artificially modified to become receptive to gene transfer with a particular vector and resistant to the environment. As a rule, barriers outside tissues (e.g. mucus) and an aggressive intercellular environment complicate gene delivery *in vivo*, which, therefore, requires more complex gene transfer procedures than transfection of tissue culture cells. This review is focused on transfection methods for mRNA vectors, which rely either on the forceful propulsion of mRNA inside the target cells (e.g. by electroporation or gene gun) or on the complexing of mRNA with other substances (e.g. polycationic transfection reagents) for delivery via endocytic pathways.

Keywords: Gene therapy, epigenetic reprogramming, gene vaccination, mRNA gene vectors, transfection methods, gene transfer

1. Introduction

1.1. Why messenger-RNA-based vectors are used in gene delivery?

DNA or RNA fragments of choice can be amplified in bacteria and eukaryotic cells by piggybacking on replicating episomes, called 'cloning vectors'. In contrast to 'cloning vectors', 'gene vectors' are the vehicles that transfer genes into cells. All gene vectors contain nucleic acids or their analogues (e.g. Peptide Nucleic Acid – PNA) as the carriers of genetic information. The complexity of gene vectors ranges from naked DNA or RNA to multi-component nano-devices with a finely ordered internal structure, which can be either virus-derived or purely synthetic. The aim of gene delivery is often the presence of specific proteins in the target cells. One way to achieve this is to transfer an immediate information source for protein biosynthesis, that is, messenger RNA (mRNA), into target cells. Presently, mRNA-based vectors are established multipurpose gene vectors applicable to a diverse range of tasks in gene therapy, gene immunisation and transgene-mediated cell-fate reprogramming [1-4].

The long-term storage of genetic information in cells is mediated by DNA, while short-term cellular memory is stored in RNA. So, if a permanent genetic change in the target cells is desirable, either DNAs or RNA-templates for reverse transcription into DNA are used as carriers of genetic information within the gene vectors. If only a non-permanent genetic change is wanted, then gene vectors containing a translatable 'sense' RNA strand ('positive strand') seem to be particularly suitable. Such vectors, whether based on mRNA generated *in vitro* or cellular mRNAs (including cellular mRNAs isolated through packaging into viral capsids), can reach ribosomes and express genes in the cytosol, without nuclear entry. There are five important implications of the extra-nuclear status of mRNA vectors.

Firstly, as mRNA does not require transfer to nucleosol for expression, mRNA-based vectors can be used in applications where a rapid and transient effect is required, e.g. wound healing or antigen-presenting. The transgene expression is fast because mRNA vectors, as opposed to DNA vectors, do not need to pass through the barrier of the nuclear envelope, which confines the nucleosol in non-dividing cells and do not need to enter the nucleus and then to exit it. In addition, no time is wasted on intra-nuclear transcription in both dividing and non-dividing cells.

Secondly, the fact that gene delivery with mRNA vectors is capable of attaining transgene expression in non-mitotic cells with a closed nuclear envelope is remarkable *per se*. Thus, mRNA vectors can be more efficient than DNA vectors for the transfection of clinically important post-mitotic cells like neurons and cardiomyocytes [5]. In fact, in non-dividing cells there is no dilution of externally delivered mRNAs and their protein products in cell divisions; this circumstance can contribute to longer persistence of mRNA-vector-mediated transgene expression in these cells in comparison to dividing cells.

Thirdly, the major mechanisms of transgene silencing, e.g. chromatin remodelling and genomic DNA methylation [6], are entirely intra-nuclear and, thus, are irrelevant for the desired expression of exogenous mRNA.

Fourthly, for the successful implementation of many therapeutic strategies, it is important that gene delivery with mRNA vectors cannot cause potentially deleterious mutations via insertional gene inactivation or undesired position effects like gene activation in the neighbourhood of a chromosomally integrated transgene. Indeed, in many cases the full long-term consequences of the genomic insertions are difficult to predict and so any permanent genetic change is often unwanted. As any gene delivery with mRNA-based vectors does not leave an undesired genomic trace, gene transfer with mRNA vectors *in vivo* benefits from the absence of the safety risks and ethical controversies of vector elements being incorporated into the human germ line and subsequently being transmitted vertically through future generations.

Fifthly, as only extra-nuclear localisation of externally delivered mRNA is required for transgene expression, 'milder' transfection conditions (e.g. shorter electric field pulses during electroporation) might be sufficient for delivery of mRNA into its 'expression *milieu*'. Indeed, 'milder' conditions increase the cell survival rate and, hence, offer higher transfection efficiency with mRNA vectors in comparison to DNA vectors [7].

Another advantage of mRNA-based vectors is the flexibility to combine several mRNAs into a single multi-gene cocktail. In addition, a number of proteins can be expressed from a single mRNA using internal ribosome entry sites (IRESes), ribosome skipping sequences or *bona fide* proteolytic signals. The ease of transgene reshuffling makes mRNA-based vectors particularly convenient in the complex tasks of epigenetic engineering, where multiple combinations of transgenes need to be screened to assess their cell-fate reprogramming effectiveness. However, on the downside, uncontrolled extracellular and intracellular decay of mRNA can be a substantial hurdle for mRNA-mediated gene transfer.

1.2. What strategies are used to deliver mRNA-based vectors to cells?

Methods for mRNA delivery are similar to DNA transfer procedures, which are well-established. Overall, there are three actors in the gene delivery play, namely, the vector, the cell and the transfer environment. The desired outcome, the efficient transfer of a gene to a target cell population and its installation as a functional transgene depends on the productive interaction of all three parties. Thus, the vector should ideally be targeted to reach the desired cells selectively and efficiently and also presented in a form that is resistant to the aggressive factors in the delivery *milieu*. At the same time, the delivery environment should be adapted to be better vector-accommodating and better cell-accommodating. The recipient cells should be subjected to a specific set of treatment procedures or artificially modified to become receptive to gene transfer with a particular vector and resistant to the environment.

In general, mRNA-based vectors can be delivered to cells in tissue culture (*in vitro*) and intracorporeally (*in vivo*). *In vitro* gene delivery is a necessary step in *ex vivo* strategies of gene immunisation [8, 9], gene therapy [10] and therapeutic cell-fate reprogramming [4]. As a rule, barriers outside tissues (e.g. mucus) and an aggressive intercellular environment complicate gene delivery *in vivo*, which, therefore, requires more complex transfection procedures than transfection *in vitro*. The standard transfection routes rely either on the forceful propulsion of mRNA inside the target cells (e.g. by electroporation or gene gun) or on the complexing of mRNA with other substances (e.g. polycationic transfection reagents) for delivery via endocytic pathways.

2. Gene delivery with mRNA-based vectors

The key parameter describing gene delivery is 'efficiency of gene transfer'. This variable can be defined as a ratio of a number of cells, which successfully received the intended genetic cargo, to the number of all cells, into which delivery of the genetic cargo was attempted. 'Successful' gene transfer normally implies not only the delivery of the genetic material *per se* but also its adequate expression in the recipient cells. Overall, 'efficiency of gene transfer' unavoidably depends on the hierarchy of multiple factors, which includes the efficiency of passage of the genetic cargo into the target cells and the efficiency of transgene expression. Instability of mRNA is a critical factor limiting the efficiency of gene transfer with mRNA-based vectors because extracellular degradation of mRNA precludes its entry into the cell and intracellular degradation of mRNA silences expression of mRNA-borne transgenes. Relative instability of mRNA is part and parcel of the general design of the living cell, as it allows the cell to change its gene expression profile depending on external stimuli and internal differentiation program. Thus, all methods of mRNA transfer into mammalian cells need to address instability as an inherent feature of mRNA. Thus, we prelude the description of the current methods of mRNA-based gene delivery with an in-depth overview of the technical means to increase the stability of mRNA.

2.1. Increasing the stability of mRNA in extracellular and intracellular environments

Comparative instability of RNA is determined by its molecular structure. In general, DNA and RNA have similar structures; they are polymers of nucleotides, composed from nucleobases, pentose sugar components and phosphate group residues. Three of the nucleobases – cytosine, adenine and guanine – are identical in RNA and DNA; the fourth nucleobase is uracil in RNA and its methylated analogue, thymine, in DNA. The sugar component in RNA is ribose and the sugar component of DNA is deoxyribose. An extra negative charge of the hydroxyl group in the RNA's ribose repels the negatively charged phosphate group and, so, makes RNA less amenable to folding into a double helix in comparison to DNA. The formation of hydrogen bonds between two neighbouring RNA strands is less efficient than between comparative DNA strands, contributing to the transiency of the existence of double-stranded RNA. Abundance of single-stranded segments in mRNA makes it poorly suitable for faithful repair, while stability of double-stranded genomic DNA in living cells is upheld through template-led enzyme-mediated repair. As a result, mRNA is vulnerable to strand breaks and spontaneous mutations.

In general, mRNA can dissipate in the form of an *in vitro* preparation, in the intercellular setting or within living cells. There are several types of degradation.

Firstly, as a substantially thread-like molecule, mRNA is susceptible to 'mechanical' degradation due to strand breaks caused by fluid shear stress or surface tension forces.

Secondly, mRNA degradation can be catalytically mediated by enzymes leading to RNA decomposition via 3′-terminal deadenylation, 5′-terminal decapping or endonucleolytic degradation. Cellular RNases are either proteins or ribozymes; the latter group is exemplified by RNase MRP and RNase P [11]. Important co-factors in enzymatic mRNA decay can be small metal ions, e.g. Mg^{2+}.

Thirdly, RNA decomposition can be catalysed by metal ions only, without enzymes. Thus, Mg^{2+} and lanthanides ions are known to accelerate RNA decay [12]. In practical terms, it is difficult to exclude a role for a trace amount of protein-based or RNA-based ribonucleases, even in ostensibly ion-led RNA degradation.

Fourthly, similarly to DNA, RNA is vulnerable to degradation in acidic conditions via 'depurination'. Depurination is the loss of adenine and guanine from the nucleic acids due to hydrolysis of their N-glycosyl linkages to ribose. Sensitivity of mRNA to low pH can compromise the transfer of mRNA vectors that are delivered to cells via endocytosis because mRNA faces degradation in acidified endosomes.

Kinetics of mRNA degradation is often described with exponential models of decay, with the 'half-life' of mRNA molecules being used as a parameter. Indeed, typical features of exponential decay can be observed during the extinction of expression of transgenes delivered to mammalian cells with mRNA vectors. Thus, the expression of transferred EGF-FLAG mRNA had reached the maximum level between 12 and 72 hours post-delivery and was very small but still detectable after 14 days [13].

While appropriate stability of many natural mRNAs was honed by natural selection, artificial mRNA vectors, e.g. new chimeric mRNAs, might be more vulnerable to attack by RNAses. The mechanism of such instability can rely on the formation of double-stranded segments within mRNA. It is thought that the co-evolution of eukaryotic cells and their viruses resulted in cellular 'friend or foe recognition systems' perceiving specific regions of double-stranded RNA as hostile. Thus, it is not unusual for double-stranded RNA to be a target for an RNAse attack, e.g. by the Dicer endoribonuclease, which is normally a part of RNAi silencing machinery. Double-stranded RNA is also a known inducer of the TLR3-mediated innate immune response, which can potentiate RNA degradation. Therefore, the emergence of non-desired segments of double-stranded RNA within molecules of mRNA gene vectors or between different molecules in mRNA vector mixtures should be considered in the design of mRNA vectors and their cocktails. Clearly, the longer the individual mRNA vector molecules and the higher the number of individual mRNA species in the vector cocktails, the higher the chance for the appearance of double-stranded RNA segments through spurious sequence homologies. Thus, the design of mRNA vectors is bound to include the search of such homologies *in silico* and minimisation of any potential unwanted double-stranded-RNA-forming regions through appropriate nucleotide changes. Some short regions of double-stranded RNA, e.g. 'stem' segments in tRNAs, do not induce adverse cell responses. Such short RNA-duplex-forming regions could be intentionally introduced into mRNA vector molecules to achieve high compactness with ensuing increased resistance to shear stress. Such compacting could be particularly relevant for long RNA molecules. In addition, extra compactness of mRNA vectors might result in their beneficial resistance to RNAse-mediated degradation because of reduced RNA access to the catalytic centres of RNAses. Suitable segments for RNA self-compression can be provided not only by short duplex-forming regions but also by G-quadruplex-forming sequences [14]. Furthermore, compacting of mRNA vectors can be achieved using peptides and proteins. For example, poly(A)-binding protein (PABP) has roles in nuclear export, enhancement of translation and mRNA stability and can be complexed with mRNA vectors to achieve their condensation. Another mRNA compacting option is the employment of cytoplasmic polyadenylation element binding protein (CPEB). Clearly, in addition to their employment in mRNA compacting, peptides and protein ligands can be used to link mRNA to elements required for efficient cell penetration and localisation within intracellular compartments capable of efficient support of protein synthesis.

Mechanical instability of mRNA vectors is more critical in the transfer systems such as gene gun, aerosol, electroporation and sonoporation, where potentially powerful shearing forces can emerge. However, encouragingly, mRNA, which is 'shaved off' along the trajectory of the gene gun particle in tissue, was shown to be functionally active [13]. Clearly, more studies of mRNA stability in extreme conditions are required.

In laboratory environment, mRNA is normally stored at -80 °C as autodegradation and other forms of degradation are substantially limited at this temperature. Freeze-thaw cycles, which can cause breaks in RNA during phase transitions, are better avoided, e.g. by splitting mRNA preparations into smaller aliquots. As many RNA degradation pathways are active only in solutions, lyophilisation (drying from the frozen state) is often used to improve storage stability of mRNA. Precautions to prevent the degradation of RNA *in vitro* by RNAses are important. RNaseZap™, a proprietary mixture of three RNase inhibitors, can be used to inactivate RNases on various surfaces. A common RNA protection agent is RNAsin, a commercial version of a placental protein with RNAse A inhibitor activity. Vials with RNA are often packaged into antistatic bags to avoid the adsorption of RNAse-contaminated dust due to electrostatic attraction. Suitable 'protective packaging' of mRNA vectors can also be applied at the molecular level with mRNAs being coated in a suitable biodegradable or soluble material within micro-droplets. Another protection option offered by nanotechnology is mRNA packaging in pleated sheets of hairpin RNA, which form 'micro-sponges' [15].

The stabilisation of mRNA is particularly important when the mRNA populations are extracted from cells; in this case, mRNA preservation with cell-permeable RNase inhibitors can be accomplished using proprietary tissue storage and RNA stabilization RNAlater™

solution (Life Technologies). Another approach for the protection of cellular mRNAs from RNAses is to use Proteinase K to destroy all the proteins in the crude preparation including RNAses. Furthermore, it is possible that defence against RNAses by RNAsin could be extended to the intracellular environment via the development of cell-permeable versions of RNAsin. Indeed, cell-permeable versions of various proteins, which were furnished with 'protein transduction domains' (PTDs), were reported in the literature [16, 17].

2.2. Methods of transfection with mRNA vectors

Procedures for mRNA delivery are analogous to DNA transfer methods, which are well-established. In general, there are three actors in the gene delivery play, namely, the vector, the cell and the transfer environment. The desired outcome, that is, the efficient delivery of a gene to a target cell population, depends on the efficient interaction of all three parties. Thus, the vector should be customised for the target cell population and presented in a form that is resistant to the aggressive factors in the delivery *milieu*. At the same time, the delivery environment should be adjusted to be more vector-friendly and more cell-friendly. The recipient cells should be subjected to a specific regimen or artificially modified to become receptive to gene transfer with a particular vector and resistant to the environment.

2.2.1. Delivery of mRNA using transfection reagents

Transfection of cells using specialised chemicals, called 'transfection reagents', is a well-established approach for the delivery of DNA to cells [18]; it is also proven to be suitable for mRNA transfer. For example, this transfection strategy was used by Weide and co-authors, who bound mRNA to a polycation protamine and used the resultant transfection-competent complexes for mRNA-mediated gene delivery [19].

In general, this type of transfection technology relies on the abrogation of the electrostatic repulsion of the negative charge of RNA and the negative charge of the cell surface. This is accomplished through complexing the RNA and the cell surface with polycations to neutralise the negative charges or, alternatively, through 'positive overcharging' of RNA-polycation complexes to cause attraction between positively charged complexes and the negatively charged cell surface. Thus, the electrostatic interaction between negatively charged phosphate groups of RNA and positively charged groups residing in the polycation 'carrier' polymer (typically amines or amidines) results in the compaction of RNA into globular complexes called polyplexes. The ensuing condensation is useful to protect mRNA from hostile factors in the transfer environment (e.g. RNAses and sheer stress). Condensation is also useful to enhance mRNA penetration into the recipient cells through the endocytosis route. Essential factors that control mRNA condensation are the local concentrations of mRNA and other components of the complexes, which can be substantially increased through 'molecular crowding' in water solutions using hydrophilic polymers like poly (N-vinyl) pyrrolidone. The important parameter of the resultant colloid is the 'electrokinetic potential' (also known as 'zeta potential') of the particles, which determines the likelihood of the undesired coagulation and flocculation of the complexes. Low colloidal stability of lipoplexes and polyplexes (aggregation of the vector particles) can be a particular problem upon systemic administration *in vivo*. Stability of the complexes can be enhanced through furnishing the surface of the vector particles with a layer of an additional polymer (e.g. a derivative of polyethylene glycol), which can also mask the particles from immune surveillance *in vivo*. Various extra-elements can be covalently attached to the polycation polymer backbone or incorporated into polyplexes through non-covalent bonds. These mRNA vector elements can include moieties promoting gene transfer and expression, such as cell-targeting peptides, membrane-penetration-enhancing PTDs, cytoskeleton attachment elements and other agents for targeted intracellular localisation. The architecture of the vector particles can be quite intricate. For example, mRNA can be contained within bubble-like 'neutral' liposomes. The liposomes can be encrusted with targeting ligands and viral membrane-fusion proteins resulting in 'virosomes' [20, 21].

Undesired binding of the transfection complexes to elements of the environment with subsequent loss of transfection activity should always be taken into account [22]. In particular, binding of vector particles to serum proteins is a known issue. Transfection reagents vary in their affinity to serum. Thus, Lipofectamine-based transfection is inhibited by serum, while FugeneHD-based transfection is not.

Many transfection reagents are toxic. For example, the toxicity of DEAE-dextran is well-known; therefore, normally transfection with DEAE-dextran requires repeated cell washing steps. Less toxic reagents can be obtained through optimised chemistry. An example of a less toxic polycation is the polysaccharide chitosan, which is produced from the shells of crustaceans or fungi. The toxicity of transfection reagents is cell-specific and should be carefully evaluated for the relevant target cell types.

A common problem that arises in mRNA delivery with transfection reagents is the degradation of mRNA, primarily through depurination, in acidified intracellular compartments such as acidified endosomes. Methods to avoid this degradation include: 1) buffering of endosomes with an externally added compound, e.g. chloroquine; 2) employment of endosome-disruption agents to enhance and accelerate mRNA escape from the endosomes. Both endosome buffering and membrane disruption can be performed by the transfection reagent itself. One example of such a multifunctional transfection reagent is polyethylenimine (PEI), a polymer, which contains protonable amines and, therefore, acts as both the acidity regulator and the agent providing the vector with an efficient escape route from endosomes into the cytosol through the 'proton-sponge' mechanism [23]. As ruptured endosomes could release aggressive proteolytic enzymes, excessive disruption of endosomes is detrimental for cell survival. Thus, transfection reagents falling into the 'golden mean' in terms of their endosome-disruption properties should be sought. Peptide elements, such as Listeriolysin O (LLO, encoded by the *hly* gene of *Listeria monocytogenes*) [24], which can produce pores in endosomes and, thus, can allow mRNA to avoid degradation in the acidic environment, are potentially useful tools to achieve high efficiency of transfection with mRNA-based vectors. Ideally, the endosomolytic activity of such peptides should be reversible, with pores forming in weak acidic conditions and then sealing back after the release of mRNA.

A number of techniques known to enhance DNA transfection are likely to be suitable for the improvement of RNA transfection. Thus, the employment of 'smart' thermo- and pH-sensitive polymers can augment transfection [25]. The candidate procedures also include transfection enhancement with laser light treatment [26], glycerol cell shock and dimethylsulphoxide (DMSO) cell shock. Another possible transfection enhancement method is magnet-assisted gene delivery. As RNA cannot move in the magnetic field by itself, in this scenario mRNA vectors need to be complexed with paramagnetic particles, which move in the magnetic field but do not become magnetized themselves. Extra-strong permanent rare-earth-metal-based magnets (samarium-cobalt or neodymium-iron-cobalt types) are currently standard tools in DNA transfection. Alternatively, devices generating a vibrating magnetic field (1Hz – 5Hz), e.g. manufactured by *Nanotherics*, can be employed [27]. One of the advantages of magnetic gene delivery is the ability to focus it and, thus, to target only selected cell populations *in vivo* [28].

2.2.2. Transfer of mRNA into cells after their treatment with a high-strength electric field

One of the common methods of mRNA-mediated gene transfer is electroporation [7, 29], which relies on the ability of a high-strength electric field to induce the formation of transient pores in cellular lipid membranes. As mRNA is negatively charged, it can be moved through these pores via electrophoresis driven by the electric field. Electroporation can be performed in carefully controlled conditions *in vitro* and also *in vivo* for the gene transfer *in situ*, including a single cell format [30]. Both adhesive and suspension cell types can be transfected using electroporation. Adhesive cells often require detachment, loading into a cuvette and re-attachment after electroporation; this procedure might reduce the cell survival rate and, consequently, reduce electroporation efficiency for adhesive cells in comparison with suspension cells.

The removal of ionic conductors prior to electroporation is important to avoid the ion-mediated electric current with the associated overheating and arcing. In addition, the purification of RNA from macromolecular substances prior to electroporation, e.g. the removal of RNA-binding proteins, is conducive for unimpeded RNA electrophoresis through the pores.

The choice of cell medium is critical for the success of mRNA delivery by electroporation *in vitro*. Electroporation buffer composition is determined by the requirements for: 1) minimal electrical conductivity; 2) optimal conditions (including pH and osmotic strength) for cell survival in a high-voltage and high-temperature environment; 3) safe *milieu* for the stability of mRNA vectors; 4) optimal parameters for mRNA transfer into the cells [31].

Buffer components should be chosen to avoid their degradation in a strong electric field and elevated temperature with the undesired release of ionic conductors. Cell-survival-supporting osmotic pressure in electroporation buffers can be achieved with non-ionic substances such as glycerol and also sugars such as sorbitol. Negatively charged cells are the subjects of electrophoresis, with some cell death occurring at the positive electrode. Cell death at the positive electrode might adversely change the electric parameters within the electroporated mixture. Therefore, minimisation of cell electrophoresis through the neutralisation of the cell surface charge by electroporation buffer components is desirable. An important parameter affecting cell survival is cell density. The presence of anti-apoptotic factors in the cell pre-treatment medium, electroporation mixture and/or cell after-treatment (recovery) medium might be useful [32]. Thus, anti-apoptotic ROCK II-kinase (Rho-kinase) inhibitors could be particularly valuable for maintaining the viability of stem cells, as some of these inhibitors (e.g. Y-27632) were shown not to affect their totipotency or pluripotency status. Alternatively, mRNA coding for electric-field-resistance, heat-resistance and/or anti-apoptotic factors could be included in the mRNA vector cocktail.

Pure mRNA or mRNA vector complexes can also be adversely affected by mRNA degradation, in particular because of overheating and mechanical shear stress due to the high strength electric field. Thus, electroporation with mRNA, if compared to electroporation with DNA, is likely to benefit from the fact that treatment by a less intense electric field for a shorter time seems to be required for mRNA vectors to reach their expression *milieu* within the cells in comparison to DNA vectors. This is because the pore formation in the plasma membrane is a sufficient membrane opening event for the successful transgene expression with mRNA vectors, while transgene expression using DNA vectors, particularly in non-dividing cells, appears also to depend on electric-field-induced pore formation in the nuclear envelope [33].

Efficient electroporation requires the optimisation of a number of electrical parameters. The fundamental variable in electroporation is the electric field strength, the magnitude of which is often measured as the number of volts applied to a centimetre of an electric circuit's length. The high strength field is often delivered as a voltage pulse with the voltage decaying through 'natural' kinetics of exponential extinction. Either resistance or capacitance parameters in the electroporation circuit can be used to control the rate of voltage drop in the 'exponential decay' protocols. The greater the resistance, the longer the decay and the larger its 'time constant', which is registered by electroporation equipment. Similarly, the greater the capacitance, the larger the 'time constant'of the decay. However, the capacitance parameter is the only one available to regulate the rate of exponential decay, when resistance is 'set to infinity' (that is, when the voltage output circuit is left open). Exponential decay transfection is thought to take advantage of the 'post-electroporation' stage when mRNA is driven by an electric field into the not-yet-closed pores in the membrane. Alternatives to the exponential decay electroporation protocols are offered by 'square' voltage pulse regimens where the voltage drops momentarily after being constant during a specified time. Both 'exponential decay' and 'square' voltage electroporation procedures could be optimised in terms of the number of pulses and duration of a pause between the pulses. Electric field strength can vary between different pulses. Thus, the initial low voltage step could be used for the preliminary 'loading' of the recipient cells' surface with mRNA. Clearly, the composition of the electroporation medium and the electrostatic details of the vectors also play an important role in the desired pre-electroporation adsorption of gene vectors on recipient cells.

Electroporation *in vitro* is accomplished either in cuvettes or in a multielectrode array format with a defined distance between the electrode plates [32]. Some commercial electroporators like BioRad *GenePulser XCell* provide a voltage versus time plot. However, ideally, current should also be recorded by an oscilloscope, providing a diagnostic signature of the electroporation experiment. Indeed, it was observed that the occurrence of rapid spontaneous current undulations during treatment of bacterial cell specimens by the electric field correlated with the efficiency of DNA delivery into the cells [34].

2.2.3. *Ultrasound-assisted delivery of mRNA*

In addition to electroporation, the formation of membrane pores can also be achieved via microcavitation induced by ultrasound in the presence of microbubbles (e.g. lipid-encased octafluoropropane gas). The transfection technique, which exploits these pores, has become known as 'microbubble-assisted sonoporation' [35] and was successfully used with mRNA vectors [36]. Sonoporation was discovered when it turned out that the microbubbles, which were used as contrast agents for ultrasound-imaging, were, in fact, potent gene transfer enhancers. Microbubbles are extremely flexible transfection tools. They can be prepared in cationic, anionic or neutral forms and can be PEGylated for increased stability *in vivo*. Microbubbles can be made more effective through their covalent attachment to the recipient cells' surface [37]. Sonoporation can be combined with chemical methods of transfection [38]. Directing the transfer of the vector particles by focusing the ultrasonic waves to the target tissue is a practical option [39, 40].

2.2.4. *Gene gun delivery of mRNA*

Delivery with a gene gun, also called bio-ballistic or biolistic gene delivery, is one of the established methods for mRNA transfer *in vivo* [13, 41]. Typically, for biolistic delivery, mRNA is precipitated with ethanol, isopropanol or $CaCl_2$/spermidine on the surfaces of the metal projectiles. The obtained mRNA-coated projectiles are then propelled by gas pressure pulse into the recipient cells. Normally, an inert gas, such as helium, is employed. The metal core of a projectile is composed of tungsten or gold. Bombardment *in vivo* normally reaches the outer 1 mm of the target tissue, which defines the range of amenable tissues. The penetration depth also depends on the gas pressure, the particle size and the type of tissue. Gas delivery pressure is an important parameter to optimise in order to achieve maximal efficiency of delivery. Gene transfer can be focused to the target area with straightforward mechanical protection of the surrounding tissue from bombardment. Some mRNA can be lost extracellularly prior to the projectiles reaching the desired recipient cells because stripping of mRNA can occur as the particles pierce the tissue [13].

2.2.5. *Delivery by injection*

Direct intracellular microinjection into cells is tedious and limits the experiment to *modus operandi* with only one cell at a time. However, microinjection continues to be a commonly used method of gene delivery with mRNA vectors to large cells like oocytes [42].

In contrast to DNA vectors, no intra-nuclear transfer of mRNA vectors is desired. This circumstance is likely to simplify the use of the multi-needle/multi-cell format for mRNA delivery. Indeed, multi-cell microinjection of nucleic acids was successfully performed with silicon microneedles [43] and carbon nanotubes [44]. Technology for manufacturing dissolvable and biodegradable microneedles is available [45, 46] and is likely to be used for gene delivery with mRNA vectors in the future.

2.2.6. *'Bactofection' and 'mycofection' for mRNA delivery*

A well-known method to deliver an mRNA–DNA mixture into cells' interior is 'bactofection', which capitalizes on the phagocytic properties of the target cells and/or the cell-invasive properties of some pathogenic bacteria. Thus, a self-destructing invasive *Listeria monocytogenes* strain was employed to deliver mRNA directly into the cytoplasm of macrophages, dendritic cells and epithelial cells [47]. In this study, the powerful T7 RNA polymerase transcription system was used to over-express mRNAs coding for EGFP protein and ovalbumin in bacterial cells, with mRNAs being adapted for translation in eukaryotic cells through the insertion of an IRES element into its 5′ untranslated portion. In order to benefit from *bona fide* caps and poly(A) tails on the delivered mRNA, which are expected to direct its efficient translation in the recipient eukaryotic cells, a yeast-based modification of bactofection was devised, which was called 'mycofection'[48]. 'Mycofection' involves the biosynthesis of the desired translation-competent mRNA in yeast and its delivery into the target cells via internalisation of mRNA-delivering yeast by the target cells. In the above study, baker's yeast, a non-invasive microorganism, was used for mRNA delivery, so the spectrum of recipient cells was restricted to the cells capable of phagocytosis. It should be noted that while, on the one hand, this restriction presents a limit to the usefulness of the yeast-based mRNA delivery system, on the other hand, it can be used for selective targeting of specific cell populations, e.g. human dendritic cells.

2.3. Methods of detection of mRNA post-delivery

The efficiency of transfection using mRNA can be evaluated, with the mRNA introduced to cells being detected both in the form of mRNA *per se* and as mRNA-encoded protein.

Methods of mRNA detection should focus on the intracellular mRNA because of the background of undelivered mRNA, which is difficult to avoid. A number of approaches are available. Total cellular RNA or poly(A)$^+$ mRNA can be fractionated using electrophoresis in an agarose or polyacrylamide gel supplemented with a chaotropic agent to remove the heterogeneity in the RNA's gel-mobility due to variations in the secondary structure of RNA molecules. Analytical approaches based on hybdridization of homologous strands of nucleic acids include both classical Northern blotting and modern microarray formats. In addition, microscopy methods, such as *in situ* hybridization, can provide important information on the intracellular localisation of the detected mRNA. An efficient strategy for highly sensitive and intracellular-location-specific detection of mRNA is the insertion of the bacteriophage MS2 stem-loop region into particular mRNAs for their recognition by the fusion protein composed of MS2 coat protein and GFP protein domains [49]. Reverse transcription polymerase chain reaction (RT-PCR) and quantitative 'real time' RT-PCR can detect and quantify very small amounts of mRNA, including in the single-cell mRNA analysis scenario.

If the proteins, encoded by mRNA vectors, have an easily tested function, the successful delivery of mRNA can be confirmed by measurement of that function. However, many therapeutically important mRNAs, such as those used in epigenetic reprogramming, code for proteins with regulatory activities, which cannot be straightforwardly tested. Antibody-based detection methods, e.g., immunostaining and Western blotting, can be used, provided a specific antibody is available. Alternatively, fusions of the target proteins with a moiety from a fluorescent protein, such as EGFP or dsRed, can be employed. Other easily detected protein domains include enzymes and antibody-tags. Commonly used short tags include FLAG, V5,

Myc, HA peptide sequences, for which antibodies are commercially available. An antibody-independent tag, HaloTag® peptide, which can be bound to fluorescent labels attached to HaloLink™ adapter, was developed by Promega. Strong ligands, including glutathione S-transferase (GST), maltose binding protein (MBP), protein A, protein G, streptavidin and His-tag moieties can be used both for the detection and preparative isolation of proteins expressed from mRNA vectors. The mRNA sequence can be designed to encode a testing domain on the N-terminus of the protein, on the C-terminus of the protein or on both the termini. As many native eukaryotic proteins are secreted into the endoplasmic reticulum with coincidental cleavage of the 'signal peptide', the placement of a testing domain on the N-terminus is often more challenging, because, firstly, it should not be cleaved off by the signal peptidase and, secondly, it should not interfere with the secretion process. Detection of proteins, 'proteomics', is currently a rapidly progressing field both in terms of improvement of its sensitivity and in terms of its expansion to the analysis of multiple samples [50].

2.4. Combined delivery of multiple gene messages using mRNA vectors

Combined delivery of multiple gene messages is often desired. Thus, future advances in gene therapy are likely to require simultaneous delivery of several curative genes. The simultaneous delivery of several messages is strictly required in current cell-fate reprogramming procedures. Immunisation with several genes for antigens is also common. Another typical gene co-transfer scenario is the combined delivery of a target gene and a marker gene. Conveniently, mRNA vectors also possess properties facilitating the delivery of several transgenes in one go. In general, the strategies for the mingling of several messages include the assembly of mRNA cocktails, construction of polycistronic mRNA vectors and engineering of mRNAs coding for fusion proteins or fusion proteins 'split-up' using the ribosome skipping mechanism.

Indeed, mRNA-based vectors are straightforward to assemble into multicomponent cocktails including bouquets of total mRNA extracted from specific cell populations. Admixture of mRNA capable of expressing a marker protein GFP was successfully used to monitor the delivery of a target gene mRNA [51]. Clearly, the same 'internal control' co-delivery strategy can be applied to the transfer of cocktails of curative, cell fate reprogramming or antigen-encoding mRNAs, which can be spiked with a marker gene mRNA.

Alternatively, several transgenes can be expressed from a single mRNA. The construction of polycistronic mRNA is often a convenient strategy to combine several reasonably short messages. The translation of the downstream cistrons in eukaryots can occur only after re-initiation at IRES sequences positioned between the cistrons. As a rule, an IRES element (e.g. borrowed from Encephalomyocarditis Virus) is embedded within a sequence of about 500 bases. The efficiency of the IRES elements can be regulated by changing the length of the inter-cistronic sequence [52]. Multiple transgenes were previously successfully assembled into a single and efficient IRES-joined transcription unit [53]. Again, a common scenario is a single transcript co-delivery of a target gene and an easily detected marker as an internal control used to gauge the level of expression of the target gene. However, one should be aware that in polycistronic gene co-delivery, the expression level of the downstream transgene is not necessarily equal to the expression level of the upstream transgene.

Another possible strategy to combine several messages for the simultaneous expression of several functions is to generate mRNA for a fusion protein, e.g. the target protein fused with a readily detectable moiety. Fusion proteins can be conveniently 'split up' into individual polypeptide chains using viral 'ribosome skipping' sequences like 2A or, alternatively, using *bona fide* proteolytic signals for resident proteases in recipient cells.

3. Future perspectives of mRNA-based gene delivery methods

There is a considerable scope for improvements of the procedures for gene delivery with synthetic mRNA. Further advancements in the field of mRNA-based gene delivery are likely to include the development of more stable, easily deliverable and gene-expression-efficient forms of mRNA vectors, incorporating specialised ligands for cell-specific targeting, cell penetration and intracellular targeting. The vector improvements, the use of potent stimulators of targeted cells' receptivity, the refinement of the mRNA cellular entry procedures and also the employment of optimised modulators of the intercellular environment are expected to increase the efficiency of gene transfer and the efficiency of body-locus-targeting, especially in clinical applications.

The potential for advancement of gene delivery with synthetic mRNAs looks strong in comparison to alternative rapid delivery methods. Indeed, high speed and other benefits of non-viral synthetic mRNA vectors are shared by: 1) virally encapsidated RNAs; 2) cell-permeable proteins. Thus, the packaging of mRNA (in positive-strand RNA viral vectors) or a template for mRNA (in vectors containing negative-strand RNA, e.g. Sendai virus-based vectors) within viral capsids is an attractive method of condensing and protecting RNA cargo destined for delivery into the cytosol of target cells. However, there are two unavoidable downsides of viral packaging in RNA transfer. Firstly, viral capsids dictate rigid size constraints for vector RNA. Secondly, this strategy tends to be tedious because the encapsidation of each RNA species requires the laborious insertion of an appropriate viral packaging sequence. Similarly, if compared to protein delivery by protein transduction into cells, gene transfer mediated by synthetic mRNAs is more advantageous since each protein to be delivered through direct cell entry requires time-consuming insertion of an effective PTD sequence. Clearly, various delivery methods can be combined. For example, as protein transduction is a very fast method of increasing the concentration of specific proteins in target cells, so, it can, in principle, be used to augment mRNA transfer. So, as cell viability currently appears to be a critical hurdle in mRNA-based gene delivery, it is possible that most significant future advances in mRNA-mediated gene transfer will be achieved through extensive employment of cell penetrating proteins capable of supporting the viability of cells before, during and after mRNA delivery procedures. The refined mRNA-based transfection techniques can also be applied to delivery of other medicinally important species of RNA, such as siRNA.

Acknowledgements

The authors are grateful to Dr Nadire N Ali, Dr Tatiana Subkhankulova (Imperial College London, UK) and Ms Lucy Tolmacheva (London City University, UK) for motivating discussions.

Author details

Oleg E. Tolmachov* and Tanya Tolmachova

*Address all correspondence to: epsilon@tinyworld.co.uk

Section of Molecular Medicine, National Heart and Lung Institute, Imperial College London, London, UK

References

[1] Yamamoto A, Kormann M, Rosenecker J, Rudolph C. Current prospects for mRNA gene delivery. *Eur J Pharm Biopharm* 2009;71(3) 484-9.

[2] Van Tendeloo VF, Ponsaerts P, Berneman ZN. mRNA-based gene transfer as a tool for gene and cell therapy. *Curr Opin Mol Ther* 2007;9(5) 423-31.

[3] Rabinovich PM, Komarovskaya ME, Ye ZJ, Imai C, Campana D, Bahceci E, Weissman SM. Synthetic messenger RNA as a tool for gene therapy. *Hum Gene Ther* 2006;17(10) 1027-35.

[4] Tolmachov OE, Tolmachova T. Design and production of mRNA-based gene vectors for therapeutic reprogramming of cell fate. *Gene Technol* 2015;4(1). http://omicsgroup.org/journals/design-and-production-of-mrnabased-gene-vectors-for-therapeutic-reprogramming-of-cell-fate-2329-6682-1000117.pdf (accessed 1 August 2015).

[5] Zou S, Scarfo K, Nantz MH, Hecker JG. Lipid-mediated delivery of RNA is more efficient than delivery of DNA in non-dividing cells. *Int J Pharm* 2010;389(1-2) 232-43.

[6] Tolmachov OE, Subkhankulova T, Tolmachova T. Silencing of Transgene Expression: A Gene Therapy Perspective. In: Martin-Molina F (ed.) *Gene Therapy - Tools and Potential Applications*. Rijeka, Croatia: InTech; 2013. p.49-68. http://www.intechopen.com/books/gene-therapy-tools-and-potential-applications/silencing-of-transgene-expression-a-gene-therapy-perspective (accessed 1 August 2015).

[7] Van Bockstaele F, Pede V, Naessens E, Van Coppernolle S, Van Tendeloo V, Verhasselt B, Philippe J. Efficient gene transfer in CLL by mRNA electroporation. *Leukemia* 2008;22(2) 323-9.

[8] Weide B, Garbe C, Rammensee HG, Pascolo S. Plasmid DNA- and messenger RNA-based anti-cancer vaccination. *Immunol Lett* 2008;115(1) 33-42.

[9] Lorenzi JC, Trombone AP, Rocha CD, Almeida LP, Lousada RL, Malardo T, Fontoura IC, Rossetti RA, Gembre AF, Silva AM, Silva CL, Coelho-Castelo AA. Intranasal vaccination with messenger RNA as a new approach in gene therapy: use against tuberculosis. *BMC Biotechnol* 2010;10(77). http://www.ncbi.nlm.nih.gov/entrez/query.fcgi?cmd=Retrieve&db=PubMed&dopt=Citation&list_uids=20961459 http://www.ncbi.nlm.nih.gov/pmc/articles/PMC2972232/pdf/1472-6750-10-77.pdf (accessed 1 August 2015).

[10] Tavernier G, Andries O, Demeester J, Sanders NN, De Smedt SC, Rejman J. mRNA as gene therapeutic: how to control protein expression. *J Control Release* 2011;150(3) 238-47.

[11] Esakova O, Krasilnikov AS. Of proteins and RNA: the RNase P/MRP family. *RNA* 2010;16(9) 1725-47.

[12] Breslow R, Huang DL. Effects of metal ions, including Mg2+ and lanthanides, on the cleavage of ribonucleotides and RNA model compounds. *Proc Natl Acad Sci U S A* 1991;88(10) 4080-3.

[13] Sohn RL, Murray MT, Schwarz K, Nyitray J, Purray P, Franko AP, Palmer KC, Diebel LN, Dulchavsky SA. In-vivo particle mediated delivery of mRNA to mammalian tissues: ballistic and biologic effects. *Wound Repair Regen* 2001;9(4) 287-96.

[14] Melko M, Bardoni B. The role of G-quadruplex in RNA metabolism: involvement of FMRP and FMR2P. *Biochimie* 2010;92(8) 919-26.

[15] Glebova KV, Marakhonov AV, Baranova AV, Skoblov M. [Therapeutic siRNAs and non-viral systems for their delivery]. Molekuliarnaia biologiia 2012;46(3) 371-86.

[16] Jo D, Nashabi A, Doxsee C, Lin Q, Unutmaz D, Chen J, Ruley HE. Epigenetic regulation of gene structure and function with a cell-permeable Cre recombinase. *Nat Biotechnol* 2001;19(10) 929-33.

[17] Gupta B, Torchilin VP. Transactivating transcriptional activator-mediated drug delivery. *Expert Opin Drug Deliv* 2006;3(2) 177-90.

[18] Mintzer MA, Simanek EE. Nonviral vectors for gene delivery. *Chem Rev* 2009;109(2) 259-302.

[19] Weide B, Pascolo S, Scheel B, Derhovanessian E, Pflugfelder A, Eigentler TK, Pawelec G, Hoerr I, Rammensee HG, Garbe C. Direct injection of protamine-protected

mRNA: results of a phase 1/2 vaccination trial in metastatic melanoma patients. *J Immunother* 2009;32(5) 498-507.

[20] Kaneda Y. Virosome: a novel vector to enable multi-modal strategies for cancer therapy. *Adv Drug Deliv Rev* 2012;64(8) 730-8.

[21] Tolmachov OE, Tolmachova TO. Artificial virosomes are an attractive tool for gene delivery in vivo. Meeting in Gene Therapy; 1994; Cold Spring Harbor, NY, USA: CSHL Press.

[22] Anderson DM, Hall LL, Ayyalapu AR, Irion VR, Nantz MH, Hecker JG. Stability of mRNA/cationic lipid lipoplexes in human and rat cerebrospinal fluid: methods and evidence for nonviral mRNA gene delivery to the central nervous system. *Hum Gene Ther* 2003;14(3) 191-202.

[23] Sonawane ND, Szoka FC, Jr., Verkman AS. Chloride accumulation and swelling in endosomes enhances DNA transfer by polyamine-DNA polyplexes. *J Biol Chem* 2003;278(45) 44826-31.

[24] Castagliuolo I, Beggiao E, Brun P, Barzon L, Goussard S, Manganelli R, Grillot-Courvalin C, Palu G. Engineered E. coli delivers therapeutic genes to the colonic mucosa. *Gene Ther* 2005;12(13) 1070-8.

[25] Lavigne MD, Pennadam SS, Ellis J, Yates LL, Alexander C, Gorecki DC. Enhanced gene expression through temperature profile-induced variations in molecular architecture of thermoresponsive polymer vectors. *J Gene Med* 2007;9(1) 44-54.

[26] Tsen SW, Wu CY, Meneshian A, Pai SI, Hung CF, Wu TC. Femtosecond laser treatment enhances DNA transfection efficiency in vivo. *J Biomed Sci* 2009;16(e36). http://www.ncbi.nlm.nih.gov/entrez/query.fcgi?cmd=Retrieve&db=PubMed&dopt=Citation&list_uids=19338665 http://www.ncbi.nlm.nih.gov/pmc/articles/PMC2669473/pdf/1423-0127-16-36.pdf (accessed 1 August 2015).

[27] Koppers-Lalic D, Hogenboom MM, Middeldorp JM, Pegtel DM. Virus-modified exosomes for targeted RNA delivery; a new approach in nanomedicine. *Adv Drug Deliv Rev* 2013;65(3) 348-56.

[28] Song HP, Yang JY, Lo SL, Wang Y, Fan WM, Tang XS, Xue JM, Wang S. Gene transfer using self-assembled ternary complexes of cationic magnetic nanoparticles, plasmid DNA and cell-penetrating Tat peptide. *Biomaterials* 2010;31(4) 769-78.

[29] Van Tendeloo VF, Ponsaerts P, Lardon F, Nijs G, Lenjou M, Van Broeckhoven C, Van Bockstaele DR, Berneman ZN. Highly efficient gene delivery by mRNA electroporation in human hematopoietic cells: superiority to lipofection and passive pulsing of mRNA and to electroporation of plasmid cDNA for tumor antigen loading of dendritic cells. *Blood* 2001;98(1) 49-56.

[30] Judkewitz B, Rizzi M, Kitamura K, Hausser M. Targeted single-cell electroporation of mammalian neurons in vivo. Nat Protoc 2009;4(6) 862-9.

[31] Met O, Eriksen J, Svane IM. Studies on mRNA electroporation of immature and mature dendritic cells: effects on their immunogenic potential. *Mol Biotechnol* 2008;40(2) 151-60.

[32] Hutson TH, Buchser WJ, Bixby JL, Lemmon VP, Moon LD. Optimization of a 96-Well electroporation assay for postnatal rat CNS neurons suitable for cost-effective medium-throughput screening of genes that promote neurite outgrowth. *Front Mole Neurosci* 2011;4(e55). http://www.ncbi.nlm.nih.gov/pubmed/22207835 http://www.ncbi.nlm.nih.gov/pmc/articles/PMC3245668/pdf/fnmol-04-00055.pdf (accessed 1 August 2015).

[33] Martinet W, Schrijvers DM, Kockx MM. Nucleofection as an efficient nonviral transfection method for human monocytic cells. *Biotechnol Lett* 2003;25(13) 1025-9.

[34] Tyurin MV, Sullivan CR, Lynd LR. Role of spontaneous current oscillations during high-efficiency electrotransformation of thermophilic anaerobes. *Appl Environ Microbiol* 2005;71(12) 8069-76.

[35] Negishi Y, Matsuo K, Endo-Takahashi Y, Suzuki K, Matsuki Y, Takagi N, Suzuki R, Maruyama K, Aramaki Y. Delivery of an angiogenic gene into ischemic muscle by novel bubble liposomes followed by ultrasound exposure. *Pharm Res* 2011;28(4) 712-9.

[36] De Temmerman ML, Dewitte H, Vandenbroucke RE, Lucas B, Libert C, Demeester J, De Smedt SC, Lentacker I, Rejman J. mRNA-Lipoplex loaded microbubble contrast agents for ultrasound-assisted transfection of dendritic cells. *Biomaterials* 2011;32(34) 9128-35.

[37] Fan Z, Liu H, Mayer M, Deng CX. Spatiotemporally controlled single cell sonoporation. *Proc Natl Acad Sci U S A* 2012;109(41) 16486-91.

[38] Kedjarune-Leggat U, Supaprutsakul C, Chotigeat W. Ultrasound treatment increases transfection efficiency of low molecular weight chitosan in fibroblasts but not in KB Cells. *PLoS One* 2014;9(3). http://www.ncbi.nlm.nih.gov/pubmed/24651870 http://www.ncbi.nlm.nih.gov/pmc/articles/PMC3961286/pdf/pone.0092076.pdf (accessed 1 August 2015).

[39] Akowuah EF, Gray C, Lawrie A, Sheridan PJ, Su CH, Bettinger T, Brisken AF, Gunn J, Crossman DC, Francis SE, Baker AH, Newman CM. Ultrasound-mediated delivery of TIMP-3 plasmid DNA into saphenous vein leads to increased lumen size in a porcine interposition graft model. *Gene Ther* 2005;12(14) 1154-7.

[40] Inoue H, Arai Y, Kishida T, Shin-Ya M, Terauchi R, Nakagawa S, Saito M, Tsuchida S, Inoue A, Shirai T, Fujiwara H, Mazda O, Kubo T. Sonoporation-mediated transduction of siRNA ameliorated experimental arthritis using 3 MHz pulsed ultrasound. *Ultrasonics* 2014;54(3) 874-81.

[41] Qiu P, Ziegelhoffer P, Sun J, Yang NS. Gene gun delivery of mRNA in situ results in efficient transgene expression and genetic immunization. *Gene Ther* 1996;3(3) 262-8.

[42] Guzeloglu-Kayisli O, Lalioti MD, Aydiner F, Sasson I, Ilbay O, Sakkas D, Lowther KM, Mehlmann LM, Seli E. Embryonic poly(A)-binding protein (EPAB) is required for oocyte maturation and female fertility in mice. *Biochem J* 2012;446(1) 47-58.

[43] Chabri F, Bouris K, Jones T, Barrow D, Hann A, Allender C, Brain K, Birchall J. Microfabricated silicon microneedles for nonviral cutaneous gene delivery. *Brit J Dermatol* 2004;150(5) 869-77.

[44] Pantarotto D, Singh R, McCarthy D, Erhardt M, Briand JP, Prato M, Kostarelos K, Bianco A. Functionalized carbon nanotubes for plasmid DNA gene delivery. *Angew Chem Int Ed Engl* 2004;43(39) 5242-6.

[45] Migalska K, Morrow DI, Garland MJ, Thakur R, Woolfson AD, Donnelly RF. Laser-engineered dissolving microneedle arrays for transdermal macromolecular drug delivery. *Pharm Res* 2011;28(8) 1919-30.

[46] Peng Q, Sun X, Gong T, Wu CY, Zhang T, Tan J, Zhang ZR. Injectable and biodegradable thermosensitive hydrogels loaded with PHBHHx nanoparticles for the sustained and controlled release of insulin. *Acta biomaterialia* 2013;9(2) 5063-9.

[47] Schoen C, Kolb-Maurer A, Geginat G, Loffler D, Bergmann B, Stritzker J, Szalay AA, Pilgrim S, Goebel W. Bacterial delivery of functional messenger RNA to mammalian cells. *Cell Microbiol* 2005;7(5) 709-24.

[48] Walch B, Breinig T, Schmitt MJ, Breinig F. Delivery of functional DNA and messenger RNA to mammalian phagocytic cells by recombinant yeast. *Gene Ther* 2012;19(3) 237-45.

[49] Chubb JR, Trcek T, Shenoy SM, Singer RH. Transcriptional pulsing of a developmental gene. *Curr Biol* 2006;16(10) 1018-25.

[50] Pleger ST, Brinks H, Ritterhoff J, Raake P, Koch WJ, Katus HA, Most P. Heart failure gene therapy: the path to clinical practice. *Circ Res* 2013;113(6) 792-809.

[51] Koste L, Beissert T, Hoff H, Pretsch L, Tureci O, Sahin U. T-cell receptor transfer into human T cells with ecotropic retroviral vectors. *Gene Ther* 2014;

[52] Attal J, Theron MC, Puissant C, Houdebine LM. Effect of intercistronic length on internal ribosome entry site (IRES) efficiency in bicistronic mRNA. *Gene Express* 1999;8(5-6) 299-309.

[53] Gonzalez-Nicolini V, Sanchez-Bustamante CD, Hartenbach S, Fussenegger M. Adenoviral vector platform for transduction of constitutive and regulated tricistronic or triple-transcript transgene expression in mammalian cells and microtissues. *J Gene Med* 2006;8(10) 1208-22.

4

Multifunctional Delivery Systems for Cancer Gene Therapy

Emma M. McErlean, Cian M. McCrudden and Helen O. McCarthy

Abstract

This chapter examines key concepts with respect to cancer gene therapy and the current issues with respect to non-viral delivery. The biological and molecular barriers that need to be overcome before effective non-viral delivery systems can be appropriately designed for oncology applications are highlighted and ways to overcome these are discussed. Strategies developed to evade the immune response are also described and targeted gene delivery is examined with the most effective strategies highlighted. Finally, this chapter proposes a new way forward based on a growing body of evidence that supports a multifunctional delivery approach involving the creation of vectors, with a unique molecular architecture designed using a bottom-up approach.

Keywords: Cancer gene therapy, Multifunctional delivery systems, Non-viral gene delivery, Bio-inspired vectors, Tumour-targeted delivery

1. Introduction

Progress in the treatment of cancer in recent times has been unprecedented as cancer survival in the UK has doubled in the last 40 years, with 50% of adult cancer patients diagnosed in 2010–2011 in England and Wales predicted to survive 10 years or more [1]. Improvements in cancer screening techniques have led to improved prognosis through early detection, with breast cancer screening estimated to prevent up to 1,300 deaths per year; women who are diagnosed with the earliest stage of breast cancer have a 90% 5-year survival rate [2]. Likewise, if diagnosed early, prostate cancer responds well to treatments such as hormone therapy, with 65–90% of men diagnosed in stage 1 or 2 likely to live at least 10 years post diagnosis [3]. Despite improvements in screening and early detection methods, conventional treatment options are not always effective. Mainstay cancer treatment options including radiotherapy, chemotherapy, and surgery are extremely arduous on patients, and often have only moderate success. Existing anticancer drugs are generally cytotoxic, but lack specificity for the target tumour, which results in severe side effects. Not only do these traditional therapies cause damage to healthy cells, they are rarely effective against all transformed cells, and sometimes lack potency entirely. Failure of treatment can result in disease recurrence, often in a more aggressive form, with chemo- and radio-resistant aggressive malignancies ensuing. Resistance to conventional therapy causes treatment failure in over 90% of patients with advanced metastatic cancer [4].

Gene therapy is an exciting research area that involves the delivery of genetic material into cells to alter their function. Diseases that arise consequential of anomalous DNA (e.g., cystic fibrosis [5, 6]) are appropriate for gene therapy intervention; as cancer's origins lie in DNA damage, this group of diseases is also particularly suitable for gene-based therapeutics [7]. The strategy of gene therapy is generally to replace or repair faulty genes by the transfer and insertion of corrective or therapeutic genes [8]. Alternatively, the strategy of gene therapy can be the supraphysiological expression of cytotoxic proteins, or the expression of proteins to affect metabolism of prodrugs, for direct or indirect cytocidal effects, respectively [9]. Silencing of problematic genes is a nascent and very popular strategy that uses RNAi therapeutics to inhibit the expression of certain undesirable genes at the post-transcriptional level [10]. Some of the most common strategies of cancer gene therapy include suicide gene therapy, tumour suppressor gene therapy, antiangiogenic therapy, and cancer immunotherapy [11].

1.1. Tumour suppressor gene therapy

Mutation of tumour suppressor genes, such as p53, has been highlighted as a mechanism of proliferation and resistance in some cancers. Functional p53 interacts with other cellular pathways including the death-receptor pathways and caspases, as well as inhibiting anti-apoptotic mediators, such as the BCL family, leading to the suppression of tumour growth [12]. For this reason, the delivery of transgenes that encode tumour suppressor genes, including genes encoding p53, IL-2, EGFR, and E1A, has received considerable attention. Promising results have been obtained, with Senzer et al. reporting the systemic administration of targeted liposomal nanoparticles with an anti-transferrin receptor targeting moiety (TfR); they delivered the p53 tumour suppressor gene in complexes known as SGT-53 for advanced solid tumours in a phase I clinical trial [13]. SGT-53 was administered to patients with a range of advanced cancer types, including cervical cancer, thyroid cancer, and colorectal cancer. Median survival was 340 days and 7 of the 11 patients treated exhibited stable disease at 6-week assessment, with one patient reclassified from inoperable to operable due to significant tumour necrosis. The authors also demonstrated the tumour targeting ability of SGT-53 with biopsies of tumour tissue and normal tissue; normal tissue showing negligible exogenous p53 levels. However, the main aim of the study was to assess safety and further studies would be required to fully assess therapeutic effects.

1.2. Suicide gene therapy

Suicide gene therapy, also known as gene-directed enzyme-producing therapy (GDEPT), involves the administration of an enzyme-encoding transgene to the tissue, with a separate administration of a relatively innocuous prodrug. Transgene expression produces the enzyme within cancerous cells and subsequently the prodrug is converted to its toxic form by this enzyme [14]. GDEPT strategies include cytosine deaminase/F-fluorocytosine (CD/5-FC), where the CD transgene metabolises 5-FC to 5-Fluorouracil (5-FU); herpes simplex virus thymidine kinase/ganciclovir (HSVtk/GCV) where HSVtk coverts GCV to its cytotoxic triphosphate derivative; and *E. coli* nitroreductase/CB1954 (NTR/CB) where NTR activates the prodrug CB1954 resulting in toxicity to tumour cells [15]. Multiple GDEPT systems have made it to clinical trials and Sangro et al. reported on a recent phase 1 clinical trial of HSVtk/GCV in the treatment of advanced hepatocellular carcinoma. Intra-tumoural injection of the TK gene in a replication deficient adenovirus vector (Ad-TK) was followed with systemic administration of GCV in 10 patients [16]. Although the main aims of the trial were to assess feasibility and safety of treatment, anti-tumour effects were also assessed. Stabilisation of tumour was observed in 60% of patients, with two patients who received the high dose treatment showing tumour necrosis and one patient surviving for 26 months. Such therapies, which may be used in addition to radiotherapy, have the advantage of being activated only in the cancerous cells due to direct intra-tumoural delivery, reducing toxic side-effects to normal cells. A 'bystander effect' where neighbouring cells receive the toxic treatment through gap junctions has also been observed, which could be beneficial for therapy as reduced amounts of treatment are needed for the same therapeutic effect; conversely, this bystander effect may limit the potential of the therapy if neighbouring healthy cells receive the toxic treatment. However, problems in vector development still need to be overcome before these treatments are to be successful [17]. Despite progression to clinical trials, no GDEPT therapy has made it to the market and the use of such treatment strategies may be limited to locally available tumour sites due to the need for intra-tumoural injection.

1.3. Anti-angiogenic therapy

In contrast to suicide gene therapy and tumour suppressor therapy, which are quite specific in focus, targeting angiogenesis may attack the root of the greater tumour establishment. There are various 'classical' protein-based angiogenesis inhibitors, including receptor tyrosine kinase inhibitors, which block the activity of vascular endothelial growth factor (VEGF), and monoclonal antibodies against VEGF-A such as bevacizumab (Avastin®). However, as angiogenesis is required for normal function in the body, such as wound healing, complete blockade of angiogenesis is not desirable. In addition, it may seem that rather than kill tumours, inhibitor therapy may merely retard further tumour growth. Moreover, the existence of various resistance mechanisms to angiogenic inhibitors, including alternative signalling pathways poses major drawbacks to such therapy. Alternatively, a gene therapy approach targeting the genes behind the pro-angiogenic factors may be more suitable [18, 19]. Doan et al. described a gene silencing approach that halts the effects of the pro-angiogenic factors VEGF and kinesin spindle protein (KSP), which play a critical role in cellular proliferation [20]. Hep3B hepatocellular carcinoma cells were treated with a cocktail of anti-VEGF and anti-KSP siRNAs, and a significant reduction in both VEGF and KSP expression was observed; in vitro, this manifested reduced proliferation of the cells, assessed by WST-1 assay and clonogenic survival assay. The results demonstrate the potential for anti-angiogenic gene therapy, but translation to in vivo studies is required to establish this further.

1.4. Cancer immunotherapy

Cancer immunotherapy is the process of harnessing the immune system to attack cancer cells. Cancer cells present antigens, known as tumour-associated antigens (TAAs) or tumour-specific antigens (TSAs) on their surface; recognition of these antigens by immune cells has been exploited in the development of cancer DNA vaccines. Cancer vaccines may be prophylactic or therapeutic in their design, which would generate an active immune response specifically to tumours while also providing memory cells to control future recurrence [21]. DNA encoding the genes for TAAs is delivered to cancer cells that subsequently express the transgenic TAA, eliciting an immune response against the tumour cells and many cancer DNA vaccines are being assessed in clinical trials [22]. Chudley et al. reported on a phase I/II clinical trial of a DNA vaccine encoding a domain (DOM) from fragment C of a tetanus toxin linked to an HLA-A2-binding epitope from prostate-specific membrane antigen (PSMA) in patients with prostate cancer [23]. Following intramuscular administration of the DNA vaccine to 30 patients, 29 had a measurable CD4+ T-cell response and PSMA-specific CD8+ T cells were detected in 16/30 patients. As a result, PSA doubling time increased significantly from 11.97 months pre-treatment to 16.82 months denoting slower progression of the disease. Staff et al. reported on a phase I clinical trial in patients with colorectal cancer with a DNA vaccine [24]. The plasmid vaccine was administered by Biojector® and encoded human carcinoembryonic antigen (CEA), which is known to be over expressed by a large number of epithelial neoplasias, including colorectal cancer. No serious adverse effects were observed with the vaccine and of the 10 patients, 8 showed no evidence of disease at follow-up. However, despite the promising trial results and 4 DNA vaccines licensed for use in animals including Oncept® for Canine Melanoma [25], no product has made it to the market in humans. Many trials use direct injection of the vaccines to tumours and efficiency may be enhanced if delivery vectors were to be used, which could maximise transduction.

To date, cancer has been the most common disease focus for gene therapy, with 64% of all ongoing gene therapy clinical trials targeting a malignancy [26]. However, the progress of gene therapy beyond clinical trials has been disappointing, with only three products currently having made it to the market, namely, Gendicine®, Oncorine®, and Glybera®. Gendicine® and Oncorine®, which deliver p53 tumour suppressor genes for the treatment of head and neck cancer, are licenced in China; while Glybera®, used for the treatment of severe lipoprotein lipase deficiency, is the only gene therapy product licensed in Europe [27]. Despite the many promising therapeutic strategies for gene therapy, the common limiting factor has been the lack of a suitable delivery vehicle that has the ability to specifically target tumour cells, whilst being non-immunogenic and non-toxic. Consequently, a vast amount of research has therefore focused on delivery systems for gene therapy. In order for the potential of gene therapy to be realised, the focus needs to be on the design of an appropriate delivery vehicle that will meet all the demands in terms of functionality and satisfaction of regulatory bodies.

2. The biological barriers to gene delivery

The safest way to deliver gene therapy is by direct administration of the therapeutic to the target site. However, this is extremely inefficient, unreliable, and feasible only in tumours in superficial sites. Generally, gene therapy approaches are delivered via the intravenous route; as nucleic acids are susceptible to degradation by nucleases and rapid clearance in systemic circulation [28], a vector is required to package, protect, and transport the genetic material to its site of action.

Viral vectors, derived from naturally evolved viruses capable of transferring their genetic material into host cells, remain the most efficient gene delivery agents [29]. However, difficulty in large scale production, limitation in size of DNA that can be carried, and concerns about mutagenesis, toxicity, and immunogenicity have hindered the progression of viral vectors [30, 31]. As a result, much research has focused on the design of non-viral vectors, which have the potential to circumvent the problems associated with viral vectors [32]. Non-viral gene delivery encompasses a wide variety of delivery systems including cationic polymers, liposomes, proteins, and peptides that have the ability to package nucleic acids and deliver them into cells [33]. However, transfection efficiency of non-viral vectors remains significantly lower than viral vectors [34], and many factors are to be considered and hurdles overcome when designing an efficient non-viral delivery system. Successful gene therapy relies largely on the development of an efficient vector that can overcome the various extracellular and intracellular barriers to deliver the genetic material to its target site [35].

2.1. Extracellular barriers

Although delivery vectors have the ability to protect the DNA from endonuclease attack, the vectors themselves may also be susceptible to recognition and clearance. In the systemic circulation, vectors may be rapidly cleared from circulation by the reticulo-endothelial system (RES), also known as the mononuclear phagocyte system (MPS) [36]. Many non-viral delivery vectors are cationic in nature, a desirable characteristic for condensing DNA and promoting cellular uptake. However, this cationic nature can be problematic for systemic administration due to interaction with blood components, such as serum proteins, which may result in opsonisation. Consequently, large aggregates are formed that cannot traverse cell membranes and may become lodged in microvascular networks or accumulate in MPS organs such as the liver or spleen [37]. Further to this, cationic systems may interact with cell membranes indiscriminately, affecting normal cells as well as cancerous cells, and strong cationic charges can induce damage of cellular membranes and apoptosis [38]. Thus, a balance must be reached in the design of a delivery vector such that the nucleic acid/vector complex has cationicity of appropriate magnitude, so as to permit proper association with target cells whilst preventing aggregation.

The circulation of gene therapy delivery systems is often cut short due to rapid hepatic metabolism and clearance, and often this clearance occurs before the particles can reach their target site to deliver the therapeutic. The use of 'stealth particles', such as those that contain polyethylene glycol (PEG), has been shown to increase the circulation time of various delivery systems by shielding the charge of the particles, reducing binding with serum proteins and aggregation, whilst evading the immune system [39]. Various strategies in evading this clearance have been employed, which will be discussed in a later section. However, if the vector can avoid clearance, extravasation from blood circulation needs to occur in order to reach the tumour cells, which can be hindered by the chaotic blood supply, poor permeability, and high interstitial pressure within the tumour [40].

2.2. Intracellular barriers

Surviving the systemic circulation and reaching the target cell is not the only hurdle faced by non-viral gene delivery systems. The nature of conventional gene therapy requires the genetic material to be transcribed by the cell, which requires delivery to the nucleus (or in the case of siRNA technology, delivery to the cytoplasm). A number of intracellular barriers exist that may impede this delivery include traversing the cell membrane, escape from the endosome, and release of the nucleic acid payload into the cytoplasm, followed by active transport to the nucleus with subsequent nuclear import.

2.2.1. Cell membrane/internalisation

Cell membranes are lipophilic anionic structures that are generally impermeable to large macromolecular anionic nucleic acids [32]. Non-viral gene delivery systems aim to complex nucleic acid cargo, thereby masking their native negative charge, to give an overall net cationic complex capable of interaction with cell membranes. Not only does this allow for electrostatic interactions between the vector and the membrane, it also condenses the DNA to a size suitable for cellular uptake (≤200 nm diameter). Various pathways of cellular uptake exist that are size dependent. For example, the cell penetrating peptide TAT, derived from the human immunodeficiency-1 virus (HIV-1) [41], enters cells via different routes depending on the size of the cargo. Larger cargoes of proteins or quantum dots that exceed the 500 Daltons restriction limit are internalised with TAT via the caveolae or macropinocytosis routes, and smaller cargoes such as peptides less than 30–40 amino acids via the clathrin route [42]. Further to this, the internalisation route may also depend on other factors such as cell type, receptors present on the cell, temperature, incubation time, concentration of the vector, and properties of the vector including cargo and linkage type [7, 43]. Different internalisation pathways also have an effect on the fate of the vector once inside the cell. As a result, much research has centred around elucidating the mechanisms involved in cellular uptake in order to improve the efficiency of gene therapy [44]. Endocytosis (clathrin-mediated, caveolae-mediated, or macropinocytosis) is thought to be the main uptake pathway for most gene delivery.

2.2.2. Clathrin-Mediated Endocytosis (CME)

CME is the most well-defined route of endocytosis and involves the internalisation of cargo via receptors on the cell membrane, such as proteoglycans, into vesicles known as clathrin coated pits, which are about 100–150 nm in diameter. These pits are transported via microtubules of the cell cytoskeleton deeper into the cell, where they form endosomes (acidic, degradative compartments that transport material back to the membrane for recycling, or to lysosomes for degradation). The term 'receptor-mediated endocytosis' is often used to describe CME, however, endocytosis via receptors does not exclusively occur via CME [45]. The addition of ligands, such as transferrin, to delivery systems has allowed for targeting to cancer cells overexpressing the transferrin receptor that binds to the ligand and facilitates internalisation via CME [46].

2.2.3. *Caveolae-Mediated Endocytosis (CvME)*

CvME is initiated by flask-shaped invaginations known as caveolae that have lipid-raft formations involving cholesterol and sphingolipids, which are around 50–200 nm in diameter. Internalisation occurs in an actin-dependent manner, forming a type of endosome known as a caveosome. Caveosomes are not as acidic or destructive as CME endosomes, but can still ultimately merge with the lysosomal machinery [47]. It has been observed that many commonly used cancer cells lines (e.g., PC-3 prostate cancer cells) lack the ability to form caveolae that may have significance for delivery systems relying on this route for internalisation [48]. Furthermore, it has been observed that caveolae may be upregulated in some cancer cells providing a possible target for delivery systems. Nguyen et al. reported that a polysorbitol-mediated transporter (PSMT) was used to deliver plasmid DNA encoding the p53 tumour suppressor gene into human cervical cancer (HeLa) cells and normal human diploid fibroblast (HDF) cells. PSMT entered cancer cells selectively via CvME with transgene expression resulting in cellular damage and apoptosis [49].

2.2.4. *Macropinocytosis*

Macropinocytosis involves the uptake of large amounts of fluid-phase materials. It occurs via an actin-driven mechanism that causes ruffling of the cell membrane to form protrusions that engulf the extracellular material into macropinosomes, which eventually merge with the endosomal pathway [50]. Anaka et al. reported that macropinocytosis was the main cellular uptake pathway of the peptide STR-CH2R4H2C when complexed with plasmid DNA and delivered to COS7 kidney fibroblast cells, attributing the position of arginine residues exposed on the surface of the complexes as the reason for this internalisation route [51].

2.2.5. *Direct internalisation*

Cationic vectors, especially those rich in arginine, have been observed to enter cells via non-endocytic routes through direct internalisation triggered by non-specific electrostatic interactions [52]. This form of internalisation is a more attractive route for non-viral gene delivery, as direct delivery into the cytoplasm avoids the endosome. In the case of arginine-rich cell penetrating peptides, an initial electrostatic interaction with the cell membrane is followed by formation of a peptide-cargo-phospholipid complex with the positively charged guanidium group of arginine bound to the phosphate groups of the phosphatidylcholine (PC) and/or sphingomyelin (SM) of the outer leaflet of the cell membrane. A 'capacitor' is then formed between the cationic arginine residues and the anionic phosphatidylserine creating an electric field strong enough to form a reversible pore, which allows the CPP-cargo to pass through the membrane [53]. Arginine-rich peptides, such as octa-arginine (R8), have therefore been utilised for gene delivery due their strong cell penetrating ability. However, little is known about this entry route, and evidence suggests that vectors can enter cells via multiple mechanisms [54]. Understanding the various routes through which vectors can enter cells can aid the gene therapist in the design of vectors; ensuring appropriate size and charge, for example, can allow for targeted internalisation via a specific mechanism.

2.3. Endosomal entrapment

Following endocytosis, vectors may be trapped in the endosomal pathway. Endosomal entrapment poses a major limiting step to efficient gene therapy. The endosomal compartment provides cells with a way of regulating what enters and leaves the cell and material within the endosome can be either recycled to the cell membrane or progressed to lysosomes. It is essential that therapeutics escape the endosome in order to avoid degradation of the nucleic acid payload [55]. Endosomal escape can be achieved by different mechanisms and typically non-viral delivery systems are designed to facilitate this. The 'proton sponge' effect is exploited by polymers that contain amine groups such as polyethylenimine (PEI) or by histidine-rich peptides, which have been used in many delivery systems for gene therapy [56]. Fusogenic peptides evoke membrane destabilisation by interacting with anionic lipids in the endosomal membrane, thereby disrupting the membrane, allowing release of the endosomal contents [57]. INF-7 peptide is an example of a synthetic fusogenic peptide derived from influenza virus hemagglutinin protein, which enhances endosomal escape. Oliviera et al. report that the addition of INF-7 peptide to Lipofectamine for delivery of anti-kRas siRNA resulted in 3.5-fold improved gene silencing effect and subsequent reduction in kRas protein expression in C26 murine colon carcinoma cells in vitro when compared to Lipofectamine/siRNA complexes alone [58].

2.4. Intracellular trafficking

Following endosomal escape, the vector and its cargo must be delivered to the correct cellular compartment, i.e., DNA delivered to the nucleus, or siRNA assembly into RNA-induced silencing complexes (RISC) in the cytoplasm [59, 60]. However, this is not without its challenges due to the restricted movement of macromolecules in the cell, slowing the mobility of vectors towards the nucleus [61], while endonucleases may degrade any naked nucleic acid [62]. The vector is therefore required to protect and transport the nucleic acid through the cytoplasm in order to reach its target organelle. Movement in the cytoplasm is restricted due to overcrowding of organelles, the cell cytoskeleton and high protein concentrations, which collectively result in a major impediment to non-viral delivery of even relatively small cargoes [63]. A network of microtubules and associated motor proteins (dyneins and kinesins) are responsible for the maintenance of correct organelle location [64] and intracellular transport of vesicles, lysosomes, and endosomes [65]. If non-viral gene delivery vectors could utilise the microtubule network within the cell, it would serve as a direct route to the nucleus and transfection efficiencies may be greatly improved. Toledo et al. presented a recombinant fusion protein based on the dynein light chain LC8 that facilitated plasmid DNA uptake into HeLa cells and transported DNA via microtubules to the nucleus for GFP transgene expression [66].

2.5. Nuclear import

In the case of DNA gene therapy, once the vector reaches the nucleus, it must gain entry and deliver its genetic payload in order for the gene to be transcribed and elicit its effect. The nucleus is protected by a bilayer known as the nuclear envelope, and entry into the nucleus through the nuclear envelope is tightly controlled by the nuclear pore complex (NPC) [67].

The NPC only allows the passive entry of molecules that do not exceed 10 nm in diameter, which limits the entry of DNA; active traversing of the nuclear envelope is hence required. The NPC therefore poses the last major hurdle to gene therapy and is a huge rate-limiting step in transfection efficiency. The addition of short amino acid sequences known as nuclear localisation signals (NLS) to vectors has been useful in trafficking and facilitating nuclear entry [68]. The nuclear localisation signal from the simian virus 40 (SV40), large tumour antigen has been used to enhance transfection efficiency in many delivery systems. Wang et al. demonstrated that the addition of SV40 NLS to R8 resulted in a transfection efficiency of up to 80% as effective as jetPEI™ (transfection reagent) with no cytotoxic effects in HeLa cells [69].

Understanding the various barriers to gene delivery allows the rational design of delivery systems that can overcome these hurdles. The ideal non-viral gene delivery vector is a multi-functional system with the ability to condense DNA effectively, overcome the various intra- and extracellular barriers and must also be non-toxic and non-immunogenic. Furthermore, vectors can be designed specifically to exploit the characteristics of cancer cells and tumours, including the enhanced permeability and retention (EPR) effect associated with tumour vasculature; where gene therapy delivery systems exploit the permeability of the tumour vasculature to localise and accumulate in the tumour through passive diffusion [70]. Other factors, including tumour microenvironment, and the aberrant expression of certain enzymes and proteins commonly associated with cancer cells may also be targeted or exploited. Figure 1 represents how a multi-functional non-viral gene delivery system may be composed.

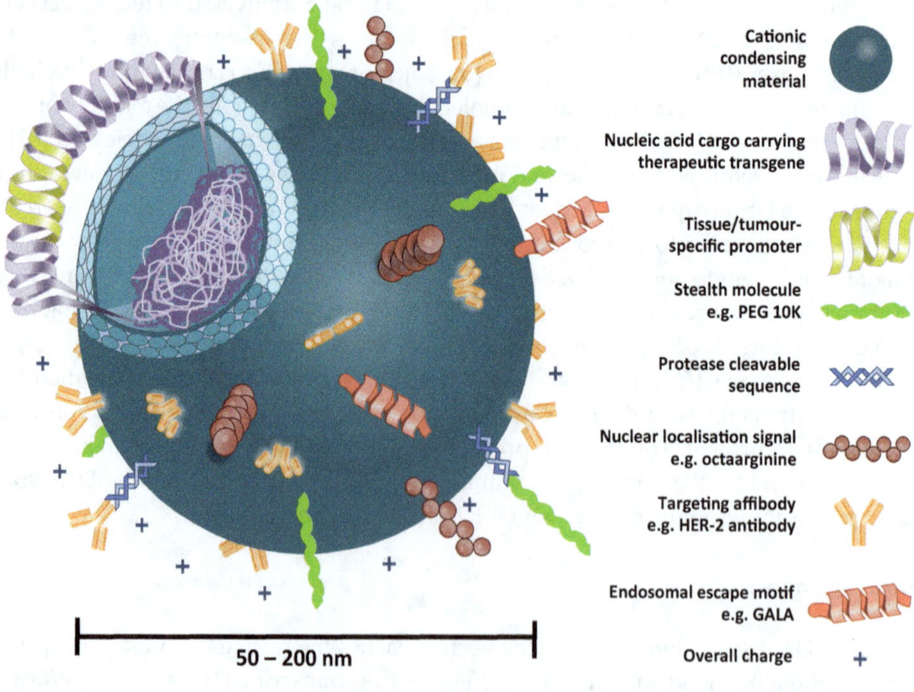

Figure 1. Schematic of a multi-functionalised vector for therapeutic transgene delivery.

Anionic plasmid DNA cargo is condensed using a cationic material such as poly-L-lysine or protamine. Vectors are functionalised with adjuncts to aid in evasion of the various barriers that are posed to gene therapy strategies, as highlighted above. The various functional groups will be discussed below.

3. Evading the immune response

When gene delivery systems are administered systemically they are usually cleared rapidly from circulation, mainly by Kupffer cells in the liver and macrophages in the spleen. This is a form of defence by the host designed to recognise and clear potentially harmful invaders from the system as quickly as possible, and involves a two-step process initiated by opsonisation with subsequent phagocytosis [71]. Opsonisation is the adsorption of foreign particles by opsonin proteins such as immunoglobulins, blood serum proteins, and complement proteins. Subsequently, macrophages may bind directly to the opsonised particle, engulf and remove it from circulation or the complement system may be activated, also leading to phagocytosis [72]. The characteristics of the particle in circulation play an important role in the recognition process and therefore are extremely important parameters to consider in the design of a delivery vector. Particles larger than the renal threshold of approximately 5,000 Daltons (usually greater than 200 nm hydrodynamic radii) are more likely to activate the complement system and are usually cleared more rapidly than their smaller counterparts. Surface charge, hydrophobicity, and the presence of certain functional groups are also important, with a more cationic nature favouring interaction with the anionic blood proteins and enhancing opsonisation [73].

Initial opsonisation of particles is critical to their subsequent removal, so if opsonisation can be reduced or avoided, then clearance may be circumvented. An extensively used method to overcome opsonisation is the utilisation of shielding groups or 'stealth' molecules that are generally long hydrophilic polymer chains. These are typically flexible and charge neutral, which can block the electrostatic and hydrophobic interactions between opsonins and the nucleic acid/vehicle complex, improving the stability of the particles in the systemic circulation. Various polymers have been used including polyacrylamide, poly(vinyl alcohol), poly(N-vinyl-2-pyrrolidone), and poly ethylene glycol (PEG) [72].

PEG is the most commonly used and effective polymer for stealth molecules; PEG is non-toxic, non-immunogenic, non-antigenic, highly water-soluble, and FDA approved. PEGylating a cationic complex shields the positive charge, thereby reducing interaction with blood components, and inhibiting clearance, allowing increased circulation time and opportunity for vectors to reach their target site. It also reduces non-specific binding to non-target cells and stabilises particles, reducing aggregation. The increased circulation time is highly desirable for passive tumour targeting, facilitated by the leaky tumour vasculature. Extravasation of vectors from the blood stream occurs with retention and accumulation in the tumour site by the EPR effect. It has been suggested, however, that repeat administrations may sensitise the immune system to PEG resulting in rapid clearance of PEGylated liposomes from circulation and formation of anti-PEG antibodies [74, 75]. However, the validity of the assays used to test for anti-PEG antibodies have been questioned over flaws and lack of specificity [76].

In order for PEG to properly oppose the attractive forces between the opsonins and the cationic particle surface, it must have a sufficient surface coverage, which is usually correlated to the molecular weight, surface chain density, and conformation of PEG. It is generally held that sufficient stealth character is achieved with a molecular weight of 2,000 Daltons or more, with loss of flexibility in shorter chains being the probable cause for lack of stealth. As molecular weight increases, the blood circulation half-life also increases. Surface chain density and conformation are also important so that adequate surface coverage is achieved to avoid gaps where opsonins may bind, while also maintaining flexibility in the PEG layer responsible for the steric hindrance properties. By fine-tuning such properties of PEG, an improved biodistribution and the pharmacokinetic profile of the therapeutic may be achieved; such tunings have led to many different PEGylation strategies being developed [72].

3.1. The PEG dilemma

A major problem with the use of PEG for cancer gene therapy is that it may hinder gene expression by impeding the entry of the delivery system into tumour cells. The initial interaction of cationic delivery systems with cell membranes relies on electrostatic association, so masking by PEG may have an unfavourable effect. Further to this, the improved stability of PEGylated particles disrupts membrane fusion and may reduce the effects of fusogenic peptides either during cell internalisation or for endosomal disruption. The term 'PEG dilemma' was coined to describe the balance that must be struck between availing of the beneficial characteristics that PEG provides while not being limited by them. Appropriate vector design must ensure that an appropriate balance is struck between the facets that make PEG an attractive supplement to a vector and those that limit its effectiveness [77].

Various strategies have been employed in order to overcome the problems posed by the PEG dilemma. Once the PEGylated vector has survived in circulation and reaches its target cell, the PEG chain becomes redundant. By removal or detachment of PEG from the surface of the vector, interaction with the cell membrane can occur and initiate internalisation. One strategy that has gained much attention is the addition of targeting ligands to PEG that bind to cell surface receptors exclusive to the target cells, limiting endocytosis of the PEGylated delivery system to the target cells [78]. However, this may involve the introduction of a charged moiety onto the PEG, reducing the effectiveness of PEG in evading clearance. The bulky PEG chain may also still hinder the gene delivery system overcoming the various intracellular barriers discussed above. Therefore, the design of a detachable or reversible PEGylation has resulted in 'smart' delivery systems that can exploit different aspects of the intracellular or extracellular tumour environment, including pH, enzyme complement, or reduction, while also functioning as a targeting tool to direct vectors to tumours [79, 80].

3.2. pH-sensitive PEG linkers

Using linkages such as ester and hydrazine bonds, which are stable in circulation but hydrolysed in acidic conditions, is a promising way of creating a detachable PEG. The acidic tumour microenvironment may cleave off the PEG chain, thereby releasing the therapeutic at the target site and allowing interaction of the cationic delivery system with cell membranes, initiating internalisation. Alternatively, the acidic pH within the endosome may also serve to cleave PEG from the delivery system after receptor-mediated endocytosis. This will unmask the vector allowing endosomal escape by, for example restoring fusogenic activity, facilitating cytosolic delivery and subsequent gene expression [79]. Fella et al. described a targeted polyplex system with PEG attached via an acid labile hydrazone linkage that afforded a 14-fold increase in transgene expression in HUH7 hepatocellular carcinoma tumours compared to the non-acid sensitive formulation. The system was able to protect the vector in the systemic circulation, facilitate entry to the cells via EGF-receptor mediated endocytosis, and exploit endosomal pH to execute the removal of PEG, which permitted release of the vector from the endosome [81].

3.3. Enzymatic cleavage of PEG

Various proteolytic enzymes are known to be secreted into the extracellular environment by cancer cells. The knowledge of specific enzymes and their substrates can then be exploited to tether PEG to a vector via an appropriate enzyme-cleavable linker. Matrix metalloproteinases (MMPs) are a family of proteases commonly secreted by tumours, degrading the extracellular matrix facilitating growth and progression of tumours [82]. Li et al. took advantage of the presence of MMP-7 proteases in the extracellular environment by functionalising polymeric nanoparticles with PEG via a MMP-7 cleavable linker for delivery of anti-luciferase siRNA. The authors reported a 2.5-fold increase in transfection efficiency in MDA-MB-231 breast cancer cells in the presence of MMP-7 in vitro compared to transfection efficiency in the absence of MMP-7 [83]. These results, however, would need to be further reinforced with in vivo studies in order to fully assess the pharmacokinetic profile of this system.

3.4. Reduction-sensitive PEG linkage

A reduction-sensitive linkage may be used to attach PEG to a vector using disulphide bonds. These bonds are susceptible to reduction by glutathione (GSH), a peptide with various functions within the cell such as antioxidant defence, metabolic processes, and regulation and maintenance of cellular redox status. The intracellular concentration of GSH is three orders of magnitude higher than in the extracellular compartment [84], which allows for reduction of the disulphide bonds and detachment of the bulky PEG chain once the functionalised vector is inside target cells. Alternatively, extracellular reduction may occur through the action of thiol-containing cell surface receptors [85]. Lei et al. described a targeted delivery system functionalised with PEG attached via a disulphide linkage. Polyethylenimine (PEI) nanoparticles that were functionalised with a reduction-sensitive linked PEG were twice as potent as their counterparts that lacked the reduction-sensitive linker in terms of GFP and RFP reporter gene delivery in vitro and in vivo in U87 glioblastoma tumours [86].

3.5. Copolymers

While the use of a cleavable linker for PEGylation has shown promise for gene delivery, issues may arise if the linker is not accessible for cleavage due to the shielding action of PEG. The nature of polymers renders them easily modifiable; changing the characteristics of the PEG polymer itself by forming crosslinks may produce a degradable copolymer suitable for controlled release [79]. Fan et al. reported on a copolymer that comprised polyethylene glycol 5000 (PEG114), Vitamin E (VE), and thioctic acid (TA), termed PEG114:VE:TA, which assembled into micelles with poly-disulfide crosslinks [87]. The copolymer resulted in improved thermodynamic and kinetic profile of the anticancer drug paclitaxel. Reduction of the disulphide crosslinks occurred in response to glutathione causing rapid disassembly of the micelles and accelerated drug release that resulted in approximately 3-fold higher plasma concentration than the non-crosslinked micelles leading to increased drug accumulation in the SKOV-3 human ovarian cancer xenograft mouse model. Although this study did not deliver gene therapy, it demonstrates the potential of modifying polymer crosslinks to achieve desirable characteristics for drug delivery.

The production of copolymers, which combine the characteristics of more than one polymer, has shown promise where a balance is struck between PEGylation and copolymer reducible characteristics. Recently, Lai et al. presented a reducible copolymer comprising poly(ethylene oxide)-b-poly(propylene oxide)-b-poly(ethylene oxide)-SS-P[Asp(DET)] (P(EPE)-SS-P[Asp(DET)]), which possesses a redox potential-sensitive disulfide linkage between the P(EPE) polymer and the cationic block P[Asp(DET)]. The copolymer was used to deliver the pGL4 DNA vector for luciferase expression, and a 2-fold increase in transfection efficiency was observed compared to delivery with non-reducible copolymer counterparts in MDA-MB-231 breast cancer cells in vitro [88]. However, much work is yet to be done to elucidate the exact characteristics and polymer design needed to produce optimal transfection efficiencies.

Systems that combine two or more mechanisms for masking delivery vectors while improving uptake have been investigated, with PEG being combined with other polymers or peptides. Huang et al. designed a multifunctional delivery system that uses a combination of an MMP-sensitive linkage, a pH-sensitive mask to quench the cationic charge of nona-arginine (R9), and PEG to improve steric stabilisation in circulation [89]. The masking peptide was pH-sensitive with an isoelectric point (pI) of 6.4, affording the masking peptide a negative charge at physiological pH, which interacts with the cationic R9 cell-penetrating peptide (CPP). However, a tumour's acidic environment neutralises the masking peptide, allowing the cationic nature of R9 to come to the fore. Cleavage of the PEG by MMP-2 allowed the CPP-cargo complex to enter cells. The authors used in vivo imaging to demonstrate the specificity of these nanoparticles to target human hepatocellular carcinoma cell (BEL-7402) xenografts.

Although PEGylation provides a means of enhancing circulation times, allowing vectors to reach their target site, reliance on the EPR effect as a means of passive targeting may not be as reliable as initially thought. The variability displayed in tumour biology as well as the disordered and discontinuous tumour vascular structure means that the accumulation of delivery vectors by the EPR effect may not give a tumour-wide distribution. Although it may give an added advantage, total reliance on the EPR effect cannot give reliable results and so there is a need for an active targeting strategy [90].

4. Targeting in non-viral systems

Early approaches to gene therapy involved direct introduction of genetic material into locally accessible tumours. While this proved useful in some cases, the invasive nature of these methods renders them impractical for internal and disseminated tumours. Therefore, a systemically administered cancer gene therapy vector that can target tumours is ideal. Traditional chemotherapeutic cytotoxic drugs cause such harsh and debilitating side effects because they affect rapidly dividing cells and do not differentiate between normal or cancerous cells. In order to avoid these off-target effects, it is necessary to target the therapeutic directly to the cancer cells without affecting normal healthy cells. Improved knowledge of cellular, metabolic, and signalling pathways essential for tumour growth has led to the identification of targets on cancer cells [91]. Different types of cancerous cells tend to have distinct characteristics, which set them apart from normal cells, meaning that a range of potential molecular targets exists that can be targeted to direct gene therapy towards tumours. Cancer cells typically overexpress certain proteins on their surface, which may be exploited through targeting strategies; commonly overexpressed proteins include integrins [92], transferrin receptors [46], epidermal growth factor receptors (EGFR) [93], folate receptors [94], and proteoglycans [95], and targeting such receptors has been found to increase the specificity and efficacy of drug delivery, while reducing side effects [96]. Active targeting using ligands that target overexpressed receptors specific to cancer cells is therefore an attractive targeting strategy for systemically administered non-viral gene delivery and much research has focused around this.

4.1. Targeting ligands

Through phage display techniques, ligands for specific receptors commonly overexpressed on cancer cells have been successfully identified and incorporated into vectors [97]. When the delivery vector reaches the tumour environment, the overexpressed receptors bind the ligand on the surface of the vector and it is subsequently internalised via receptor-mediated endocytosis. This strategy serves to both target the cells and facilitate uptake by cells, but the endocytic pathway used can depend on the targeting ligand and cell type [98]. RGD peptide is a commonly used peptide targeting ligand. It is a tripeptide of Arg-Gly-Asp that was derived from fibronectin, which mediates cell attachment. RGD peptide is involved in cell adhesion to cell surface integrins [99]. Integrin receptors, such as $\alpha v\beta 3$ integrin and related αv-integrins, are commonly upregulated on the surface of angiogenic endothelial cells and can have a profound effect on the ability of tumours to survive and progress through regulation of stemness, metastasis, and resistance [100]. This activity makes integrins valuable for targeting aggressive cancers and various strategies have been used to incorporate RGD into non-viral delivery systems for targeting angiogenic tumours [101]. Kim et al. presented a tumour-targeting, RGD-conjugated, bio-reducible polymer for the delivery of vascular endothelial growth factor (VEGF) siRNA. The RGD-functionalised vectors showed 20–59% higher cellular uptake in MCF-7 breast cancer cells and PANC-1 pancreatic cancer cells compared to non-targeted vectors. In addition, MCF-7 and PANC-1 cancer cells had significantly reduced VEGF gene expression (51–71%) and cancer cell viability (35–43%) compared with control [102]. Nie et al. described a dual functionalised system that boasts two targeting ligands, namely RGD and B6 peptide, which target transferrin receptors. Transfection efficiency of the dual targeting system resulted in 8- and 4-fold higher luciferase reporter gene expression compared to single targeted control formulations with either B6 or RGD in DU145 and PC3 prostate cancer cells, respectively [103].

When formulating a targeted non-viral gene delivery system, there are a number of factors to be considered that may have an effect on the overall efficiency of the delivery system, such as ligand density and positioning on the surface of the vector, vector size, and choice of targeting ligand [90]. Vector ligand density should be optimised to ensure efficient binding to receptors. Furthermore, the binding of a ligand to its substrate may facilitate binding of neighbouring receptors in a thermodynamically favourable way [104]. In addition, the strategies used to link the targeting moieties to vectors, as well as many other factors including relative specificity, expression of target receptors, and physiological factors need to be considered in order to improve effectiveness and avoid interference or loss of biological activity [105].

One such problem with active targeting is that it is dependent on the expression of certain receptors by tumour cells. In breast cancer, oestrogen, progesterone, and human epidermal growth factor (HER) receptors have been identified and targeted. However, 15% of breast cancers, termed triple negative, are defined by a lack of these receptors. Absence of these receptors makes such cancers difficult to target and treat, hence patients with triple-negative disease have poorer prognoses [106]. Therefore, there is a need for a more general targeting strategy that targets the common characteristics of cancer cells and is not reliant on the expression of any one receptor. This would also broaden the scope of disease states that may be treated using any individual gene therapy strategy, making them more marketable for the pharmaceutical industry. Additionally, drug resistance can develop if mutation of cancer cells affects the expression of the target receptors. The receptors may be down-regulated resulting in reduced targetability and subsequent reduced cellular uptake of the vectors, or conversely up-regulation of receptors could render the vector inefficient. Receptors may also be expressed in different isoforms, altering their recognition of the targeting moiety [107]. Moreover, heterogeneity of tumours may result in different levels of receptor expression within a single tumour [108].

Although ligand-targeted vectors have proven to be safe and efficacious in preclinical models, it has not yet been unambiguously proven that targeting ligands contribute to the efficacy of vectors, and it seems that targeting ligands do not cause localisation within the target tissue, but rather provide benefits in terms of internalisation to target cells and retention at the target site once the delivery system has arrived [109]. While this method of targeting may enhance non-viral gene delivery systems, it has not completely met expectations and other targeting strategies have been explored.

4.2. Targeting at the transcriptional level

In an attempt to overcome these problems with the targeting of proteins expressed by cancer cells, it has been suggested that targeting the upstream genetic causes of dysregulated genes may be more successful [110]. Regulation of gene expression at the transcriptional level for cancer gene therapy can occur in a cell-specific manner with a focus on tissue-specific and tumour-specific promoters, or alternatively the use of inducible promoters, which allow gene expression to be controlled exogenously by factors such as heat or radiation. The major drawback with tissue-specific promoters, however, is that toxic gene expression occurs in all cells in the tissue, both healthy and cancerous, which limits use of this method to tissues that are not critical to the survival of the patient such as thyroid or prostate [111]. Use of inducible promoters to drive transgene expression requires the activation by exogenous factors, but the tumour specificity that this strategy affords may be useful in supplementing the potency of other therapies, such as the use of a radiation-inducible promoter for enhancement of iNOS transgene expression [112]; this dual approach to therapy can limit toxic effects in normal cells. However, for simplicity, we will focus solely on tumour-specific promoters.

The complex interplay of various factors involved in gene expression is often altered in cancer cells, and through exploiting this genetic signature of cancer, reduced off target effects and toxicity should result. Certain genes are upregulated in cancer through the over activation of transcription factors, which activate the upstream promoter of these genes. This can then be exploited to give tumour-specific targeting by using promoters that are activated by transcription factors known to be overexpressed in cancer cells to drive expression of the transgene in tumour cells only. Tumour-specific promoters are sub-categorized as follows: cancer specific promoters, tumour-type specific promoters, tumour microenvironment-related promoters, and tumour vasculature-related promoters, and are extensively reviewed by [113] and [114].

4.2.1. Cancer-specific promoters

The identification of genes that are expressed in cancer cells only may lead to targeting of cancer gene therapy in a broad sense regardless of cancer type. One such example is telomerase, involved in telomere maintenance, which is considered crucial in the progression and immortalisation of cancer cells and is expressed in the vast majority of cancers [115]. Telomerase expression is regulated by the human telomerase reverse transcriptase subunit promoter (hTERTp), which was recently used by Xie et al. in a non-viral delivery system. The hTERTp promoter was used to drive expression of a transgene amplification vector VISA (VP16-GAL4-WPRE integrated systemic amplifier) to target a phosphoprotein that is enriched in astrocytes (PEA-15) in advanced breast tumours. PEA-15 is known to affect signal-regulated kinase (ERK) in the cytoplasm, thereby inhibiting cell proliferation and inducing apoptosis [116]. Transgene expression was found to be highly specific, inducing cancer-cell killing in breast cancer cell lines (T47D, MCF-7, MDA-MB-231, MDA-MB-468, MDA-MB-361, MDA-MB-453, BT474, 4T1, SKBR-3) in vitro without affecting normal mammary epithelial cells (184A1 and MCF-10A). Furthermore, an in vivo study in a MDA-MB-231 xenograft mouse model demonstrated that the expression of PEA-15 driven by the hTERTp driven VISA vector prolonged mouse survival more effectively than PEA-15 driven by cytomegalovirus (CMV) promoter whilst showing no acute toxicities. The authors demonstrated that the use of the hTERT promoter achieved targeting and selective cell kill in triple negative MDA-MB-231 breast cancer cells, a selectivity that was lacking when transgene expression was promoted by the CMV promoter [116].

Survivin is a protein that functions in the inhibition of apoptosis, therefore, its overexpression in cancer cells can facilitate uninhibited growth. It is known to be upregulated in cancer cells and expression is controlled by various transcription factors including nuclear factor kappa B (NF-kB), Runx2 and the Ras family that bind to the survivin promoter, triggering expression [117, 118]. The survivin promoter (pSURV) has therefore been incorporated into gene delivery systems to drive transgene expression preferentially in cancer cells. Qu et al. used pSURV to drive the expression of the herpes simplex virus thymidine kinase (HSVtk) gene for suicide gene therapy. The authors used pSURV/GFP to demonstrate that gene expression occurred in HepG2 hepatocellular carcinoma cells, while no gene expression was observed in LO2 normal human liver cells. Apoptotic rates of up to 55% were achieved in HepG2 cells with pSURV/HSVtk demonstrating the possibility of this system for suicide gene therapy. However, further in vivo studies need to be carried out to properly assess the targeting ability of this system [119].

4.2.2. *Tumour-type specific promoters*

Many different types of cancer overexpress various genes, which are characteristic of that tumour type, and the promoters responsible for this expression can then be exploited for tumour-type specific targeting. Osteocalcin is a protein normally found in the bone matrix but has been found to be elevated in cancers such as ovarian and prostate cancer and is associated with the progression and formation of bone metastases; McCarthy's group used the human osteocalcin promoter (hOC) for tumour-limited gene expression. It has been shown that hOC has strong promoter activity in cancer cells, with transcription factors such as Runx2 involved in gene upregulation [120, 121]. In this case, hOC was used to drive the expression of inducible nitric oxide synthase expression in PC-3 and DU145 prostate cancer cells. The authors demonstrated significant delay in tumour growth with no toxic side effects in vivo, highlighting the potential for hOC to target prostate cancer tumours [122]. The advantage of using this tumour-type specific promoter is that it may facilitate the targeting of the primary tumour, as well as disseminated metastatic lesions that are often the most aggressive and hardest to treat forms of cancer. Figure 2 represents the targeting strategy of a tumour-type specific promoter that is activated in cancerous cells but not in normal cells.

Figure 2 summarises active internalisation of gene delivery vector and initiation of transgene expression in a non-transformed and a transformed cell. Gene delivery vectors are commonly functionalised using an antibody that targets HER-2 [123], while the human osteocalcin promoter has been employed to drive inducible nitric oxide synthase gene expression in prostate and breast cancer cells [122].

4.2.3. *Tumour microenvironment-related promoters*

The tumour microenvironment provides a unique environment that provides ideal conditions for growth and progression of tumours. Hypoxic conditions are often associated with chemo- and radio-resistance in tumours, and hypoxia is thought to be a key element for the cancer stem cell niche [124]. Various genes have been identified to be upregulated in the hypoxic environment with hypoxia response elements (HREs) working in concert with transcription factors, such as HIF-1, to activate transcription in response to hypoxia. Fujioka et al. reported

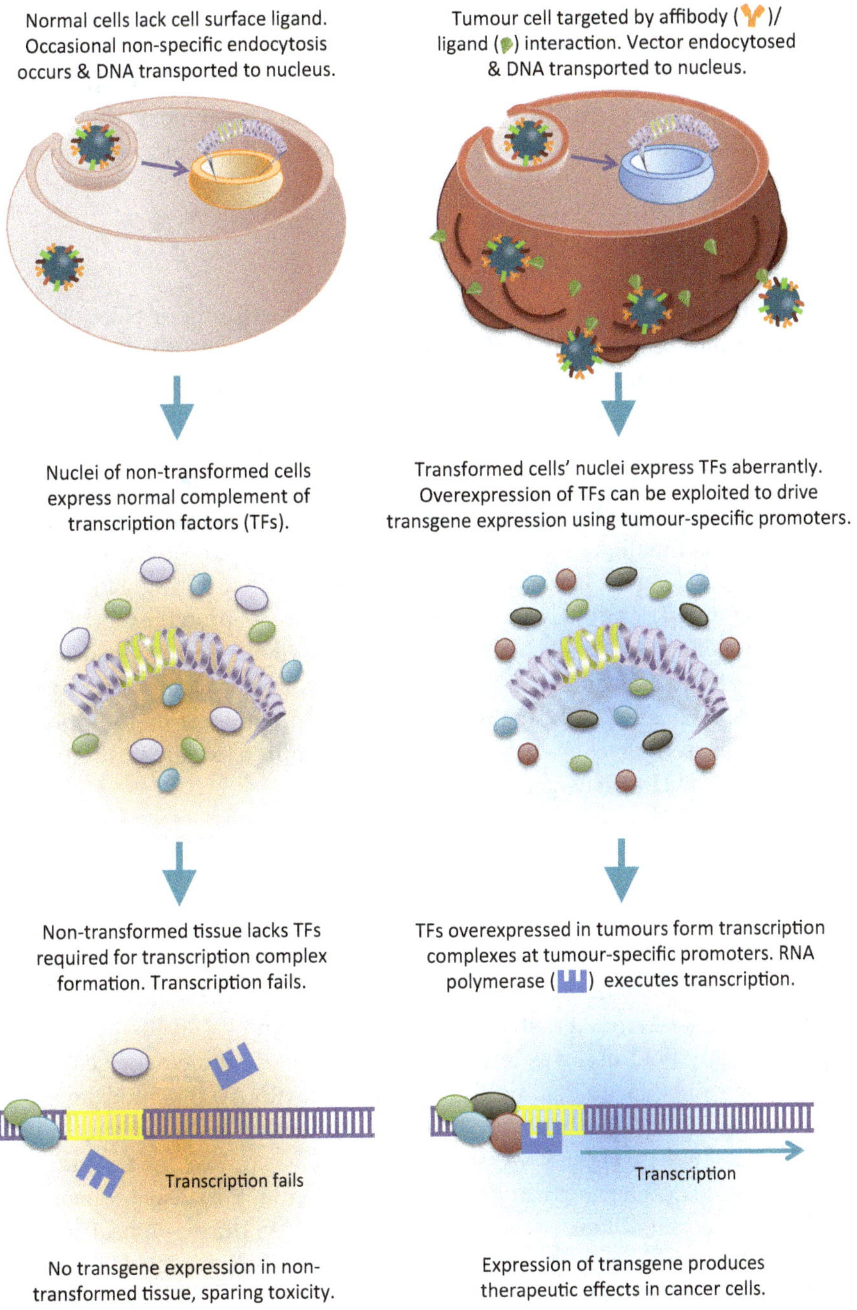

Figure 2. Targeted therapeutic transgene expression using affibodies and a tumour-specific promoter.

the construction of a vector combining a hypoxia response promoter with the CMV promoter (HRE-CMV) that resulted in a 2-fold increase in apoptotic gene expression compared to expression driven by CMV alone. In vivo, BCL-2 shRNA activity driven by the HRE-CMV promoter in hypoxic colon 26 tumours resulted in tumour volume reduction that was significantly greater than when bcl-2 shRNA was driven by CMV alone [125]. Although this study demonstrates the action of the HRE promoter for treatment in hypoxic tumours, the authors used intra-tumoural injections to deliver the vector, which does not give an indication of the tumour targeting specificity of this strategy.

4.2.4. Tumour vasculature-related promoters

The ability of tumours to trigger angiogenesis for increased tumour blood supply has been associated with more aggressive tumours, metastases, and poor prognosis. Identification of the genes involved in this process has led to the use of promoters that can be exploited for targeting. One such example is VEGF, which has been shown to have a major role in tumour angiogenesis by activating tyrosine kinase receptors VEGFR1 (Flt-1) and VEGFR2 (kinase insert receptor (KDR) in humans/Flk-1 in mice). KDR was found to be overexpressed in activated endothelial cells of newly formed vessels and strongly associated with invasion and metastasis in human malignant diseases [126]. Wang et al used the KDR promoter to drive thymidine kinase (TK) gene expression, which activated the prodrug ganciclovir (GCV) for suicide gene therapy. The authors demonstrated that the KDR promoter and TK/GCV showed a targeted killing effect on transfected human umbilical vein endothelial cells (HUVEC). Cells transfected with KDR-TK were 2- to 5-fold more sensitive to GCV compared to non-transfected HUVEC and HepG2 cells [127]. Again, however, confirmation of these impressive in vitro results in an in vivo setting using systemic delivery is required to validate tumour targetability and efficacy of the suicide gene/prodrug system.

5. RNA interference

Most of the strategies of cancer gene therapy discussed so far have involved introduction of therapeutic transgenes. An alternative strategy that is gaining considerable attention in the cancer gene therapy field involves inhibiting expression of problematic genes. Inhibition of gene expression can be facilitated by RNA interference (RNAi) that binds to mRNA. RNAi, discovered by Fire and Mello in 1998 [128], can be defined as a mechanism of gene-silencing produced by small RNAs. These RNAs include endogenous miRNA and exogenous siRNA or shRNA and their gene silencing activity is highly dependent on gene sequence [129]. These small RNAs then recruit cellular proteins, such as the RNA-induced silencing complex (RISC), to elicit their effect either through degradation of the mRNA or blocking the translation of mRNA [130, 131]. RNAi interference is therefore a highly attractive approach to cancer gene therapy and is currently a major research focus.

5.1. siRNA and shRNA

siRNA is a short (usually 21-bp) double-stranded RNA with phosphorylated 5′ ends and hydroxylated 3′ ends with two overhanging nucleotides. siRNA exerts its effect by directly incorporating into RISC, where its guide-strand binds to and cleaves the complementary mRNA with a perfect match. The cleaved mRNA is subsequently released and the siRNA guide-strand-bound RISC is free to bind to another mRNA and start a new round of cleavage [132]. However, the short half-life of siRNA has resulted in production of shRNA, which has been developed as an alternative RNA molecule. Transcription of shRNA occurs in the nucleus from an expression vector that bears a short double-stranded DNA sequence with a hairpin loop. This shRNA transcript is then processed by RNase enzymes and incorporated into RISC in the cytoplasm [133].

The use of siRNA and shRNA to silence unfavourable genes that are overexpressed in cancer has gained much attention. Multidrug resistance (MDR) genes, responsible for resistance to chemotherapeutics have been problematic in the treatment of cancer and associated with poor prognosis. By silencing these genes using siRNA, it has been possible to improve response to conventional treatments. For example, Chen et al. used siRNA to silence the MDR1 gene in doxorubicin resistant MCF-7 breast cancer cells, which resulted in 85–90% reduction in MDR1 gene expression and subsequently sensitisation of 70% of cells to doxorubicin [134]. Another approach is to target and silence pro-angiogenic genes such as the Notch pathway. Yang et al. used a non-viral delivery system to deliver siRNA for silencing the Notch-1 gene in breast cancer and found that transfected MDA-MB-231 cells exhibited significantly decreased expression of Notch-1, inhibited cell proliferation, and increased cell apoptosis [135]. One advantage of using siRNA to down-regulate overexpressed proteins is that non-specific delivery is often less toxic than the delivery of plasmid DNA that encodes genes such as IL-2 and TNF-alpha. However, to limit any toxicity that does exist, many groups have added targeting ligands to the delivery systems to increase tumour specificity [136].

5.2. MicroRNA

MicroRNAs (miRNA) are highly conserved short non-coding RNAs that negatively regulate a wide range of physiological processes at the post-transcriptional level including apoptosis, proliferation, and migration [137]. Initially, miRNA is transcribed in the nucleus as a primary transcript (pri-miRNA), which is processed to give a two-nucleotide overhang at its 3′ and is termed a pre-miRNA. Pre-miRNA is subsequently exported to the cytoplasm where it is further cleaved and mature miRNA is loaded into RISC to elicit its effect [138]. miRNAs can be either oncogenic or tumour suppressive in nature and as a result, may be overexpressed (e.g., miR-132, miR-20, and miR-17-92 family) or underexpressed (e.g., miR-34a and miR-126) in cancer cells making them targets for cancer gene therapy. A vast amount of information has been obtained in recent years on many different miRNAs and their role in cancer and with cancer stem cells, and by characterising their function, it may be possible to exploit them in cancer gene therapy [139, 140].

A single miRNA may have several varied targets to which it could bind and bring about gene silencing. miRNA-34a, known to be down-regulated in various cancers, has been shown to be a potent tumour suppressor that has various targets including the Notch pathway, BCL-2, survivin, c-Myc, and c-Met transcription factors [141]. Hu et al. demonstrated the value of miR-34a-mediated tumour suppression with the in vivo systemic administration of a non-viral miR-34a delivery system. Nanoparticles were used to deliver the miR-34a using a tumour-targeting and penetrating bifunctional CC9 peptide (CRGDKGPDC) conjugated to β-cyclodextrin-polyethylenimine in a PANC-1 pancreatic cancer xenograft model; the miR-34a-loaded particles significantly inhibited tumour growth and induced cancer cell apoptosis [142]. Conversely, the inhibition of some miRNAs using complementary miRNA antagonist oligonucleotides (anti-miRNAs) can be an attractive gene therapy strategy to neutralise miRNA function. miR-132 acts as an angiogenic switch at the endothelium, inducing tumour neovascularization. Anand et al. reported the systemic administration of anti-miR-132 containing liposomes incorporating an integrin $\alpha v\beta 3$-targeting cyclic RGD peptide to inhibit angiogenesis [143]. The authors demonstrated that anti-miR-132 blocked the action of mi-132 on angiogenesis induced by a VEGF-secreting ID-8 ovarian carcinoma in mice, and significantly reduced tumour burden and angiogenesis in an MDA-MB 231 xenograft model of human breast carcinoma when compared to treatment with scrambled miR-132. There is a huge potential of miRNA therapeutics for cancer. However, miRNA gene therapy is still in its infancy and more research is required to elucidate the exact pathways and possible targets available.

The active targeting of cancer gene therapy is hugely important for efficiency and safety. Yet despite the plethora of characteristics that can be targeted, active targeting remains elusive in many non-viral gene delivery systems. A move towards a combination of targeting strategies in one delivery system may hold promise for improved specificity using non-viral vectors.

6. The future: Molecular engineering

Strategies involving PEGylation and the use of targeting ligands have shown great promise for cancer gene therapy in overcoming certain hurdles, but in order to maximise the efficiency of non-viral delivery, vectors must have the ability to overcome all the barriers to gene delivery. Recent research in the field has focused on the development of vectors for nucleic acid delivery that efficiently evade the barriers to gene delivery highlighted above, and provoke adequate transgene expression in vivo following systemic delivery.

6.1. Multifunctional Envelope-type Nano Devices (MENDs)

Harashima et al. presented a multifunctional envelope-type nano device (MEND) that was produced on the concept of 'programmed packaging' with a rational design to overcome barriers to delivery and assembly into nano-sized vectors. Generally, a MEND comprises a DNA core condensed using a cationic polymer such as poly-L-lysine (PLL), which is wrapped in a separate lipid envelope fortified with various functional attachments including targeting ligands, PEG, and groups facilitating cellular uptake and endosomal escape [144]. One of the first MEND systems described consisted of a PLL DNA condensing core, surrounded by a lipid envelope, and functionalised with stearylated octaarginine (R8) to promote cellular uptake to deliver anti-luciferase siRNA [145]. The gene silencing effect of the MEND was found to be comparable to that of the transfection reagent Lipofectamine 2000, without any detectable cytotoxicity and further optimisation of this system to include protamine as the DNA condensing agent resulted in a 70% silencing effect in transfected COS7 fibroblast cells.

The nature of the MEND system renders it relatively easy to modify in order to optimise transfection efficiency. When the lipid component of egg phosphatidylcholine (EPC) and cholesterol were replaced with the fusogenic lipids DOPE and cholesteryl hemisuccinate (CHEMS), respectively, an overall 2-fold improvement was observed due to the optimisation of the lipid component [146]. Furthermore, functionalization of MEND with octa-arginine R8 (R8-MEND) for enhanced cellular uptake resulted in a transfection efficiency of more than 80% in HeLa cells [147]. The addition of pH-sensitive endosomal escape motifs to MEND, such as INF7 derived from the HA2 protein of the influenza virus envelope, has also proven beneficial, and the combination of INF7 with R8 resulted in the production of R8/INF7/MEND. In vivo administration of R8/INF7/MEND to ICF mice produced luciferase expression 240-fold higher in liver and 115-fold higher in spleen than that of R8-MEND alone, demonstrating the importance of optimising functionality of the MEND system [148].

In a similar approach, the pH-sensitive fusogenic peptide GALA was incorporated into a MEND system as an endosomal escape enhancer in a system that comprised of R8 and an MMP-cleavable PEG functionality. Increased gene silencing effect was observed for delivery of anti-luciferase siRNA in HeLa-luc cells in vitro when compared to an unmodified MEND [149]. In addition to this, an in vivo study using a HT1080-luc xenografted model demonstrated that the cleavable PEGylated GALA/R8/MEND exhibited efficient luciferase gene knockdown in comparison to PEG-MEND, which was unable to cause any gene knockdown.

Incorporation of targeting motifs has also proved useful in MEND systems. The addition of RGD peptide to MEND, which is a targeting ligand for integrins, resulted in significant tumour growth delay in OS-RC-2 human renal carcinoma bearing mice when RGD-MEND was used to deliver anti-VEGF siRNA in vivo [150]. GALA peptide was also used as a targeting ligand for sialic acid-terminated sugar chains on pulmonary endothelium as reported by Kusumoto et al. [151]. Following intravenous administration of GALA-MEND delivering antiCD31 siRNA in vivo, approximately 50% inhibition of lung metastasis in a Murine melanoma B16-F10 mouse model was observed when compared with control groups. Examples of MENDs and the various functionalities that have been employed are detailed in Table 1.

Name	Condensing material and nucleic acid cargo	Lipid Envelop	Endosomolytic component	Nuclear localisation component	Other functional groups	Activity
R8/INF7-MEND	Protamine (plasmid DNA for luciferase transgene expression)	Egg phosphatidylcholine (EPC), cholesterol (Chol), 1,2-dioleoyl-sn-glycero-3-phosphocholine	INF7 peptide derived from N-terminal domain of the HA2 protein influenza virus envelope	Protamine	-	Luciferase transgene expression levels 240-fold higher in liver and 115-fold higher in spleen

Name	Condensing material and nucleic acid cargo	Lipid Envelop	Endosomolytic component	Nuclear localisation component	Other functional groups	Activity
		(DOPC), and dioleoylphosphatidyl ethanolamine (DOPE)				than that of the R8-MEND *in vivo* [148].
GALA/ PPD-MEND	Stearylated octahistidine (STR-H8) (anti-luciferase siRNA condensation)	DOPE, 1,2-dioleoyl-3-trimethylammonium-propane(DOTAP), Chol	pH-responsive fusogenic GALA peptide derived from HA2	N/A	(MMP-cleavable PEG)	Intratumoural injection of PPD/ GALA- MEND HT1080-luc into human fibrosarcoma mouse xenografts resulted in more efficient luciferase gene silencing compared with unmodified MENDs *in vivo* [149].
RGD-MEND	Protamine (anti VEGF siRNA)	YSK05 (pH dependent cationic lipid), 1-Palmitoyl-2-oleoyl-sn-glycero-3-phosphoethanolamine (POPE), Chol	YSK05 (YSK05 consists of two linoleyl fatty acid chains and a tertiary amino group, which are responsible for pH-responsive fusiogenicity in endosomes)	N/A	Cyclo (RGADPK) (cRGD) peptide ligand for $\alpha V\beta 3$ integrin PEG	Significant tumour growth delay was observed in OS-RC-2 human renal carcinoma bearing mice when RGD-MEND was used to deliver anti-VEGF siRNA *in vivo* [150].
GALA-MEND	Polyethylenimine (PEI) (anti-CD31 siRNA)	EPC, Chol	GALA peptide	N/A	GALA peptide (ligand for sialic acid-terminated sugar chains on pulmonary endothelium) PEG	Murine melanoma B16-F10 lung metastasis significantly inhibited by approx. 50% compared with control groups

Name	Condensing material and nucleic acid cargo	Lipid Envelop	Endosomolytic component	Nuclear localisation component	Other functional groups	Activity
						following intravenous administration of GALA-MEND delivering anti-CD31 siRNA *in vivo* [151].

Table 1. MEND non-viral delivery systems, their components and applications to gene therapy

The potential of controlled intracellular delivery using the MEND system was also highlighted by Toriyabe et al. who used stearylated-octahistidne (STR-H8) as a pH-responsive component to facilitate the efficient release of siRNA in the cytoplasm [152]. STR-H8 was used to complex anti-luciferase siRNA and delivered using a conventional R8/GALA functionalised MEND. The authors demonstrated that luciferase gene knockdown was significantly higher in HeLa-GL3 cells treated with the STR-H8 MEND than with a MEND containing stearylated octaarginine (STR-R8) to condense the siRNA. This may be explained by more efficient de-condensation and release of siRNA from STR-H8 in the cytoplasm, which was confirmed by a RiboGreen assay showing siRNA release efficiency from STR-H8 was much higher than siRNA release from STR-R8 at pH7.4 (intracellular pH). It is clear, therefore, that PEGylation and unpackaging of DNA are important considerations in the development of MEND systems, and with further optimisation and characterisation, MENDs have great promise as effective non-viral gene delivery agents.

6.2. Bio-inspired systems

Viral vectors still remain the most efficient gene therapy delivery vehicles with no non-viral delivery system producing comparable gene delivery potencies. Viruses have evolved naturally to infect and transfer their genetic material into host cells [153]. Understanding the various mechanisms by which viruses elicit delivery of genetic material has led to exploitation of viral peptide motifs by gene therapists and molecular engineers [154]. Functional peptide motifs derived from viruses have been engineered and incorporated into a wide range of bio-inspired non-viral delivery systems with great success, thereby benefiting from the viruses' expertise, while circumventing immunogenicity and safety concerns associated with viruses [35, 154]. Peptides are an attractive alternative to polymer and lipid-based non-viral vectors as they are less toxic, easily synthesised, and only weakly activate the complement system therefore enhancing safety [155]. The main peptides of interest are generally classified according to their function, i.e., DNA condensing peptides, cell penetrating peptides, endosomolytic peptides, and nuclear location sequences [156].

6.3. DNA-condensing peptides

Cationic peptides containing lysine or arginine residues interact electrostatically with the negatively charged phosphate backbone of DNA, condensing and packaging DNA into complexes with a net positive charge, which protects DNA from degradation and allows interaction with cell membranes [157]. Examples include histones, including H2A, which are natural basic proteins [158], μ (mu) peptide derived from adenovirus [159], and TAT peptide from HIV-1 [160]. Condensing peptides alone have a limited role because they cannot overcome many of the barriers to gene delivery; although some peptides, such as TAT, have cell penetrating properties, which makes them more attractive options in vector development [161]. However, the unpredictable nature of interactions between peptides and nucleic acids remains an issue and further research is needed for optimisation of vectors [157].

6.4. Cell Penetrating Peptides (CPPs)

Cell penetrating peptides (CPPs) are generally short peptides that have the ability to cross the cell membrane via various mechanisms including endocytic pathways or through direct translocation, without the need for receptors or other carriers [162]. Such peptides have been shown to deliver various cargoes to a range of cell types; peptide sequences are easily modifiable to optimise properties such as cargo transport or subcellular targeting [163]. Natural peptides exhibiting this penetrating activity include Penetratin (RQIKIYFQNRRMKWKK), derived from the third helix of the homeodomain of Antennapedia [164], and TAT (GRKKRRQRRR) derived from HIV-1 [41]. Both have regions of basic amino acids and an alpha-helical conformation with the ability to translocate a cargo across cell membranes, which highlights the potential application of CPPs in gene therapy. Novel CPPs have since been derived and include peptides with a wide range of structures and characteristics; however, generally CPPs are cationic/basic, amphipathic, or hydrophobic in nature [156].

Amphipathic peptides are composed of both hydrophobic and hydrophilic domains in primary or secondary conformation. The secondary structure produces an alpha-helical structure with the hydrophobic residues such as leucine, glycine, or tryptophan localised on one face of the helix and the hydrophilic residues such as lysine, arginine, or histidine localised on the other. This amphipathic structure has been shown to be essential for passage across the cell membranes [165]. Structural changes of amphipathic peptides contribute to their binding affinity for cell membranes, and insertion of hydrophobic portions of the peptide into the membrane are important for interaction with the lipid membrane and subsequent uptake [54]. However, although amphipathic peptides have shown much promise, not all CPPs rely on this amphipathic nature for internalisation. For example, in the case of Penetratin, it is the positive charges rather than the helical structure that is responsible for cell penetration [166]. Therefore, increasingly, attention has been paid to developing simple linear peptides rich in cationic amino acids such as arginine. Cationic CPPs are composed mainly of basic amino acid residues including arginine, lysine, and histidine [167] and electrostatically bind to various anionic species present on the extracellular surface of the cell membranes, e.g., lipid head groups or proteoglycans such as heparin sulphate [168].

It has been reported that peptides containing arginine residues have stronger cell penetrating ability than peptides comprising lysine and histidine, with the guanidine moiety possessed by arginine being held as crucial for cell entry [169]. As a result, arginine-rich peptides have been extensively researched in order to characterise their activity [170–172]. The discovery that the basic portion of TAT responsible for the cell penetrating activity is rich in arginine residues prompted much research into the characterisation of mechanisms involved in the cellular entry of arginine-rich peptides [41]. It has been elucidated that the exact peptide sequence involved is not as crucial as the length of sequence and number of arginine residues incorporated, with between 6 and 15 arginine residues required for optimum activity [54]. In a study carried out by Wender et al., it was observed that truncated versions of TAT with arginine residues replaced with alanine exhibited reduced cellular uptake, but a 9-mer oligoarginine peptide (R9) was 20-fold more efficient than TAT [173]. Further to this, Mitchell et al. used peptides composed of multiple arginine residues termed oligoarginines, labelled with fluorescein to demonstrate that negligible cell uptake was exhibited with fewer than 6 arginine residues, but that when peptides of 7 arginines or more were tested, fluorescence increased as a function of peptide length up to 15 arginine residues, beyond which no increase in fluorescence was observed. Peptides containing more than 15 arginine residues can still penetrate cells, although this happens at a reduced efficiency and with toxicity to cells [169].

CPPs have the ability to enter any cell they come in contact with and this lack of specificity is problematic for gene therapy [174]. The use of 'smart' delivery vectors with 'activatable' CPPs (ACPs) has been explored, where a CPP is connected to a neutralising polyanion via a cleavable linker, reducing the overall charge and non-specific electrostatic uptake by cells. Enzymes produced in cancerous cells, such as MMPs, can then cleave the linker and allow the CPP to enter cancer cells [175]. For example, Mei et al. reported an ACP that includes a masking sequence of anionic E8 (sequence: EEEEEEEE) to shield the cationic nature of R8 [176]. The mask was linked to R8 by a MMP-2 sensitive linker; when the ACP nanoparticles were in the tumour environment, which overexpresses MMP-2, the mask was cleaved exposing R8 to tumour cells allowing tumour specific uptake. The authors used in vivo imaging to demonstrate this, while also showing lower ACP nanoparticle distribution in other tissues.

Another strategy for targeting and cell specificity has focused on the use of cell-penetrating-homing peptides (CPHPs) [97, 177] that combine targeting and cell penetration abilities. Kondo et al. described a CPHP known as RLW (peptide sequence: RLWMRWYSPRTRAYG) found through systematic selection from a random peptide library that had the ability to selectively target and penetrate A549 non-small cell lung cancer cells via an unknown mechanism thought to involve specific RLW ligand receptors on A549 cells [178]. Gao et al. demonstrated that when RLW was anchored onto poly(ethyleneglycol)-poly(ε-caprolactone) (PEG-PCL) nanoparticles loaded with infrared dye (DiR) cellular uptake was 2-fold higher in A549 cells than in umbilical vein endothelial cells in vitro [179]. Further to this, in vivo imaging showed the RLW nanoparticles targeted A549 xenografts specifically over U87 xenografts, with only low levels seen in normal organs in comparison to PEG-PCL nanoparticles functionalised with R8, which evoked DiR accumulation in all tissues. The specificity of CHCPs is a great asset; however, elucidation of the exact mechanism of how CHCPs work and a broader spectrum of activity may be more attractive so that a peptide may be used to treat more than one cancer type.

The cargo being carried by the vector must also be considered when designing a vector, as CPPs interact with various cargoes in different ways. For example, TAT mediates internalisation by at least two distinct pathways. Large cargoes, e.g., proteins, enter via caveolae endocytosis and macropinocytosis leading to endosomal entrapment, whereas small cargoes, e.g., peptides, enter slowly by endocytosis and rapidly by transduction by an unknown mechanism that gives direct access to the cytosol [42]. As endosomal entrapment is a major barrier to transfection, CPPs have been functionalised with endosomolytic peptides. Liou et al. described a fusion peptide that combines R9 for cell penetration and hemagglutinin-2 (HA2) for endosomal escape; the resulting vector was tagged with red fluorescent protein (RFP) for imaging purposes [180]. Significantly more RFP was detected in vitro when A549 human lung carcinoma cells were treated with the R9-HA2 peptide in comparison to R9 alone.

Problems with CPPs, such as humoral immune response induction, as seen in studies with Penetratin [181], and stability need to be addressed. Amino acids exist in different isoforms with variable susceptibility to degradation by proteases in serum. The L-isoform found in abundance in nature is sensitive to degradation, but the D-isoform is more resistant due to the altered stereochemistry that affects protease recognition. The use of the D-isoform of amino acids has therefore been suggested as a modification to render CPPs protease-resistant, enhancing stability [182]. However, further characterisation of the structure-activity relationship of individual CPPs is needed to allow the tailoring of specific CPPs to particular intracellular targets, optimising efficiency and reducing side effects [183].

6.5. Endosomolytic peptides

The harsh endosomal environment can lead to degradation of peptides and their cargo, as CPPs, such as TAT and oligoarginines, lack the ability to escape the endosome unaided, resulting in poor transfection efficiencies [184]. Histidine-rich peptides are usually endosomolytic in nature and can facilitate endosomal escape through the proton sponge where the protonation of imidazole groups in histidine-rich peptides facilitates buffering of the endosome causing endosomes to swell and burst, releasing their contents [185, 186]. Another mechanism employed by histidine-rich peptides is the 'flip-flop' effect, which may operate depending on the number of histidine residues or their arrangement in a peptide [187]. In a study conducted by Lo et al., the addition of 10 histidine residues to TAT increased luciferase transgene expression up to 7,000-fold in the human glioma cell line U251 in vitro [188]. Bafilomycin A1, a known inhibitor of the proton sponge effect for endosomal escape, in turn inhibited transfection significantly, supporting the idea that the activity of histidine as an endosomal escape motif could improve the transfection efficiency of TAT. However, in vivo administration of the TAT-histidine peptide/DNA complexes to deliver the luciferase reporter gene into the brain of rats showed 5-fold lower expression than was achieved using PEI 25 kDa/DNA complexes, suggesting more work needs to be done to ensure in vitro results translate to the in vivo setting. One example of a histidine-rich peptide that has shown great promise is H5WYG, derived from the HA2 subunit of haemaglutinin (HA) protein of the influenza virus. H5WYG causes endosomal escape through the proton sponge effect, when the histidine residues become protonated at around pH 6. H5WYG is unaffected by the presence of serum that gives it an added advantage of being suitable for in vivo gene delivery [189]. Asseline et al. reported a 2-fold increase in luciferase mRNA levels when H5WYG was added to an antisense oligonucleotide (2′-Ome RNA705) targeting aberrant splicing of luciferase pre-mRNA in HeLa pLuc705 cells [190].

Fusogenic peptides have also been of great importance in facilitating endosomal escape [191]. Pore formation may be mediated by cationic amphiphilic peptides that bind to the lipid bilayer of the endosomal membrane, causing internal stress or tension leading to pore formation. Fusogenic peptides are known to adopt an amphipathic α-helical structure when pH drops to around 5 within the endosome, causing interaction with the phospholipid membrane and endosomal disruption [156, 192]. This fusogenic activity also allows these peptides to interact with cell membranes and facilitate internalisation, giving some fusogenic peptides a dual function with ability to package nucleic acid to avoid degradation and be delivered into the cytoplasm of the cell. One such example is RALA (WEARLARALARALARHLARALARALRACEA), a 30 amino acid fusogenic peptide with a cationic nature [193]. It is composed of a hydrophilic arginine (R) region that facilitates condensation of anionic complexes, e.g., DNA; a hydrophobic leucine (L) region that interacts with lipid membranes; and an alanine (A)-rich region that gives the peptide amphipathicity. This structure allows RALA to maintain α-helical conformation at low pH, enabling endosomal escape. The design of RALA was informed by the understanding of two similar peptides, namely GALA (WEAALAEALAEALAEHLAEALAEALEALAA) and KALA (WEAKLAKALAKALAKHLAKALAKALKACEA), peptides that were in turn derived from the HA2 subunit of the influenza virus, with GALA being the first cell penetrating amphipathic peptide demonstrated to possess fusogenic activity [192]. However, GALA carries an overall negative charge and therefore cannot be used for delivery of DNA alone. KALA was derived by substituting the glutamic acid (E) in GALA with lysine (K); the resulting derivative was positively charged, and thereby more suitable for delivery of DNA. This E to K substitution resulted in improved interaction with negatively charged cell membranes and allowed condensation of negatively charged DNA cargoes [194]. RALA was derived by substituting lysine residues with arginine (R), which conferred a lower toxicity [172, 193].

6.6. Nuclear Localisation Sequences (NLSs)

Intracellular trafficking of nucleic acid cargo and entry into the nucleus is crucial for transgene expression. The use of nuclear localisation sequences (NLS) has proved beneficial in improving the efficiency of vectors. NLSs help traffic vectors towards the nucleus and facilitate entry through the nuclear envelope in association with the importin pathway [62]. Classical nuclear localisation signals, such as the NLSs from simian virus 40 (SV40), large tumour antigen (PKKKRKV), and Rev peptide (RRNRRRRWRERQRQ), consist of short stretches of basic amino acids [195]. Such NLSs have the ability to bind DNA in order to facilitate nuclear entry. Elder et al. used atomistic molecular dynamics to investigate the effect of peptide chemistry and sequence on DNA binding behaviour, focusing on the NLS from SV40 [196]. By analysing the conformational entropy and free energy of binding, the authors found that replacing arginine with lysine reduced binding strength by eliminating arginine–DNA interactions, but placing arginine in a less sterically hindered location has little effect on polycation–DNA binding strength. This strong binding ability of arginine is important for an NLS because nucleic acids need to be bound and protected from degradation by nucleases in the cytosol before reaching the nucleus.

Several other proteins derived from viruses are excellent at traversing the intracellular network and facilitating nuclear import [197]. The TAT, Rev, and Rex proteins of the retroviruses contain arginine-rich NLSs, which have the ability to shuttle to and from the nucleus. Herpes simplex virus (HSV) type 1 tegument proteins, known as VP13/14, are also arginine-rich and act in a similar way [198, 199]. The arginine-rich portion of these proteins is responsible for the nuclear import, with leucine-rich portions, known as nuclear export signals (NES), being responsible for the shuttling between the nucleus and cytoplasm. Arginine-rich NLSs have been shown to use importin β pathway with no involvement of importin α pathway [200]. Importin β is not only involved in nuclear import but is also a potential adaptor for movement along microtubules, which may enhance trafficking of arginine-rich peptides to the nucleus, as well as entry to the nucleus [201]. Identification of exact binding sites and utilisation of such mechanisms may be the key to improving transfection efficiencies for peptide delivery vectors.

Incorporation of such sequences has proven to be useful in vector design. Hatefi et al. demonstrated that the addition of Rev (RRNRRRRWRERQRQ) to their fusion peptide KALA-2H1-NLS-TP facilitated cargo delivery to the nucleus by utilising microtubules for nuclear localisation [186]. Non-classical NLSs, such as M9 from human mRNA binding protein hnRNP A1, have also shown promise for non-viral vector functionalisation [202]. These NLSs lack stretches of basic amino acids and do not enter the nucleus via the importin pathway. M9 binds to the transportin receptor that results in nuclear localisation and has shown the ability to transport the vector towards the nucleus by shuttling between the nucleus and cytoplasm [203–205]. These properties make M9 an attractive NLS for gene delivery [65]. A number of viruses are known to exploit host microtubule machinery to facilitate access to the nucleus [206], but little is known about the exact mechanisms and binding domains used by viruses, and further study is required to elucidate exact peptide sequences involved that may be incorporated into non-viral vectors for rational design to achieve enhanced transfection efficiencies [207]. For example, the motif sequence contained in the adenoviral capsid hexon (E3-14.7K peptide: VVMVGEKPITITQHSVETEG) was conjugated to plasmid DNA and promoted microtubule-mediated transport of the DNA, resulting in 2.5-fold increase in transfection efficiency in HeLa cells compared to plasmid DNA only [208]. Incorporation of this sequence into a non-viral vector may therefore improve transfection efficiency.

Problems have been encountered where binding of an NLS with DNA renders the NLS unable to bind to the importins that allow passage through the NPC. Using a basic NLS to condense and deliver DNA alone has not been successful because they do not bind DNA strongly enough and the complexes are generally broken down in the cytoplasm [209]. Covalent conjugation of an NLS to DNA has been problematic as this may render the NLS or the DNA non-functional, as demonstrated when covalent bonding of SV40 did not increase nuclear localisation of pDNA [68]. Various binding strategies have been used to improve this, as well as using condensing agents such as histones that also possess nuclear localisation properties [210], but generally, NLSs are used to supplement other delivery systems rather than as stand-alone vectors.

6.7. Designer Biomimetic Vectors (DBVs)

An exciting approach to the multifunctional vector has been the introduction of recombinant production of bio-inspired fused protein sequences, each coding for a discrete motif with an explicit barrier evasion function [211]. Termed designer biomimetic vectors, these vectors are rationally designed to incorporate several motifs with distinct functions, and could be a step towards the production of 'artificial viruses'. The previous strategies discussed involving different components of a multi-functional system being conjugated together by various attachments may not be ideal for production of gene delivery systems. Simple conjugation of certain peptides has also led to alteration in the function of the peptides [212], therefore conjugating all the desired components together may be problematic. Production of DBVs using recombinant DNA technology allows the fusion of discrete motifs in a relatively simple process that should not affect the functional operation of the motifs. This would circumvent any problems involved with complex conjugation reactions to attach different components and ultimately could be more cost effective and reproducible in a large scale industrial setting. The production process involves introduction of plasmids, which have been engineered to contain the desired motifs for the protein, into competent bacterial cells. The bacteria then utilise the plasmid to produce the fusion proteins, which are subsequently extracted and purified. The use of this recombinant DNA technology allows the specific design of the vector at the molecular level, which can be tailored to enhance and optimise gene delivery [213]. Examples of multi-functional recombinant vectors are detailed in Table 2.

Name	Nucleic acid condensation	Endosomolytic component	Nuclear localisation	Targeting motif	Other	Activity
Tetra-H2A(TH)	Four tandem repeats of human histone H2A peptide (TH)	GALA peptide	N/A (anti-luciferase siRNA delivery)	Anisamide (AA) to target cancer cells that overexpress sigma receptor	PEGylated, cathepsin D cleavage sites in the TH for digestion in endosome compartment, DOTAP and Chol Lipid envelope surrounding TH	TH produced a higher silencing efficiency in HT60-luc cells *in vitro* and *in vivo* than the NPs assembled with protamine as the nucleic acid condensing agent [218].
KALA-2H1-NLS-TP	Two repeating units of histone H1 (2H1)	KALA peptide	NLS from Rev protein of HIV virus	ZR-75-1 targeting peptide (RVCFLWQ DGRCVF)	-	Transfection efficiency of luciferase comparable to PEI 25 kDa with preferential targeting to ZR-75-1

Name	Nucleic acid condensation	Endosomolytic component	Nuclear localisation	Targeting motif	Other	Activity
						breast cancer cells [186].
FP–(DCE)$_n$–NLS–CS–TM FP– (DCE)*n*–CS–TM	Arginine-histidine (RH) with general structure (RRXRRXHHXHHX)n	Arginine-histidine (RH)	M9 (included in FP–(DCE)$_n$–NLS–CS–TM for DNA delivery; absent in FP–(DCE)*n*–CS–TM for siRNA delivery)	HER2 targeting affibody to target SKOV-3	-	Significant cell death observed in SKOV-3 cells treated in vitro with FDT/BCL2-siRNA in combination with FDNT/pSR39 plus GCV [216,217].
DBV	μ peptide derived from adenovirus	H5WYG	Rev	HER2 affibody	Targeting moiety attached via cathepsin substrate (CS) for cleavage in the endosome	DBV-mediated iNOS gene delivery resulted in a maximum of 62% cell killing and less than 20% clonogenicity in ZR-75-1 breast cancer cells *in vitro* [215].

Table 2. Recombinant multifunctional non-viral delivery systems, their components, and application in gene therapy

Recently the Gandehari and Hatefi groups have reported the design and development of recombinant fusion proteins for targeted gene delivery [34, 211]. The DBVs are produced by fusing the desired motif sequences, usually composed of a DNA condensing motif (DCM), endosomal disruption motif (EDM) and nuclear localisation motif (NLS) [34, 214]. Sadeghian et al. described a fusion protein comprised of two repeats of histone H1 for DNA condensation, H5WYG pH responsive fusogenic peptide for endosomal escape and the simian virus 40 (SV40) large T-antigen NLS for a nuclear localization [211]. The fusion peptide was complexed with the pGL3 plasmid for luciferase expression to form nanoparticles; the nanoparticles transfected Chinese hamster ovary (CHO) cells efficiently in vitro. However, this system lacked a targeting motif that is highly desirable in the design of gene delivery system.

Soltani et al. recently described a delivery system known as KALA-2H1-NLS-TP, which is composed of two repeating units of histone H1 (2H1) to efficiently condense DNA into nano-sized particles, a synthetic pH-dependent endosome disrupting motif (KALA) to promote escape from endosomes, a cyclic targeting peptide (TP) selected from a phage display library to target antigens on the surface of ZR-75-1 breast cancer cells, and an NLS from the Rev protein of HIV to facilitate translocation of DNA towards the cell nucleus [186]. The authors demonstrated that the recombinant vector had a high rate of gene transfection efficiency compared to vectors that lacked one or more functional motifs, and targeted the ZR-75-1 cells. Besides the ability to target, the developed multifunctional vector was able to disrupt endosomal membranes, reach the nucleus by utilizing microtubules, and transfect efficiently while showing no detectable toxicity. McCarthy et al. presented similar results using a DBV for the delivery of iNOS gene therapy targeted to breast cancer [215].

Canine et al. described a biopolymer termed FP–(DCE)$_n$–NLS–CS–TM that contains repeating units of arginine and histidine to condense pDNA and lyse endosome membranes (DCE), a HER-2 targeting affibody to target cancer cells (TM), a pH responsive fusogenic peptide (FP) H5WYG to destabilize endosome membranes and enhance endosomolytic activity of histidine residues, and a nuclear localization signal (NLS) M9 to enhance translocation of pDNA towards the cell nucleus. A cathepsin D enzyme substrate (CS) was also engineered in between targeting motif and NLS to facilitate dissociation of the targeting motif from the biopolymer inside late endosomes where cathepsin D is abundant [216]. The authors demonstrated the functioning of each motif in the polymer resulting in successful transfection of SKOV-3 and GFP transgene expression.

The production of these recombinant vectors renders it relatively easy to change their characteristics by sequence modification. Canine et al. further demonstrated that by modifying the sequence of the biopolymer FP–(DCE)$_n$–NLS–CS–TM, it was possible to fine tune the vector for either delivery of plasmid DNA to the nucleus or delivery of siRNA to the cytoplasm [217]. It was reported that inclusion of the M9 NLS rendered the biopolymer (FP–(DCE)$_n$–NLS–CS–TM) suitable for delivery of plasmid DNA to the nucleus but not for delivery of siRNA. However, exclusion of the NLS from the biopolymer (FP– (DCE)*n*–CS–TM) rendered it more suitable for delivery of siRNA to the cytoplasm but not for nuclear delivery of plasmid DNA in SKOV-3 human ovarian cancer cells. This study demonstrates the possibility of not only targeting specific cells for gene delivery, but also the ability to target intracellular compartments depending on the nature of the therapeutic to be delivered.

Wang et al. presented a novel recombinant protein tetra-H2A (TH) derived from histone H2A that was developed to replace protamine as a conditionally reversible, nucleic acid condensing agent. The recombinant protein comprised of four tandem repeats of human histone H2A peptide, interspersed with cathepsin D cleavage sites and a pH-responsive fusogenic peptide GALA to facilitate the endosome escape of the cargo. The recombinant protein, tetra-H2A (TH), was able to condense siRNA into a stable complex that was in turn coated in a cationic lipid with a high degree of PEGylation, forming Lipid-tetra-H2A-Hyaluronic acid (LHH) nanoparticles [218]. This design was developed in order to mimic lipid-enveloped viruses to replicate the transfection abilities of viruses in vivo. The histone-containing polymer demonstrated an enhanced intracellular release of the cargo and an increased anti-luciferase siRNA silencing efficiency in vitro compared with the protamine-containing polymer in H460-luc human lung carcinoma cells. Furthermore, in vivo gene silencing by tumour-targeted anti-luciferase siRNA was evaluated in H460-luc xenograft-bearing mice with the histone-containing nanoparticles loaded with anti-luciferase siRNA resulting in ~66% silencing of luciferase expression, significantly higher than that of the protamine-mediated knockdown (34%). This study demonstrates the importance of efficient release of the genetic payload for efficient gene therapy; through optimisation of each component of the multifunctional vector, it may be possible to maximise transfection efficiency. However, these vectors are still in the early stage of development and much research is needed. Many of these findings serve only to confirm the theory behind the design of the vector, and further in vivo work with therapeutic transgenes is ultimately required.

7. Conclusion

There is a huge potential for cancer gene therapy, which, in some respect, has yet to be realised. However, the lack of gene therapy products making it onto the market is disappointing when one considers the number of research groups involved and clinical trials underway. It seems that until a suitable delivery system for cancer gene therapy becomes available, the potential of this field will never be reached. The difficulty in this is the number of hurdles to overcome and the extremely high standards of safety and efficiency expected by regulatory authorities. Nevertheless, the development of multifunctional systems and a move towards the creation of artificial viruses may finally help cancer gene therapy to progress to a viable and successful cancer treatment.

Author details

Emma M. McErlean, Cian M. McCrudden and Helen O. McCarthy*

*Address all correspondence to: h.mccarthy@qub.ac.uk

School of Pharmacy, Queen's University Belfast, UK

References

[1] Cancer Research UK. Cancer survival statistics [Internet]. Available from: http://www.cancerresearchuk.org/cancer-info/cancer.

[2] Cancer Research UK. Breast cancer screening [Internet]. [cited 2015 Feb 9]. Available from: http://www.cancerresearchuk.org/about-cancer/type/breast-cancer/about/screening/who-is-screened-for-breast-cancer.

[3] NHS Choices. Cancer of the prostate [Internet]. [cited 2015 Feb 9]. Available from: http://www.nhs.uk/Conditions/Cancer-of-the-prostate/Pages/Treatment.aspx.

[4] Longley DB, Johnston PG. Molecular mechanisms of drug resistance. J Pathol. 2005;205(Cml):275–92.

[5] Armstrong DK, Cunningham S, Davies JC, Alton EWFW. Gene therapy in cystic fibrosis. Arch Dis Child. 2014;99(5):465–8.

[6] Ibraheem D, Elaissari A, Fessi H. Gene therapy and DNA delivery systems. Int J Pharm [Internet]. Elsevier B.V.; 2014;459(1-2):70–83. Available from: http://dx.doi.org/10.1016/j.ijpharm.2013.11.041.

[7] Godbey WT, Mikos AG. Recent progress in gene delivery using non-viral transfer complexes. J Control Release. 2001;72:115–25.

[8] Mulligan RC. The Basic Science of Gene Therapy. Science (80-). 1993;260(5110):926–32.

[9] Walther W, Schlag PM. Current status of gene therapy for cancer. Curr Opin Oncol. 2013;25(6):659–64.

[10] Guo W, Chen W, Yu W, Huang W, Deng W. Small interfering RNA-based molecular therapy of cancers. Chin J Cancer. 2013;32:488–93.

[11] Wysocki PJ, Mackiewicz-Wysocka M, Mackiewicz A. Cancer gene therapy—state-of-the-art. Reports Pract Oncol Radiother. 2002;7(4):149–55.

[12] Ternovoi V V, Curiel DT, Smith BF, Siegal GP. Adenovirus-mediated p53 tumor suppressor gene therapy of osteosarcoma. Lab Invest. 2006;86:748–66.

[13] Senzer N, Nemunaitis J, Nemunaitis D, Bedell C, Edelman G, Barve M, et al. Phase I study of a systemically delivered p53 nanoparticle in advanced solid tumors. Mol Ther. 2013;21(5):1096–103.

[14] Altaner C. Prodrug cancer gene therapy. Cancer Lett. 2008;270:191–201.

[15] Zhang J, Kale V, Chen M. Gene-directed enzyme prodrug therapy. AAPS J. 2015;17(1):102–10.

[16] Sangro B, Mazzolini G, Ruiz M, Ruiz J, Quiroga J, Herrero I, et al. A phase I clinical trial of thymidine kinase-based gene therapy in advanced hepatocellular carcinoma. Cancer Gene Ther. 2010;17:837–43.

[17] Vajda A, Marignol L, Foley R, Lynch TH, Lawler M, Hollywood D. Clinical potential of gene-directed enzyme prodrug therapy to improve radiation therapy in prostate cancer patients. Cancer Treat Rev. 2011;37(8):643–54.

[18] Gardlik R, Celec P, Bernadic M. Targeting angiogenesis for cancer (gene) therapy. Bratisl Lek Listy. 2011;112(8):428–34.

[19] Persano L, Crescenzi M, Indraccolo S. Anti-angiogenic gene therapy of cancer: Current status and future prospects. Mol Aspects Med. 2007;28:87–114.

[20] Doan CC, Le LT, Hoang SN, Do SM, Le D Van. Simultaneous silencing of VEGF and KSP by siRNA cocktail inhibits proliferation and induces apoptosis of hepatocellular carcinoma Hep3B cells. Biol Res. 2014;47:1–15.

[21] Aly HAA. Cancer therapy and vaccination. J Immunol Methods. 2012;382(1-2):1–23.

[22] Senovilla L, Vachelli E, Garcia P, Eggermont A, Hervé Fridman W, Galon J, et al. Trial Watch: DNA vaccines for cancer therapy. Oncoimmunology. 2013;3(April):e28185.

[23] Chudley L, McCann K, Mander A, Tjelle T, Campos-Perez J, Godeseth R, et al. DNA fusion-gene vaccination in patients with prostate cancer induces high-frequency CD8+ T-cell responses and increases PSA doubling time. Cancer Immunol Immunother. 2012;61:2161–70.

[24] Staff C, Mozaffari F, Haller BK, Wahren B, Liljefors M. A Phase I safety study of plasmid DNA immunization targeting carcinoembryonic antigen in colorectal cancer patients. Vaccine [Internet]. Elsevier Ltd; 2011;29(39):6817–22. Available from: http://dx.doi.org/10.1016/j.vaccine.2010.12.063.

[25] Kumaragurubaran K, Kaliaperumal K. DNA vaccine: The miniature miracle. Vet World. 2013;6:228–32.

[26] Ginn SL, Alexander IE, Edelstein ML, Abedi MR, Wixon J. Gene therapy clinical trials worldwide to 2012—an update. J Gene Med. 2013;15(2):65–77.

[27] Wirth T, Parker N, Ylä-Herttuala S. History of gene therapy. Gene. 2013;525(2):162–9.

[28] Niidome T, Huang L. Gene therapy progress and prospects: Nonviral vectors. Gene Ther. 2002;9:1647–52.

[29] Morille M, Passirani C, Vonarbourg A, Clavreul A, Benoit J-P. Progress in developing cationic vectors for non-viral systemic gene therapy against cancer. Biomaterials. 2008;29(24-25):3477–96.

[30] Templeton NS. Cationic liposome-mediated gene delivery in vivo. Bioscience Reports. 2002. p. 283–95.

[31] Wilson JM. Lessons learned from the gene therapy trial for ornithine transcarbamylase deficiency. Mol Genet Metab. 2009;96(4):151–7.

[32] Wang T, Upponi JR, Torchilin VP. Design of multifunctional non-viral gene vectors to overcome physiological barriers: Dilemmas and strategies. Int J Pharm. 2012;427(1):3–20.

[33] Tros de Ilarduya C, Sun Y, Düzgüneş N. Gene delivery by lipoplexes and polyplexes. Eur J Pharm Sci. 2010;40:159–70.

[34] Hatefi A, Megeed Z, Ghandehari H. Recombinant polymer-protein fusion: A promising approach towards efficient and targeted gene delivery. J Gene Med. 2006;8(4): 468–76.

[35] De Laporte L, Cruz Rea J, Shea LD. Design of modular non-viral gene therapy vectors. Biomaterials. 2006;27(7):947–54.

[36] Ogris M, Brunner S, Schüller S, Kircheis R, Wagner E. PEGylated DNA/transferrin-PEI complexes: Reduced interaction with blood components, extended circulation in

blood and potential for systemic gene delivery. Gene Ther. 1999;6(October 1998):595–605.

[37] Laga R, Carlisle R, Tangney M, Ulbrich K, Seymour LW. Polymer coatings for delivery of nucleic acid therapeutics. J Control Release. 2012;161(2):537–53.

[38] Moghimi SM, Symonds P, Murray JC, Hunter a. C, Debska G, Szewczyk A. A two-stage poly(ethylenimine)-mediated cytotoxicity: Implications for gene transfer/therapy. Mol Ther. 2005;11(6):990–5.

[39] Veronese FM, Pasut G. PEGylation, successful approach to drug delivery. Drug Discov Today. 2005;10(21):1451–8.

[40] Danquah MK, Zhang XA, Mahato RI. Extravasation of polymeric nanomedicines across tumor vasculature. Adv Drug Deliv Rev. 2011;63(8):623–39.

[41] Vives E, Brodin P, Lebleu B. A Truncated HIV-1 Tat Protein Basic Domain Rapidly Translocates through the Plasma Membrane and Accumulates in the Cell Nucleus. J Biol Chem. 1997;272(25):16010–7.

[42] Cahill K. Cell-Penetrating Peptides, Electroporation, and Drug Delivery. IET Syst Biol. 2010;4.

[43] Brooks H, Lebleu B, Vivès E. Tat peptide-mediated cellular delivery: Back to basics. Adv Drug Deliv Rev. 2005;57(4):559–77.

[44] Xiang S, Tong H, Shi Q, Fernandes JC, Jin T, Dai K, et al. Uptake mechanisms of non-viral gene delivery. J Control Release. 2012;158(3):371–8.

[45] El-Sayed A, Harashima H. Endocytosis of gene delivery vectors: From clathrin-dependent to lipid raft-mediated endocytosis. Mol Ther. 2013;21(6):1118–30.

[46] Daniels TR, Bernabeu E, Rodríguez JA, Patel S, Kozman M, Chiappetta DA, et al. The transferrin receptor and the targeted delivery of therapeutic agents against cancer. Biochim Biophys Acta - Gen Subj. 2012;1820(3):291–317.

[47] Rewatkar PV, Parton RG, Parekh HS, Parat M-O. Are caveolae a cellular entry route for non-viral therapeutic delivery systems? Adv Drug Deliv Rev. 2015.

[48] Hill MM, Bastiani M, Luetterforst R, Kirkham M, Kirkham A, Nixon SJ, et al. PTRF-Cavin, a Conserved Cytoplasmic Protein Required for Caveola Formation and Function. Cell. 2008;132(1):113–24.

[49] Nguyen KCT, Muthiah M, Islam MA, Kalash RS, Cho CS, Park H, et al. Selective transfection with osmotically active sorbitol modified PEI nanoparticles for enhanced anti-cancer gene therapy. Colloids Surfaces B Biointerfaces. 2014;119:126–36.

[50] Kerr MC, Teasdale RD. Defining macropinocytosis. Traffic. 2009;10(2):364–71.

[51] Anaka KT, Anazawa TK, Gawa TO, Uda YS, Akashima YT, Ukuda TF, et al. A Novel, Bio-Reducible Gene Vector Containing Arginine and Histidine Enhances Gene Transfection and Expression of Plasmid DNA. 2011;59(2):202–7.

[52] Brock R. The uptake of arginine-rich cell-penetrating peptides: Putting the puzzle together. Bioconjug Chem. 2014;25(5):863–8.

[53] Cahill K. Molecular electroporation and the transduction of oligoarginines. Phys Biol. 2009;7:16001.

[54] Schmidt N, Mishra A, Lai GH, Wong GCL. Arginine-rich cell-penetrating peptides. FEBS Lett. 2010;584(9):1806–13.

[55] Billiet L, Gomez JP, Berchel M, Jaffrès PA, Le Gall T, Montier T, et al. Gene transfer by chemical vectors, and endocytosis routes of polyplexes, lipoplexes and lipopolyplexes in a myoblast cell line. Biomaterials. 2012;33(10):2980–90.

[56] Midoux P, Pichon C, Yaouanc JJ, Jaffrès PA. Chemical vectors for gene delivery: A current review on polymers, peptides and lipids containing histidine or imidazole as nucleic acids carriers. Br J Pharmacol. 2009;157(January):166–78.

[57] Hafez IM, Cullis PR. Roles of lipid polymorphism in intracellular delivery. Adv Drug Deliv Rev. 2001;47:139–48.

[58] Oliveira S, van Rooy I, Kranenburg O, Storm G, Schiffelers RM. Fusogenic peptides enhance endosomal escape improving siRNA-induced silencing of oncogenes. Int J Pharm. 2007;331:211–4.

[59] Panyam J, Labhasetwar V. Biodegradable nanoparticles for drug and gene delivery to cells and tissue. Adv Drug Deliv Rev. 2003;55:329–47.

[60] Mao S, Sun W, Kissel T. Chitosan-based formulations for delivery of DNA and siRNA. Adv Drug Deliv Rev. 2010;62(1):12–27.

[61] Zhang X-X, McIntosh TJ, Grinstaff MW. Functional lipids and lipoplexes for improved gene delivery. Biochimie. 2012;94(1):42–58.

[62] Dean DA, Strong DD, Zimmer WE. Nuclear entry of nonviral vectors. Gene Ther. 2005;12(11):881–90.

[63] Moseley GW, Leyton DL, Glover DJ, Filmer RP, Jans DA. Enhancement of protein transduction-mediated nuclear delivery by interaction with dynein/microtubules. J Biotechnol. 2010;145(3):222–5.

[64] Alieva IB. Role of microtubule cytoskeleton in regulation of endothelial barrier function. Biochem Biokhimiia. 2014;79(9):964–75.

[65] Vale RD. The molecular motor toolbox for intracellular transport. 2003;112:467–80.

[66] Toledo MAS, Janissen R, Favaro MTP, Cotta MA, Monteiro GA, Prazeres DMF, et al. Development of a recombinant fusion protein based on the dynein light chain LC8 for non-viral gene delivery. J Control Release. 2012;159(2):222–31.

[67] Hébert E. Improvement of exogenous DNA nuclear importation by nuclear localization signal-bearing vectors: A promising way for non-viral gene therapy. Biol Cell. 2003;95(2):59–68.

[68] Escriou V, Carrière M, Scherman D, Wils P. NLS bioconjugates for targeting therapeutic genes to the nucleus. Adv Drug Deliv Rev. 2003;55:295–306.

[69] Wang H-Y, Chen J-X, Sun Y-X, Deng J-Z, Li C, Zhang X-Z, et al. Construction of cell penetrating peptide vectors with N-terminal stearylated nuclear localization signal for targeted delivery of DNA into the cell nuclei. J Control Release. 2011;155(1):26–33.

[70] Maeda H, Wu J, Sawa T, Matsumura Y, Hori K. Tumor vascular permeability and the EPR effect in macromolecular therapeutics: A review. J Control Release. 2000;65:271–84.

[71] Moghimi SM, Hunter AC, Murray JC. Long-Circulating and Target-Specific Nanoparticles: Theory to Practice. 2001;53(2):283–318.

[72] Owens DE, Peppas NA. Opsonization, biodistribution, and pharmacokinetics of polymeric nanoparticles. Int J Pharm. 2006;307:93–102.

[73] Moghimi SM, Hunter a C, Murray JC. Nanomedicine: Current status and future prospects. FASEB J. 2005;19:311–30.

[74] Ishida T, Maeda R, Ichihara M, Irimura K, Kiwada H. Accelerated clearance of PEGylated liposomes in rats after repeated injections. J Control Release. 2003;88:35–42.

[75] Ishida T, Ichihara M, Wang X, Yamamoto K, Kimura J, Majima E, et al. Injection of PEGylated liposomes in rats elicits PEG-specific IgM, which is responsible for rapid elimination of a second dose of PEGylated liposomes. J Control Release. 2006;112:15–25.

[76] Schellekens H, Hennink WE, Brinks V. The immunogenicity of polyethylene glycol: Facts and fiction. Pharm Res. 2013 Jul;30(7):1729–34.

[77] Hatakeyama H, Akita H, Harashima H. The polyethyleneglycol dilemma: Advantage and disadvantage of PEGylation of liposomes for systemic genes and nucleic acids delivery to tumors. Biol Pharm Bull. 2013;36(6):892–9.

[78] Wang M, Thanou M. Targeting nanoparticles to cancer. Pharmacol Res. 2010;62(2): 90–9.

[79] Romberg B, Hennink WE, Storm G. Sheddable coatings for long-circulating nanoparticles. Pharm Res. 2008;25(1):55–71.

[80] Pasut G, Veronese FM. State of the art in PEGylation: The great versatility achieved after forty years of research. J Control Release. 2012;161(2):461–72.

[81] Fella C, Walker GF, Ogris M, Wagner E. Amine-reactive pyridylhydrazone-based PEG reagents for pH-reversible PEI polyplex shielding. Eur J Pharm Sci. 2008;34(4-5): 309–20.

[82] Yadav L, Puri N, Rastogi V, Satpute P, Ahmad R, Kaur G. Matrix metalloproteinases and cancer—roles in threat and therapy. Asian Pac J Cancer Prev. 2014;15(3):1085–91.

[83] Li H, Yu SS, Miteva M, Nelson C, Werfel T, Giorgio TD, et al. Matrix Metalloproteinase Responsive, proximity-activated polymeric nanoparticles for siRNA delivery. Adv Funct Mater. 2013;23(24):3040–52.

[84] Lushchak V. Glutathione Homeostasis and functions: Potential targets for medical interventions. J Amino Acids. 2011;2012.

[85] Moriarty-Craige SE, Jones DP. Extracellular thiols and thiol/disulfide redox in metabolism. Annu Rev Nutr. 2004 Jan;24:481–509.

[86] Lei Y, Wang J, Xie C, Wagner E, Lu W, Li Y, et al. Glutathione-sensitive RGD-poly(ethylene glycol)-SS-polyethylenimine for intracranial glioblastoma targeted gene delivery. J Gene Med. 2013;15(8-9):291–305.

[87] Fan W, Wang Y, Dai X, Shi L, Mckinley D, Tan C. Reduction-responsive Crosslinked Micellar Nanoassemblies for Tumor-targeted Drug Delivery. Pharm Res. 2014;

[88] Lai TC, Kataoka K, Kwon GS. Bioreducible polyether-based pDNA ternary polyplexes: Balancing particle stability and transfection efficiency. Colloids Surfaces B Biointerfaces. 2012;99:27–37.

[89] Huang S, Shao K, Kuang Y, Liu Y, Li J, An S, et al. Tumor targeting and microenvironment-responsive nanoparticles for gene delivery. Biomaterials. 2013;34:5294–302.

[90] Bertrand N, Wu J, Xu X, Kamaly N, Farokhzad OC. Cancer nanotechnology: The impact of passive and active targeting in the era of modern cancer biology. Adv Drug Deliv Rev. 2014;66:2–25.

[91] Torchilin VP, Lukyanov AN. Peptide and protein drug delivery to and into tumors: Challenges and solutions. Drug Discov Today. 2003;8(6):259–66.

[92] Goodman SL, Picard M. Integrins as therapeutic targets. Trends Pharmacol Sci. 2012;33(7):405–12.

[93] Mendelsohn J. The epidermal growth factor receptor as a target for cancer therapy. Endocr Relat Cancer. 2001;8(1):3–9.

[94] Lu Y, Low PS. Folate-mediated delivery of macromolecular anticancer therapeutic agents. Adv Drug Deliv Rev. 2002;54(5):675–93.

[95] Iozzo RV, Sanderson RD. Proteoglycans in cancer biology, tumor microenvironment and angiogenesis. J Cell Mol Med. 2011;15(5):1013–31.

[96] Curnis F, Gasparri A, Sacchi A, Longhi R, Corti A. Coupling tumor necrosis factor-α with αV integrin ligands improves its antineoplastic activity. Cancer Res. 2004;64:565–71.

[97] Svensen N, Walton JGA, Bradley M. Peptides for cell-selective drug delivery. Trends Pharmacol Sci. 2012;33(4):186–92.

[98] Medina-Kauwe LK, Xie J, Hamm-Alvarez S. Intracellular trafficking of nonviral vectors. Gene Ther. 2005;12(24):1734–51.

[99] D'Souza SE, Ginsberg MH, Plow EF. Arginyl-glycyl-aspartic acid (RGD): A cell adhesion motif. Trends Biochem Sci. 1991;16(7):246–50.

[100] Seguin L, Desgrosellier JS, Weis SM, Cheresh DA. Integrins and cancer: Regulators of cancer stemness, metastasis, and drug resistance. Trends Cell Biol. 2015;1–7.

[101] Park J, Singha K, Son S, Kim J, Namgung R, Yun C-O, et al. A review of RGD-functionalized nonviral gene delivery vectors for cancer therapy. Cancer Gene Ther. 2012;19(11):741–8.

[102] Kim HA, Nam K, Kim SW. Tumor targeting RGD conjugated bio-reducible polymer for VEGF siRNA expressing plasmid delivery. Biomaterials. 2014;35(26):7543–52.

[103] Nie Y, Schaffert D, Rödl W, Ogris M, Wagner E, Günther M. Dual-targeted polyplexes: One step towards a synthetic virus for cancer gene therapy. J Control Release. 2011;152(1):127–34.

[104] Mammen M, Choi S-K, Whitesides GM. Polyvalent Interactions in Biological Systems: Implications for Design and Use of Multivalent Ligands and Inhibitors. Angew Chemie Int Ed. 1998;37(20):2754–94.

[105] Muro S. Challenges in design and characterization of ligand-targeted drug delivery systems. J Control Release. 2012;164(2):125–37.

[106] Turner N, Moretti E, Siclari O, Migliaccio I, Santarpia L, D'Incalci M, et al. Targeting triple negative breast cancer: Is p53 the answer? Cancer Treat Rev. 2013;39(5):541–50.

[107] Muzykantov VR, Torchilin VP. Biomedical aspects of drug targeting. 2002.

[108] Brenner MK, Gottschalk S, Leen AM, Vera JF. Is cancer gene therapy an empty suit? Lancet Oncol. 2013;14(11):e447–56.

[109] Van der Meel R, Vehmeijer LJC, Kok RJ, Storm G, van Gaal EVB. Ligand-targeted particulate nanomedicines undergoing clinical evaluation: current status. Adv Drug Deliv Rev. 2013;65(10):1284–98.

[110] Pandolfi PP. Transcription therapy for cancer. Oncogene. 2001;20(24):3116–27.

[111] Lu Y. Transcriptionally regulated, prostate-targeted gene therapy for prostate cancer. Adv Drug Deliv Rev. 2009;61(7-8):572–88.

[112] Worthington J, McCarthy HO, Barrett E, Adams C, Robson T, Hirst D. Use of the radiation-inducible WAF1 promoter to drive iNOS gene therapy as a novel anti-cancer treatment. J Gene Med. 2004;6(6):673–80.

[113] Harrington KJ, Linardakis E, Vile RG. Transcriptional control: An essential component of cancer gene therapy strategies? Adv Drug Deliv Rev. 2000;44:167–84.

[114] Robson T, Hirst DG. Transcriptional Targeting in Cancer Gene Therapy. J Biomed Biotechnol. 2003;2003:110–37.

[115] Kyo S, Takakura M, Fujiwara T, Inoue M. Understanding and exploiting hTERT promoter regulation for diagnosis and treatment of human cancers. Cancer Sci. 2008;99(8):1528–38.

[116] Xie X, Tang H, Liu P, Kong Y, Wu M, Xiao X, et al. Development of PEA-15 using a potent non-viral vector for therapeutic application in breast cancer. Cancer Lett [Internet]. 2015;356(2 Pt B):374–81. Available from: http://linkinghub.elsevier.com/retrieve/pii/S0304383514005710.

[117] Mita AC, Mita MM, Nawrocki ST, Giles FJ. Survivin: Key regulator of mitosis and apoptosis and novel target for cancer therapeutics. Clin Cancer Res. 2008;14(16):5000–5.

[118] Lim M, Zhong C, Yang S, Bell AM, Cohen MB, Roy-burman P. Runx2 regulates survivin expression in porstate cancer cells. Lab Invest. 2010;90(2):222–33.

[119] Qu L, Wang Y, Gong L, Zhu J, Gong R, Si J. Suicide gene therapy for hepatocellular carcinoma cells by survivin promoter-driven expression of the herpes simplex virus thymidine kinase gene. Oncol Rep. 2013;29(4):1435–40.

[120] Coleman R, Brown J, Terpos E, Lipton A, Smith MR, Cook R, et al. Bone markers and their prognostic value in metastatic bone disease: Clinical evidence and future directions. Cancer Treat Rev. 2008;34(7):629–39.

[121] McCarthy HO, Coulter JA, Worthington J, Robson T, Hirst D. Human osteocalcin: A strong promoter for nitric oxide synthase gene therapy, with specificity for hormone refractory prostate cancer. J Gene Med. 2007;9(6):511–20.

[122] Coulter JA, Page NL, Worthington J, Robson T, Hirst DG, McCarthy HO. Transcriptional regulation of inducible nitric oxide synthase gene therapy: Targeting early stage and advanced prostate cancer. J Gene Med. 2010;12(9):755–65.

[123] Alexis F, Basto P, Levy-Nissenbaum E, Radovic-Moreno AF, Zhang L, Pridgen E, et al. HER-2-targeted nanoparticle-affibody bioconjugates for cancer therapy. ChemMedChem. 2008;3(12):1839–43.

[124] Peitzsch C, Perrin R, Hill RP, Dubrovska A, Kurth I. Hypoxia as a biomarker for radioresistant cancer stem cells. Int J Radiat Biol. 2014;90(August):1–17.

[125] Fujioka T, Matsunaga N, Okazaki H, Koyanagi S, Ohdo S. Hypoxia-response plasmid vector producing bcl-2 shRNA enhances the apoptotic cell death of mouse rectum carcinoma. J Pharmacol Sci. 2010;113:353–61.

[126] Shibuya M. Differential roles of vascular endothelial growth factor receptor-1 and receptor-2 in angiogenesis. J Biochem Mol Biol. 2006;39(5):469–78.

[127] Wang Y, Xu HX, Lu M De, Tang Q. Expression of thymidine kinase mediated by a novel non-viral delivery system under the control of vascular endothelial growth factor receptor 2 promoter selectively kills human umbilical vein endothelial cells. World J Gastroenterol. 2008;14(2):224–30.

[128] Fire A, Xu S, Montgomery MK, Kostas SA, Driver SE, Mello CC. Potent and specific genetic interference by double-stranded RNA in Caenorhabditis elegans. Nature. 1998;391(6669):806–11.

[129] Wang Z, Rao DD, Senzer N, Nemunaitis J. RNA interference and cancer therapy. Pharm Res. 2011;28:2983–95.

[130] Hutvagner G. Small RNA asymmetry in RNAi: Function in RISC assembly and gene regulation. FEBS Lett. 2005;579:5850–7.

[131] Mansoori B, Shotorbani SS, Baradaran B. RNA Interference and its Role in Cancer Therapy. Adv Pharm Bull. 2014;4(4):313–21.

[132] Robb GB, Brown KM, Khurana J, Rana TM. Specific and potent RNAi in the nucleus of human cells. Nat Struct Mol Biol. 2005;12(2):133–7.

[133] Yu J-Y, DeRuiter SL, Turner DL. RNA interference by expression of short-interfering RNAs and hairpin RNAs in mammalian cells. Proc Natl Acad Sci U S A. 2002;99(9): 6047–52.

[134] Chen Y, Bathula SR, Li J, Huang L. Multifunctional nanoparticles delivering small interfering RNA and doxorubicin overcome drug resistance in cancer. J Biol Chem. 2010;285(29):22639–50.

[135] Yang H, Li Y, Li T, Xu M, Chen Y, Wu C, et al. Multifunctional core/shell nanoparticles cross-linked polyetherimide-folic acid as efficient Notch-1 siRNA carrier for targeted killing of breast cancer. Sci Rep. 2014;4:7072.

[136] Kullberg M, McCarthy R, Anchordoquy TJ. Systemic tumlur-specific gene delivery. J Control Release. 2013;172(3):730–6.

[137] Yue J. MiRNA and vascular cell movement. Adv Drug Deliv Rev. 2011;63(8):616–22.

[138] Bartel DP. MicroRNAs: Genomics, biogenesis, mechanism, and function. Cell. 2004;116(2):281–97.

[139] Hao J, Zhao S, Zhang Y, Zhao Z, Ye R, Wen J, et al. Emerging role of microRNAs in cancer and cancer stem cells. J Cell Biochem. 2014;115(4):605–10.

[140] Garofalo M, Croce CM. Role of microRNAs in maintaining cancer stem cells. Adv Drug Deliv Rev. 2015;81:53–61.

[141] Misso G, Teresa M, Martino D, Rosa G De, Farooqi AA, Lombardi A, et al. Mir-34: A New Weapon Against Cancer? 2014;(August):1–16.

[142] Hu QL, Jiang QY, Jin X, Shen J, Wang K, Li YB, et al. Cationic microRNA-delivering nanovectors with bifunctional peptides for efficient treatment of PANC-1 xenograft model. Biomaterials. 2013;34(9):2265–76.

[143] Anand S, Majeti BK, Acevedo LM, Murphy EA, Mukthavaram R, Scheppke L, et al. MicroRNA-132-mediated loss of p120RasGAP activates the endothelium to facilitate pathological angiogenesis. Nat Med. 2010;16(8):909–14.

[144] Kogure K, Akita H, Harashima H. Multifunctional envelope-type nano device for non-viral gene delivery: Concept and application of Programmed Packaging. J Control Release. 2007;122:246–51.

[145] Moriguchi R, Kogure K, Akita H, Futaki S, Miyagishi M, Taira K, et al. A multifunctional envelope-type nano device for novel gene delivery of siRNA plasmids. Int J Pharm. 2005;301:277–85.

[146] Hatakeyama H, Akita H, Harashima H. A multifunctional envelope type nano device (MEND) for gene delivery to tumours based on the EPR effect: A strategy for overcoming the PEG dilemma. Adv Drug Deliv Rev. 2011;63(3):152–60.

[147] Nakamura Y, Kogure K, Futaki S, Harashima H. Octaarginine-modified multifunctional envelope-type nano device for siRNA. J Control Release. 2007;119:360–7.

[148] El-Sayed A, Masuda T, Khalil I, Akita H, Harashima H. Enhanced gene expression by a novel stearylated INF7 peptide derivative through fusion independent endosomal escape. J Control Release. 2009;138(2):160–7.

[149] Hatakeyama H, Ito E, Akita H, Oishi M, Nagasaki Y, Futaki S, et al. A pH-sensitive fusogenic peptide facilitates endosomal escape and greatly enhances the gene silencing of siRNA-containing nanoparticles in vitro and in vivo. J Control Release. 2009;139(2):127–32.

[150] Sakurai Y, Hatakeyama H, Sato Y, Hyodo M, Akita H, Ohga N, et al. RNAi-mediated gene knockdown and anti-angiogenic therapy of RCCs using a cyclic RGD-modified liposomal-siRNA system. J Control Release. 2014;173:110–8.

[151] Kusumoto K, Akita H, Ishitsuka T, Matsumoto Y, Nomoto T. A Lipid Envelop-Type Nano Particle Incorporating a Multifunctional Peptide for the Systemic siRNA Delivery to the Pulmonary Endothelium. ACS Nano. 2013;7(9):7534–41.

[152] Toriyabe N, Hayashi Y, Harashima H. The transfection activity of R8-modified nanoparticles and siRNA condensation using pH sensitive stearylated-octahistidine. Biomaterials. 2013;34(4):1337–43.

[153] El-Aneed A. An overview of current delivery systems in cancer gene therapy. J Control Release. 2004;94(1):1–14.

[154] Chailertvanitkul VA, Pouton CW. Adenovirus: A blueprint for non-viral gene delivery. Curr Opin Biotechnol. 2010;21(5):627–32.

[155] Fabre JW, Collins L. Synthetic peptides as non-viral DNA vectors. Curr Gene Ther. 2006 Aug;6(4):459–80.

[156] Mann A, Thakur G, Shukla V, Ganguli M. Peptides in DNA delivery: Current insights and future directions. Drug Discov Today. 2008;13(3-4):152–60.

[157] Saccardo P, Villaverde A, González-Montalbán N. Peptide-mediated DNA condensation for non-viral gene therapy. Biotechnol Adv. 2009;27(4):432–8.

[158] Kaouass M, Beaulieu R, Balicki D. Histonefection: Novel and potent non-viral gene delivery. J Control Release. 2006;113:245–54.

[159] Murray KD, Etheridge CJ, Shah SI, Matthews DA, Russell W, Gurling HM, et al. Enhanced cationic liposome-mediated transfection using the DNA-binding peptide mu (mu) from the adenovirus core. Gene Ther. 2001;8:453–60.

[160] Soundara Manickam D, Bisht HS, Wan L, Mao G, Oupicky D. Influence of TAT-peptide polymerization on properties and transfection activity of TAT/DNA polyplexes. J Control Release. 2005;102(1):293–306.

[161] Vandenbroucke RE, De Smedt SC, Demeester J, Sanders NN. Cellular entry pathway and gene transfer capacity of TAT-modified lipoplexes. Biochim Biophys Acta. 2007;1768(3):571–9.

[162] Heitz F, Morris MC, Divita G. Twenty years of cell-penetrating peptides: From molecular mechanisms to therapeutics. 2009;(October 2008):195–206.

[163] Deshayes S, Morris MC, Divita G, Heitz F. Cell-penetrating peptides: Tools for intracellular delivery of therapeutics. Cell Mol Life Sci. 2005;62(16):1839–49.

[164] Derossi D, Joliot A, Chassaing G, Prochiantztn A. The third helix of the Antennapedia homeodomain translocates through biological membranes. J Biol Chem. 1994;10444–50.

[165] Cells GT, Ohmori N, Niidome T, Kiyota T, Lee S, Sugihara G, et al. Importance of Hydrophobic Region in Amphiphilic Structures of a -Helical Peptides for Their. 1998;265(245):259–65.

[166] Scheller A, Oehlke J, Wiesner B, Dathe M, Krause E, Beyermann M, et al. Structural requirements for cellular uptake of alpha-helical amphipathic peptides. J Pept Sci. 1999;5:185–94.

[167] Bolhassani A. Potential efficacy of cell-penetrating peptides for nucleic acid and drug delivery in cancer. Biochim Biophys Acta. 2011;1816(2):232–46.

[168] Gonçalves E, Kitas E, Seelig J. Binding of oligoarginine to membrane lipids and heparan sulfate structural and thermodynamic characterization of a cell-penetrating peptide. - 2005 - Gonçalves, Kitas, Seelig.pdf. Biochemistry. 2005. p. 2692–702.

[169] Mitchell DJ, Kim DT, Steinman L, Fathman CG, Rothbard JB. Polyarginine enters cells more efficiently than other polycationic homopolymers. J Pept Res. 2000;56:318–25.

[170] Chang M, Huang Y-W, Aronstam R, Lee H-J. Cellular Delivery of Noncovalently-Associated Macromolecules by Cell- Penetrating Peptides. Curr Pharm Biotechnol. 2014;15(3):267–75.

[171] Nakase I, Takeuchi T, Tanaka G, Futaki S. Methodological and cellular aspects that govern the internalization mechanisms of arginine-rich cell-penetrating peptides. Adv Drug Deliv Rev. 2008;60(4-5):598–607.

[172] Futaki S, Nakase I, Tadokoro A, Takeuchi T, Jones AT. Arginine-rich peptides and their internalization mechanisms. Biochem Soc Trans. 2007;35(Pt 4):784–7.

[173] Wender PA, Mitchell DJ, Pattabiraman K, Pelkey ET, Steinman L, Rothbard JB. The design, synthesis, and evaluation of molecules that enable or enhance cellular uptake: Peptoid molecular transporters. Proc Natl Acad Sci U S A. 2000;97(24):13003–8.

[174] Koren E, Torchilin VP. Cell-penetrating peptides: Breaking through to the other side. Trends Mol Med. 2012;18(7):385–93.

[175] Olson ES, Aguilera TA, Jiang T, Ellies LG, Nguyen TQ, Wong E, et al. In vivo characterization of activatable cell penetrating peptides for targeting protease activity in cancer. Integr Biol. 2009;1(5-6):382–93.

[176] Mei L, Zhang Q, Yang Y, He Q, Gao H. Angiopep-2 and activatable cell penetrating peptide dual modi fi ed nanoparticles for enhanced tumor targeting and penetrating. Int J Pharm. 2014;474(1-2):95–102.

[177] Martín I, Teixidó M, Giralt E. Building cell selectivity into CPP-mediated strategies. Pharmaceuticals. 2010.

[178] Kondo E, Saito K, Tashiro Y, Kamide K, Uno S, Furuya T, et al. Tumour lineage-homing cell-penetrating peptides as anticancer molecular delivery systems. Nat Commun. 2012;3:951.

[179] Gao H, Zhang Q, Yang Y, Jiang X, He Q. Tumor homing cell penetrating peptide decorated nanoparticles used for enhancing tumor targeting delivery and therapy. Int J Pharm. 2015;478(1):240–50.

[180] Liou JS, Liu BR, Martin AL, Huang YW, Chiang HJ, Lee HJ. Protein transduction in human cells is enhanced by cell-penetrating peptides fused with an endosomolytic HA2 sequence. Peptides. 2012;37(2):273–84.

[181] Bitler BG, Schroeder JA. Anti-cancer therapies that utilize cell penetrating peptides. Recent Pat Anticancer Drug Discov. 2010 Jun;5(2):99–108.

[182] Verdurmen WPR, Bovee-Geurts PH, Wadhwani P, Ulrich AS, Hällbrink M, Van Kuppevelt TH, et al. Preferential uptake of L-versus D-amino acid cell-penetrating peptides in a cell type-dependent manner. Chem Biol. 2011;18:1000–10.

[183] Zhang X-X, Eden HS, Chen X. Peptides in cancer nanomedicine: drug carriers, targeting ligands and protease substrates. J Control Release. 2012;159(1):2–13.

[184] Melikov K, Chernomordik L V. Arginine-rich cell penetrating peptides: From endosomal uptake to nuclear delivery. Cell Mol Life Sci. 2005;62(23):2739–49.

[185] Cho YW, Kim J-D, Park K. Polycation gene delivery systems: Escape from endosomes to cytosol. J Pharm Pharmacol. 2003;55(6):721–34.

[186] Soltani F, Sankian M, Hatefi A, Ramezani M. Development of a novel histone H1-based recombinant fusion peptide for targeted non-viral gene delivery. Int J Pharm. 2013;441(1-2):307–15.

[187] Mason AJ, Leborgne C, Moulay G, Martinez A, Danos O, Bechinger B, et al. Optimising histidine rich peptides for efficient DNA delivery in the presence of serum. J Control Release. 2007;118(1):95–104.

[188] Lo SL, Wang S. An endosomolytic Tat peptide produced by incorporation of histidine and cysteine residues as a nonviral vector for DNA transfection. Biomaterials. 2008 May;29(15):2408–14.

[189] Midoux P, Kichler A, Boutin V, Maurizot JC, Monsigny M. Membrane permeabilization and efficient gene transfer by a peptide containing several histidines. Bioconjug Chem. 1998;9(2):260–7.

[190] Asseline U, Gonçalves C, Pichon C, Midoux P. Improved nuclear delivery of antisense 2′-Ome RNA by conjugation with the histidine-rich peptide H5WYG. J Gene Med. Jan;16(7-8):157–65.

[191] Han K, Yang J, Chen S, Chen J-X, Liu C-W, Li C, et al. Novel gene transfer vectors based on artificial recombinant multi-functional oligopeptides. Int J Pharm. 2012;436(1-2):555–63.

[192] Varkouhi AK, Scholte M, Storm G, Haisma HJ. Endosomal escape pathways for delivery of biologicals. J Control Release. 2011;151(3):220–8.

[193] McCarthy HO, McCaffrey J, McCrudden CM, Zholobenko A, Ali AA, McBride JW, et al. Development and characterization of self-assembling nanoparticles using a bio-inspired amphipathic peptide for gene delivery. J Control Release. 2014;189:141–9.

[194] Li W, Nicol F, Szoka FC. GALA: A designed synthetic pH-responsive amphipathic peptide with applications in drug and gene delivery. Adv Drug Deliv Rev. 2004;56(7):967–85.

[195] Kalderon D, Roberts B, Richardson W, Smith A. A short amino acid sequence able to specify nuclear localisation. Cell. 1984;39:499–509.

[196] Elder RM, Jayaraman A. Molecular Simulations of Polycation – DNA Binding Exploring the E ff ect of Peptide Chemistry and Sequence in Nuclear Localization Sequence Based Polycations. 2013.

[197] Whittaker G. Virus nuclear import. Adv Drug Deliv Rev. 2003;55:733–47.

[198] Donnelly M, Elliott G. Nuclear localization and shuttling of herpes simplex virus tegument protein VP13/14. J Virol. 2001;75(6):2566–74.

[199] Pollard VW, Malim MH. THE HIV-1 Rev Protein: Overview of the Retroviral Life Cycle. Annu Rev Microbiol. 1998;491–532.

[200] Palmeri D, Malim MH. Importin beta can mediate the nuclear import of an arginine-rich nuclear localization signal in the absence of importin alpha. Mol Cell Biol. 1999;19(2):1218–25.

[201] Van der Aa MAEM, Mastrobattista E, Oosting RS, Hennink WE, Koning GA, Crommelin DJA. The Nuclear Pore Complex: The Gateway to Successful Nonviral Gene Delivery. Pharm Res. 2006;23(3):447–59.

[202] Iijima M, Suzuki M, Tanabe A, Nishimura A, Yamada M. Two motifs essential for nuclear import of the hnRNP A1 nucleocytoplasmic shuttling sequence M9 core. FEBS Lett. 2006;580:1365–70.

[203] Pollard VW, Michael WM, Nakielny S, Siomi MC, Wang F, Dreyfuss G. A novel receptor-mediated nuclear protein import pathway. Cell. 1996;86(6):985–94.

[204] Piñol-Roma S, Dreyfuss G. Shuttling of pre-mRNA binding proteins between nucleus and cytoplasm. Nature. 1992;355(6362):730–2.

[205] Nakielny S, Siomi MC, Siomi H, Michael WM, Pollard V, Dreyfuss G. Transportin: Nuclear transport receptor of a novel nuclear protein import pathway. Exp Cell Res. 1996;229(2):261–6.

[206] Zhang W, Greene W, Gao S-J. Microtubule- and dynein-dependent nuclear trafficking of rhesus rhadinovirus in rhesus fibroblasts. J Virol. 2012;86(1):599–604.

[207] Hsieh MJ, White PJ, Pouton CW. Interaction of viruses with host cell molecular motors. Curr Opin Biotechnol. 2010;21(5):633–9.

[208] Pigeon L, Gonçalves C, Gosset D, Pichon C, Midoux P. An E3-14.7K peptide that promotes microtubules-mediated transport of plasmid DNA increases polyplexes transfection efficiency. Small. 2013 Nov;9(22):3845–51.

[209] Ludtke JJ, Zhang G, Sebestyén MG, Wolff JA. A nuclear localization signal can enhance both the nuclear transport and expression of 1 kb DNA. J Cell Sci. 1999 Jun; 112(Pt 12):2033–41.

[210] Pouton C, Wagstaff K. Targeted delivery to the nucleus. Adv drug Deliv.... 2007;59(8):698–717.

[211] Sadeghian F, Hosseinkhani S, Alizadeh A, Hatefi A. Design, engineering and preparation of a multi-domain fusion vector for gene delivery. Int J Pharm. 2012;427(2): 393–9.

[212] Chaloin L, Vidal P, Heitz A, Van Mau N, Méry J, Divita G, et al. Conformations of primary amphipathic carrier peptides in membrane mimicking environments. Biochemistry. 1997;36(37):11179–87.

[213] McCarthy HO, Wang, Yuhua, Mangipudi S, Hatefi A. Advances with the use of bio-inspired vectors towards creation of artifical viruses. Expert Opin Drug Deliv. 2010;7(4):497–512.

[214] Wang Y, Mangipudi SS, Canine BF, Hatefi A. A designer biomimetic vector with a chimeric architecture for targeted gene transfer. J Control Release. 2009;137(1):46–53.

[215] McCarthy HO, Zholobenko AV, Wang Y, Canine B, Robson T, Hirst DG, et al. Evaluation of a multi-functional nanocarrier for targeted breast cancer iNOS gene therapy. Int J Pharm. 2011;405(1-2):196–202.

[216] Canine BF, Wang Y, Hatefi A. Biosynthesis and characterization of a novel genetically engineered polymer for targeted gene transfer to cancer cells. J Control Release. 2009;138(3):188–96.

[217] Canine BF, Wang Y, Ouyang W, Hatefi A. Development of targeted recombinant polymers that can deliver siRNA to the cytoplasm and plasmid DNA to the cell nucleus. J Control Release. 2011;151(1):95–101.

[218] Wang Y, Zhang L, Guo S, Hatefi A, Huang L. Incorporation of histone derived recombinant protein for enhanced disassembly of core-membrane structured liposomal nanoparticles for efficient siRNA delivery. J Control Release. 2013;172:179–89.

5

Gene Delivery into the Central Nervous System (CNS) Using AAV Vectors

Koichi Miyake, Noriko Miyake and Takashi Shimada

Abstract

Application of gene therapies is a promising approach to the treatment of various neurological disorders, including Parkinson's disease, amyotrophic lateral sclerosis (ALS), and lysosomal storage disorders, which are not treatable by any other means. However, the blood–brain barrier (BBB) is a key obstacle to gene delivery to the central nervous system (CNS). Adeno-associated virus (AAV) vectors have emerged as a promising tool for gene delivery to the CNS, thanks to their safety and ability to transduce non-dividing neuronal cells. In this chapter, we discuss strategies for delivering genes across the BBB, focusing especially on potential routes of administration of AAV vectors and promising applications of AAV vectors to the treatment of CNS disorders.

Keywords: Adeno-associated virus vector, central nervous system, routes of administration, lysosomal storage disorders

1. Introduction

Because it is often difficult to treat central nervous system (CNS) disorders using standard pharmacological methods, other, more effective, strategies are being sought. Among these alternatives, gene therapy appears to be a promising approach to treating various neurological disorders, including Parkinson's disease, amyotrophic lateral sclerosis, Huntington disease, Alzheimer's disease, and lysosomal storage disorders, which are not treatable by any other methods. However, the efficacy of gene therapies in clinical trials has been limited by physiological barriers unique to the CNS, as well as by the post-mitotic state of many of the cellular targets in the brain and spinal cord. The blood–brain barrier (BBB) in particular is a key obstacle to gene delivery to the CNS.

Adeno-associated virus (AAV) is a member of the family Parvoviridae that has been widely used as a vector for gene delivery. AAV is a small, non-enveloped single-stranded DNA virus with a genome of approximately 4.7 kb [1]. The AAV genome consists of three open reading frames (ORFs) flanked by two inverted terminal repeats (ITRs). It is a dependovirus because it requires helper functions from other viruses such as adenovirus or herpes simplex virus for its replication. AAV is a suitable gene transfer tool because of its safety due to a lack of pathogenicity, its ability to transduce both dividing and non-dividing cells, and its minor immune response. Among the more than 100 nonredundant AAV genotypes that have been identified, 12 AAV serotypes with unique properties have been used to produce most expression vectors [2].

AAV vectors are powerful tools that are able to mediate gene transfer to the CNS, thanks to their safety and ability to transduce non-dividing neuronal cells. Consequently, they hold great potential for use in therapeutic gene delivery strategies for the treatment of neurological disorders. Although a breakthrough treatment has remained elusive, current approaches are now considerably safer and potentially much more effective than in the past. In this chapter, we discuss how to administer vectors across the BBB, focusing especially on potential routes for administration of AAV vectors and promising strategies for application of AAV vectors in CNS disorders.

2. AAV vectors for CNS disorders

2.1. Advantages of AAV vectors for gene transfer to CNS

A variety of both viral and non-viral vectors have been applied to the effort to transfer genes into the CNS. Among these gene transfer methods, AAV vectors have emerged as a particularly promising tool for gene delivery. There are many advantages to using AAV vectors for transduction of the CNS [3]. First, AAV is itself not pathogenic and has received a P1 and P1A recombinant DNA safety classification. It is therefore easy to use AAV vectors without specific facilities. Second, because AAV vectors have the ability to transduce non-dividing cells, they are a suitable means for delivering transgenes to non-dividing neuronal cells [4]. Third, long-term expression of transgenes with little immunogenicity or toxicity can be achieved using AAV vectors. It was reported that there was a gradual decline in the number of transduced cells when the cytomegalovirus (CMV) immediate-early promoter was used [5]. However, with the use of cellular or hybrid promoters, such as the chicken beta-actin/CMV promoter, transgene expression was sustained. Indeed, we found that following administration to mice of an AAV vector in which the CAG promoter drove the green fluorescent protein (GFP) gene, GFP expression was sustained for more than one and a half years, or nearly the entire life span of the mice [6]. In addition, we are now using several AAV vector serotypes (mainly from AAV serotype 1 to 12), depending on the target. On the other hand, a disadvantage of AAV vectors is the size limitation of the transgene. Since AAVs package a ~4.7-kb genome, it is better to have 4.7 kb between the inverted terminal repeats at the 5′ and 3′ ends [7].

2.2. How to cross the BBB?

To apply gene therapy to the treatment of CNS disorders, there are two immediate problems that must be solved: One is how to cross the BBB, which is a physical and biochemical barrier that precisely regulates the ability of endogenous and exogenous substances to accumulate within brain tissue [8, 9], and the second is how to distribute the transgene to the entire brain. In some cases, we have to treat the whole brain, including the peripheral nervous system (PNS). To transfer genes across the BBB, there are two main approaches: brain-directed local therapy and less invasive systemic therapy. Table 1 shows possible approaches of gene delivery to CNS using AAV vectors.

1. Brain-directed gene transfer
1) Intracranial injection of AAV vector
2. Systemic gene transfer
1) Intravenous injection of AAV vector
2) Intracerebroventricular injection of AAV vector
3) Intrathecal injection of AAV vector

Table 1. Possible approaches of gene delivery to CNS using AAV vectors

3. Local gene delivery to the CNS using AAV vectors

Brain-directed local injection of AAV vectors is a straightforward approach to gene transfer to the CNS. We compared the transduction efficiency of several AAV vector serotypes encoding the luciferase gene (AAV/Luc) after intracranial injection in mice. Fig. 1 shows the resultant transduction efficiencies determined using an in vivo imaging system (IVIS). Efficient transduction was achieved using the AAV9/Luc or AAV10/Luc vectors compared to the AAV1/Luc or AAV8/Luc vectors, and sustained expression was detected for at least 6 months after injection. Notably, however, following injection of a small amount of AAV1/Luc or AAV9/Luc vectors (2 μl) into the striatum, expression of the transgene was detected in the liver after 2 weeks of injection (Fig. 1A). Therefore, although expression of the transgene was absent at 6 months after injection, one must be aware of the potential for the occurrence of unexpected transduction following directed local injection of an AAV vector.

Fig. 2 shows another comparison of transduction efficiency after local administration to the CNS, this time using AAV vectors encoding GFP (AAV/GFP). As expected, the AAV9/GFP vector exhibited the greatest ability to transduce neuronal cells 2 weeks after injection. Surprisingly, however, nearly the same high transduction efficiency was detected 2 months after injection of the AAV2/GFP vector. Although a long time is needed to achieve strong expression with AAV2, since there is no limitation for the patient, the use of AAV2 is one option for highly efficient CNS transduction.

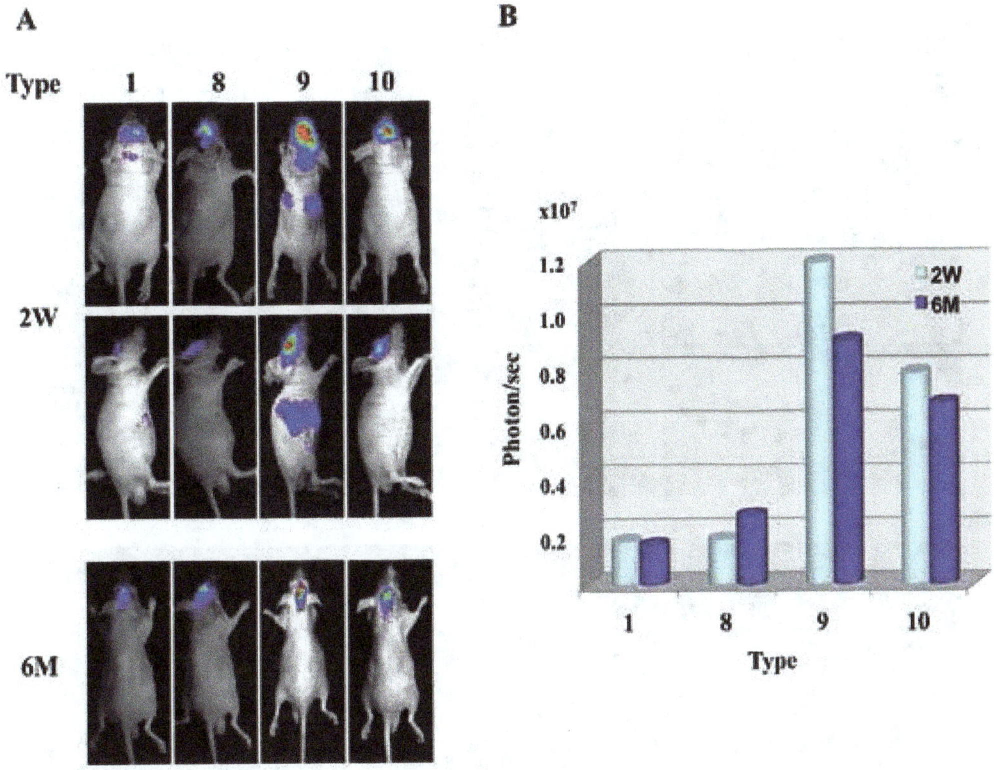

Figure 1. Brain-directed injection of AAV vectors encoding the luciferase gene (AAV/Luc). (A) Approximately 2.0 x 10^{10} vector genomes (vg) of recombinant AAV/Luc vectors (serotypes 1, 8, 9, and 10) were injected into the right striatum over a period of 5 min using a Hamilton syringe with a 33-G blunt-tip needle. Bioluminescent images of mice were obtained using a Xenogen IVIS imaging system at 2 weeks and 6 months post administration. (B) Comparative measurement of AAV/Luc transduction *in vivo* in the brain area 2 weeks and 6 months after injection.

Finally, Fig. 3 shows results obtained with direct intracranial injection of AAV1/GFP vectors into the hippocampus (CA3). Although we injected AAV1/GFP vectors into the right hippocampus (CA3), GFP expression was detected on both sides of the brain, indicating that GFP is efficiently transported to the left side through long axons. This axonal transport is an advantage of direct injection [10, 11].

4. Systemic gene delivery to CNS using AAV vectors

Although in some cases axonal transport may be useful for widespread transduction with AAV vectors, most often local injection of AAV vectors provides transgene expression only to limited regions in the CNS. Consequently, to obtain global transduction of the CNS, multiple intracerebral injections are needed. But this strategy is invasive, and safety becomes a problem. To overcome this problem, an ideal approach for efficient and safe transduction to CNS is systemic administration.

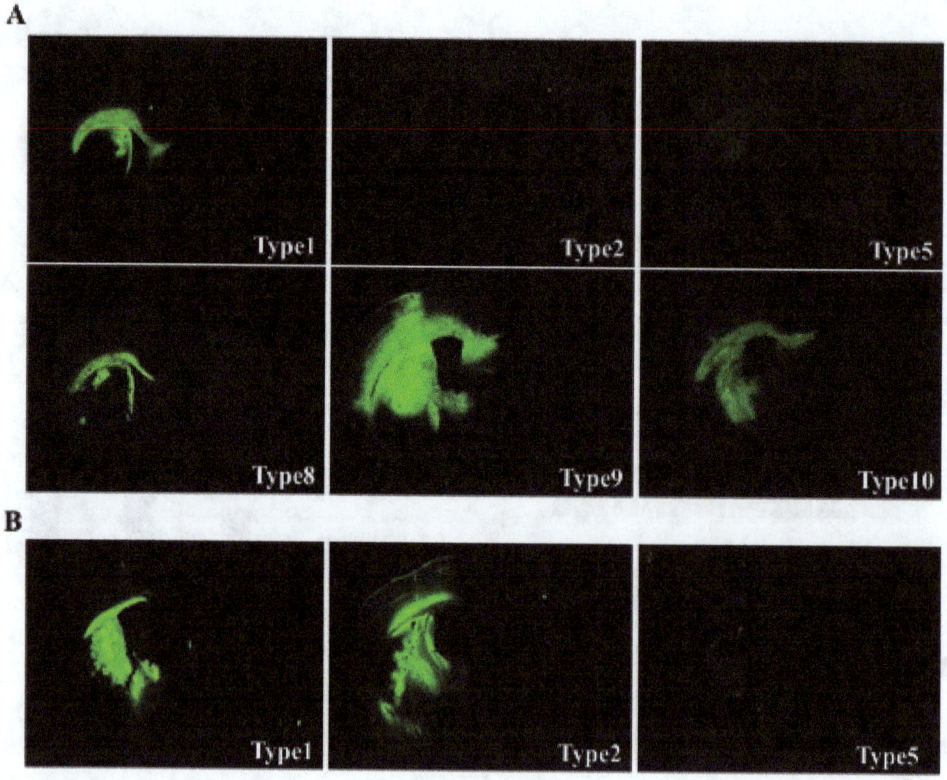

Figure 2. Brain-directed injection of AAV vectors encoding green fluorescent protein gene (AAV/GFP). Approximately 2.0×10^{10} vg of AAV/GFP vectors (serotypes 1, 2, 5, 8, 9, and 10) were injected into the right striatum over a period of 5 min using a Hamilton syringe with a 33-G blunt-tip needle. Expression of GFP was analyzed using fluorescent microscopy at 2 weeks (A) and 2 months (B) post administration.

4.1. Systemic administration of AAV vectors for gene transfer to CNS

4.1.1. Systemic administration of AAV vectors during the neonatal period

Systemic administration of AAV vectors is a promising approach for widespread organ transduction, though the BBB is an obstacle to the transduction of the CNS. To overcome this problem, one possibility is to administer the vector during the neonatal period, when the BBB is immature. We injected AAV/GFP vectors (serotypes 1, 8, 9, and 10: 1.5×10^{11} vg each) into the jugular veins of neonatal mice and then used diaminobenzidine (DAB) staining to examine GFP expression. GFP signals were detected throughout the entire brain after injection of any of these serotypes. Efficient gene transfer was obtained by AAV9/GFP or AAV10/GFP vector injection (Fig. 4A). Fig. 4B shows immunohistochemical staining of GFP in the brain by systemic neonatal injection of AAV9/GFP vectors. GFP expression was detected throughout the brain, including the olfactory bulb, cerebral cortex, hippocampus, and brainstem, and the spinal cord was also transduced efficiently. However, after the use of the AAV8/GFP vector, widespread transduction in the brain was detected 2 weeks after injection. Moreover, global

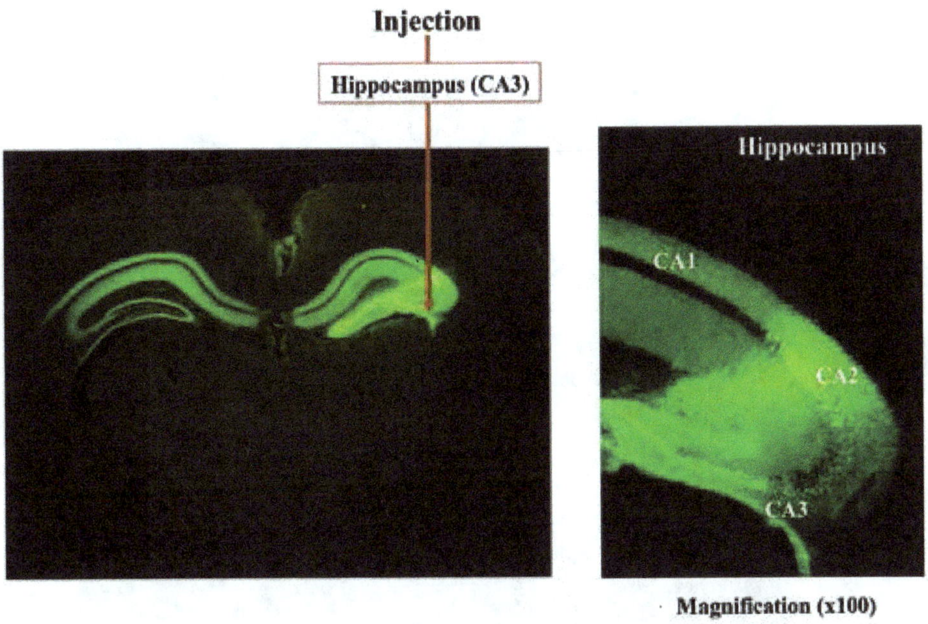

Figure 3. Brain-directed injection of AAV1/GFP vectors into hippocampus (CA3). The CA3 regions of the hippocampus of 7-month-old mice were injected with AAV1/GFP vectors (8.0 x 10^9 vg) and examined 5 months later. Using a fluorescent microscope, slices of the hippocampal regions were analyzed for GFP expression.

expression of GFP was sustained for at least 18 months (Fig. 4C). Immunohistochemical staining revealed the presence of GFP within GFAP-positive astrocytes, NeuN-positive neurons, and Calbindin-positive Purkinje cells [6]. These findings suggest that systemic neonatal administration of AAV is an effective means of delivering transgenes to target neuronal systems.

4.1.2. Systemic administration of AAV vectors after the neonatal period

It is our experience that AAV vectors are able to pass through the BBB for at least 2 weeks after birth, but within 6 weeks, all AAV vectors lose the ability to cross the BBB [6]. Therefore, to transduce the CNS of adult mice, double-stranded (or self-complementary) AAV vectors (dsAAV) must be used [12]. When we injected single-stranded (ss) AAV9 or dsAAV9 vectors encoding GFP into the tail veins of 8-week-old mice and assessed GFP expression immunohistochemically, minimal expression was detected in mice administered ssAAV9, whereas efficient GFP expression was achieved throughout the entire brain using dsAAV9 (Fig. 5). Thus, systemic administration of the dsAAV9 vector appears to be an effective means of transducing the CNS in adult mice. It was demonstrated that combined injection of AAV vectors with mannitol [13, 14] or use of ultrasound-targeted microbubble destruction [15] enhances gene expression in the brain after systemic injection of AAV vectors. Therefore, to improve gene delivery in the brain, systemic administration of the dsAAV9 vector, along with these strategies, may be a powerful tool for transduction to the CNS.

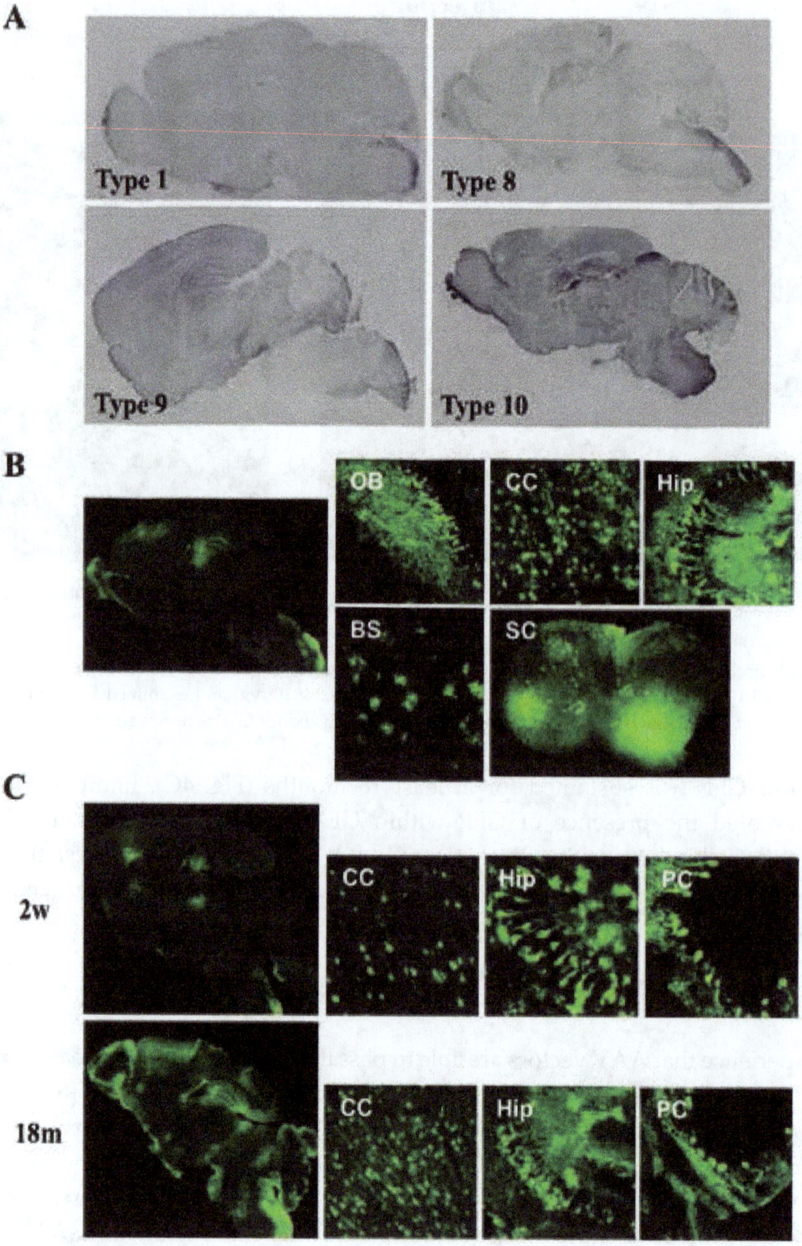

OB, olfactory bulb; CC, cerebral cortex; Hip, hippocampus; PC, Purkinje cells in the cerebellum; BS, brain stem; SC, spinal cord.

Figure 4. Direct comparison of AAV serotypes to transduce CNS by neonatal systemic injection. (A) After serotype-1, -8, -9, or -10 AAV/GFP vectors were intravenously injected into neonatal C57BL/6 mice, cerebral GFP expression was analyzed by DAB staining 4 weeks after injection. Representative brain images showing immunohistochemistry using an anti-GFP antibody after AAV9/GFP (B) and AAV8/GFP (C) injection.

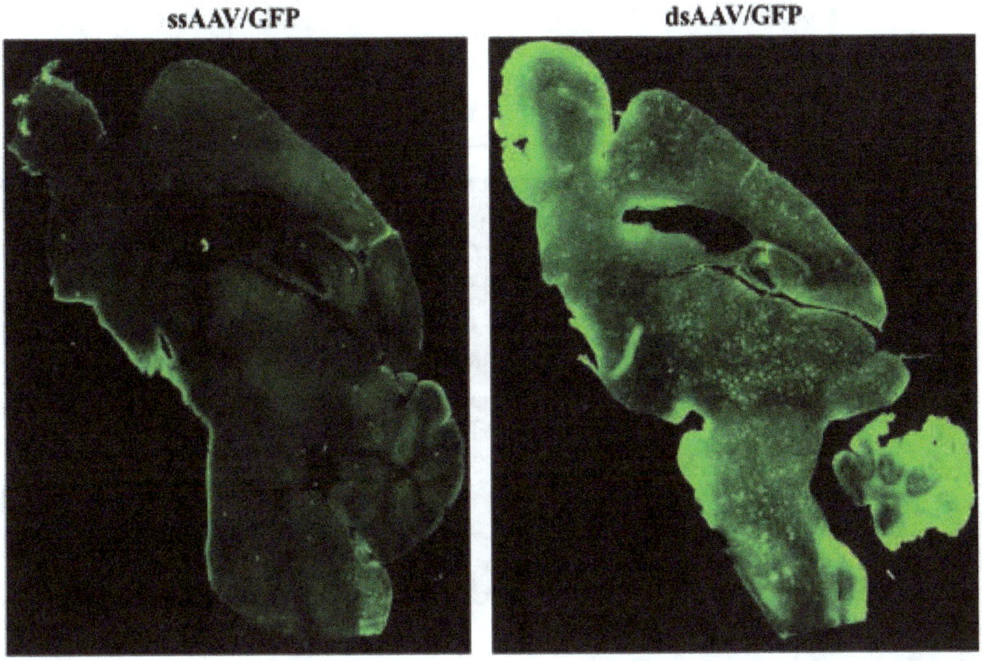

Figure 5. Immunohistochemical staining of brain sections of adult mice following systemic injection of ssAAV9/GFP or dsAAV9/GFP vectors. After 7.0 x 10^{12} vg of AAV9/GFP vectors were injected via tail veins of adult (7-week-old) mice, expression of GFP was analyzed using fluorescent microscopy at 5 weeks post administration.

4.2. Intracerebroventricular and intrathecal injection of AAV vectors

Another strategy for achieving global gene transfer into the CNS through systemic administration is vector delivery into the cerebrospinal fluid (CSF). There are two approaches to delivering an AAV vector into the CSF: intracerebroventricular injection and intrathecal injection. To evaluate the feasibility of intracerebroventricular injection, AAV1/GFP vectors were injected into the right lateral ventricle. Following the injection, GFP expression was broadly distributed in the choroid plexus and ependymal cells throughout the cerebral ventricles (Fig. 6A). Coronal brain sections revealed widespread diffusion of AAV1 from the injection site to the contralateral, anterior lateral and third ventricles, as well as the fourth ventricles via the cerebral aqueduct [16]. GFP expression was mainly confined to the choroid plexus and ependymal cells, with little or no detection of GFP in the brain parenchyma or spinal cord. Similarly, when we administered the AAV1/GFP vector intrathecally, GFP expression was broadly distributed throughout the brain (Fig. 6B). In addition, large numbers of nerve fibers in the dorsal spinal cord and the neuronal cell bodies in the dorsal root ganglia were also efficiently transduced [17]. Thus, it can be concluded that both intracerebroventricular and intrathecal injection of AAV vectors are useful for transduction of the CNS, especially if one wants to also transduce the peripheral nervous system.

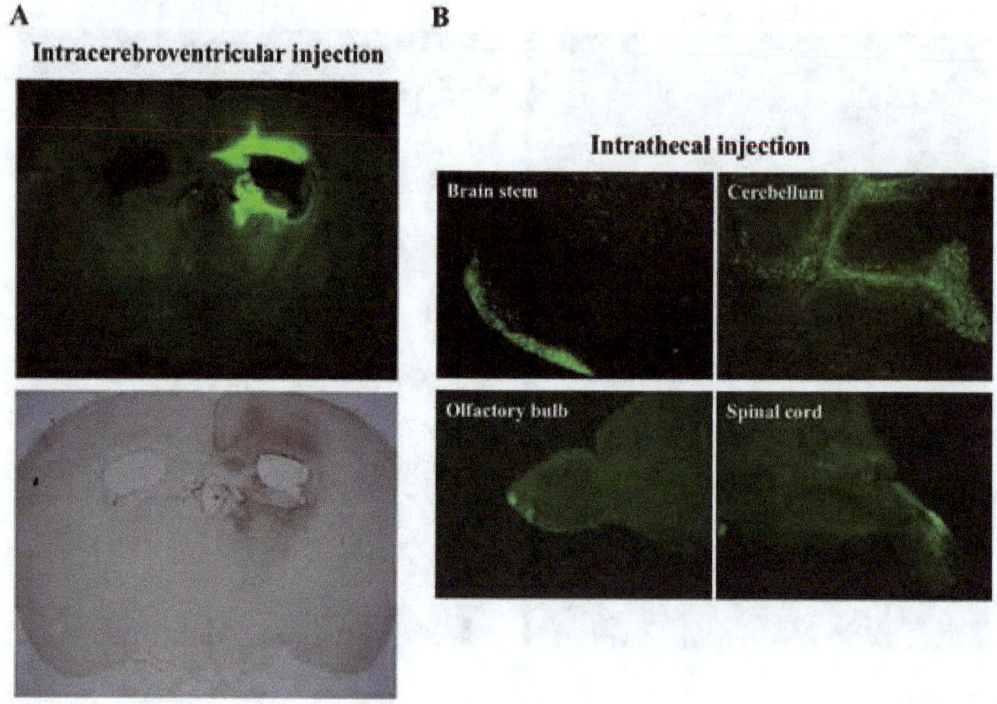

Figure 6. Expression of GFP in the brain after intracerebroventricular or intrathecal injection of AAV vectors. (A) After injection of AAV1/GFP vectors into the right lateral ventricle, GFP expression in the brain was analyzed by fluorescence microscopy (upper panel) or immunostaining with DAB staining (lower panel). (B) AAV1/GFP vectors were injected into the posterior cistern of 8-week-old mice and the brains were examined 8 weeks after injection. GFP expression was monitored by fluorescence microscopy.

5. Application of AAV vectors to CNS disorders

As summarized above, AAV vectors are an effective means of delivering genes into the CNS, thanks to their ability to transduce post-mitotic neurons and mediate efficient and stable transduction. Indeed, the utility of directly delivered AAVs has been demonstrated in numerous preclinical studies, and they are currently being used in clinical trials of treatments for Alzheimer's disease [18, 19], Parkinson's disease [20, 21], Canavan's disease [22], and Batten's disease [23, 24], among others. We also evaluated the utility of brain directed [25], intracerebroventricular [16], intrathecal [17], and intravenous neonatal administration [26] of AAV vectors for the treatment of metachromatic leukodystrophy (MLD), an inherited lysosomal storage disease with severe neurological symptoms. When we injected AAV9 vectors expressing human arylsulfatase A (AAV9/ASA) into the jugular vein of newborn MLD model mice, efficient ASA expression was detected throughout the entire brain (Fig. 7A) and peripheral nervous system (Fig. 7C), suppressing the accumulation of sulfatides in both CNS (Fig. 7B) and PNS (Fig. 7D). Moreover, the treated mice showed a greater ability to traverse narrow balance beams than untreated mice [26]. These data clearly demonstrate that MLD model mice can be effectively treated through systemic administration of AAV9/ASA vector to neonates. Thus, neonatal gene therapy is one approach with the potential to overcome the limitation imposed by the BBB on treating genetic disorders of the CNS. Other advantages of systemic gene transfer to neonates with genetic disease over treatment of adults are as follows: (1) because the immune system is immature, recipients are immunologically tolerant of the vector; (2) it may prevent early onset of genetic diseases; (3) neonates can be effectively treated with a smaller amount of vectors than adults; and (4) nearly all organs are efficiently transduced. Systemic neonatal gene therapy thus appears to be a promising method for treating systemic genetic diseases with neurological symptoms.

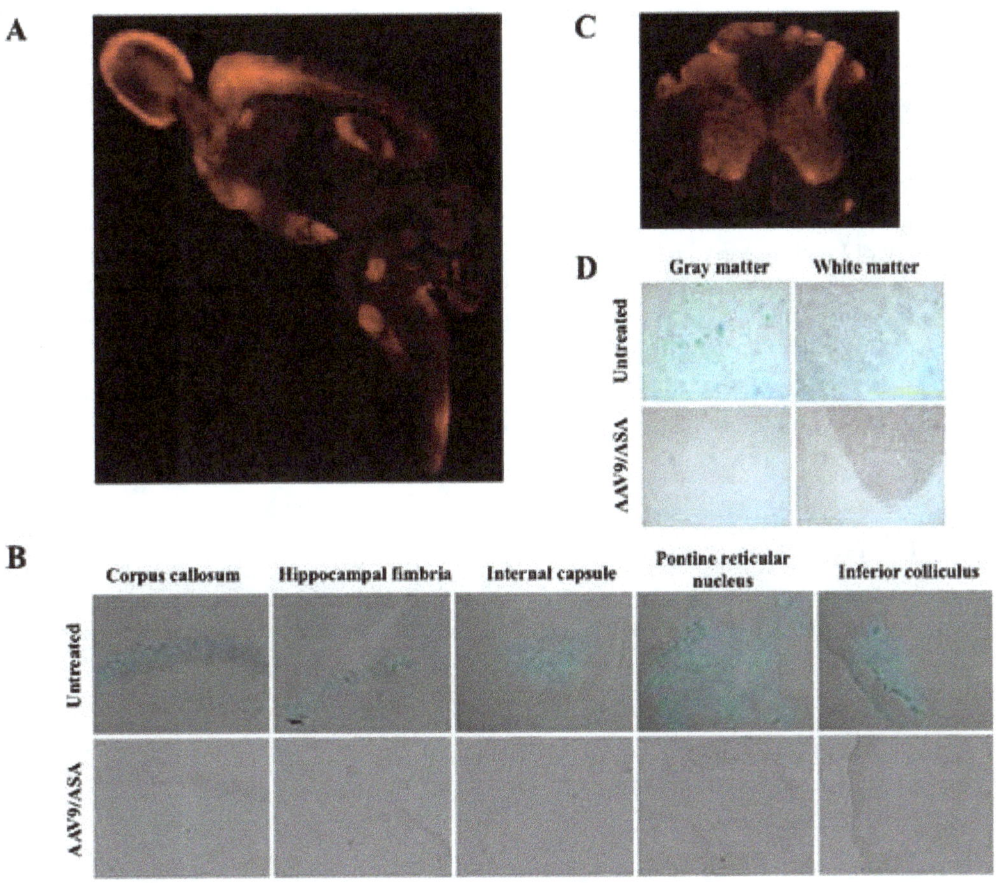

Figure 7. Correction of sulfatide storage by neonatal systemic injection of AAV9/ASA vectors. After injection of AAV9/ASA into the jugular vein of newborn MLD mice, ASA expression in the brain (A) and spinal cord (C) was analyzed by immunohistochemistry using an anti-ASA antibody at 15 months after injection. Correction of sulfatide storage in the brain (B) and spinal cord (D) was analyzed by alcian blue staining.

6. Summary and future developments

In summary, AAV vectors are a promising tool to transduce both the CNS and the spinal cord. Following a single systemic injection, AAV vectors cross the BBB and mediate widespread gene transduction throughout the brain, including the cerebral cortex, cerebellum, olfactory bulb, and brain stem. Recently, to obtain more efficient transduction, a new AAV vector serotype [27] or tyrosine mutant capsid [2] was developed. In addition, Rafi et al. succeeded in treating a mouse model of Krabbe disease (twitcher mice) by administering a combination of intracerebroventricular, intracerebellar, and intravenous injections of AAV vectors to neonates [28]. This suggests that administration of AAV vectors via several routes could prove highly useful for efficient and long-term overexpression or downregulation of genes throughout the CNS and spinal cord and could be a useful means of treating genetic neurological diseases.

Acknowledgements

We thank Dr. James Wilson (University of Pennsylvania), Dr. R. Jude Samulski (University of North Carolina), Dr. Robert M. Kotin (National Institutes of Health), Dr. David W. Russell (University of Washington), Dr. Arun Srivastava (University of Florida College of Medicine), and Dr. A. Dusty Miller (Fred Hunchins Cancer Research Center) for kindly providing AAV packaging or vector plasmids. We also thank Dr. Toshiyuki Kurai, Dr. Naotaka Iwamoto, Dr. Yoshiyuki Yamazaki, Dr. Yukihiko Hirai, and Dr. Yuki Oue for the joint research and helpful discussions. This work was supported in part by grants from the Ministry of Health and Welfare of Japan and the Ministry of Education, Science and Culture of Japan.

Author details

Koichi Miyake*, Noriko Miyake and Takashi Shimada

*Address all correspondence to: kmiyake@nms.ac.jp

Department of Biochemistry and Molecular Biology, Division of Gene Therapy, Research Center for Advanced Medical Technology, Nippon Medical School, Japan

References

[1] Grieger, J.C. and R.J. Samulski, Adeno-associated virus vectorology, manufacturing, and clinical applications. Methods Enzymol, 2012. 507: pp. 229–54.

[2] Zolotukhin, I., et al., Improved Adeno-associated Viral Gene Transfer to Murine Glioma. J Genet Syndr Gene Ther, 2013. 4(133).

[3] Gray, S.J., Gene therapy and neurodevelopmental disorders. Neuropharmacology, 2013. 68: pp. 136–42.

[4] Weinberg, M.S., R.J. Samulski, and T.J. McCown, Adeno-associated virus (AAV) gene therapy for neurological disease. Neuropharmacology, 2013. 69: pp. 82–8.

[5] Gray, S.J., et al., Preclinical differences of intravascular AAV9 delivery to neurons and glia: a comparative study of adult mice and nonhuman primates. Mol Ther, 2011. 19(6): pp. 1058–69.

[6] Miyake, N., et al., Global gene transfer into the CNS across the BBB after neonatal systemic delivery of single-stranded AAV vectors. Brain Res, 2011. 1389: pp. 19–26.

[7] Skubis-Zegadlo, J., A. Stachurska, and M. Malecki, Vectrology of adeno-associated viruses (AAV). Med Wieku Rozwoj, 2013. 17(3): pp. 202–6.

[8] Tajes, M., et al., The blood-brain barrier: structure, function and therapeutic approaches to cross it. Mol Membr Biol, 2014. 31(5): pp. 152–67.

[9] Aronovich, E.L. and P.B. Hackett, Lysosomal storage disease: gene therapy on both sides of the blood-brain barrier. Mol Genet Metab, 2015. 114(2): pp. 83–93.

[10] Castle, M.J., et al., Adeno-associated virus serotypes 1, 8, and 9 share conserved mechanisms for anterograde and retrograde axonal transport. Hum Gene Ther, 2014. 25(8): pp. 705–20.

[11] Castle, M.J., et al., Long-distance axonal transport of AAV9 is driven by dynein and kinesin-2 and is trafficked in a highly motile Rab7-positive compartment. Mol Ther, 2014. 22(3): pp. 554–66.

[12] McCarty, D.M., P.E. Monahan, and R.J. Samulski, Self-complementary recombinant adeno-associated virus (scAAV) vectors promote efficient transduction independently of DNA synthesis. Gene Ther, 2001. 8(16): pp. 1248–54.

[13] Burger, C., et al., Systemic mannitol-induced hyperosmolality amplifies rAAV2-mediated striatal transduction to a greater extent than local co-infusion. Mol Ther, 2005. 11(2): pp. 327–31.

[14] Mastakov, M.Y., et al., Combined injection of rAAV with mannitol enhances gene expression in the rat brain. Mol Ther, 2001. 3(2): pp. 225–32.

[15] Huang, Q., et al., Effective gene transfer into central nervous system following ultrasound-microbubbles-induced opening of the blood-brain barrier. Ultrasound Med Biol, 2012. 38(7): pp. 1234–43.

[16] Yamazaki, Y., et al., Targeted gene transfer into ependymal cells through intraventricular injection of AAV1 vector and long-term enzyme replacement via the CSF. Sci Rep, 2014. 4: pp. 5506.

[17] Iwamoto, N., et al., Global diffuse distribution in the brain and efficient gene delivery to the dorsal root ganglia by intrathecal injection of adeno-associated viral vector serotype 1. J Gene Med, 2009. 11(6): pp. 498–505.

[18] Pillai, J.A. and J.L. Cummings, Clinical trials in predementia stages of Alzheimer disease. Med Clin North Am, 2013. 97(3): pp. 439–57.

[19] Rafii, M.S., et al., A phase1 study of stereotactic gene delivery of AAV2-NGF for Alzheimer's disease. Alzheimers Dement, 2014. 10(5): pp. 571–81.

[20] Mittermeyer, G., et al., Long-term evaluation of a phase 1 study of AADC gene therapy for Parkinson's disease. Hum Gene Ther, 2012. 23(4): pp. 377–81.

[21] Bartus, R.T., et al., Safety/feasibility of targeting the substantia nigra with AAV2-neurturin in Parkinson patients. Neurology, 2013. 80(18): pp. 1698–701.

[22] McPhee, S.W., et al., Immune responses to AAV in a phase I study for Canavan disease. J Gene Med, 2006. 8(5): pp. 577–88.

[23] Souweidane, M.M., et al., Gene therapy for late infantile neuronal ceroid lipofuscinosis: neurosurgical considerations. J Neurosurg Pediatr, 2010. 6(2): pp. 115–22.

[24] Worgall, S., et al., Treatment of late infantile neuronal ceroid lipofuscinosis by CNS administration of a serotype 2 adeno-associated virus expressing CLN2 cDNA. Hum Gene Ther, 2008. 19(5): pp. 463–74.

[25] Kurai, T., et al., AAV1 mediated co-expression of formylglycine-generating enzyme and arylsulfatase a efficiently corrects sulfatide storage in a mouse model of metachromatic leukodystrophy. Mol Ther, 2007. 15(1): pp. 38–43.

[26] Miyake, N., et al., Long-term correction of biochemical and neurological abnormalities in MLD mice model by neonatal systemic injection of an AAV serotype 9 vector. Gene Ther, 2014. 21(4): pp. 427–33.

[27] Lawlor, P.A., et al., Efficient gene delivery and selective transduction of glial cells in the mammalian brain by AAV serotypes isolated from nonhuman primates. Mol Ther, 2009. 17(10): pp. 1692–702.

[28] Rafi, M.A., et al., Extended normal life after AAVrh10-mediated gene therapy in the mouse model of Krabbe disease. Mol Ther, 2012. 20(11): pp. 2031–42.

6

AAV Biology, Infectivity and Therapeutic Use from Bench to Clinic

Melisa A. Vance, Angela Mitchell and Richard J. Samulski

Abstract

Adeno-associated virus (AAV) has been isolated from numerous vertebrate species since 1966. Besides its wide and promiscuous tropism, AAV infection does not result in considerable toxicity or pathogenicity and is capable of achieving adequate and long-term levels of gene transfer, especially following generation of the AAV recombinant variant: rAAV. Due to these properties, rAAV has gained special attention as a viral vector for gene therapy in the last decade. Currently, there are 130 clinical trials taking place worldwide for several diseases testing the safety and efficacy profiles of rAAV. During preclinical and clinical studies, several challenges have arisen in terms of reaching the full therapeutic potential of rAAV, such as efficient delivery of the virus in a targeted and specific manner to a desired tissue. Importantly, the development of immune responses towards the viral capsids poses an obstacle to rAAV applicability in the clinical setting. Numerous approaches have been developed in order to tailor an optimized therapeutic virus for treating specific diseases, including the use of different AAV serotypes or the creation of recombinant capsid variants with distinctive transduction and immunological profiles. This chapter reviews current information on rAAV clinical trials and the potential for combining rAAV platform with other technologies, such as induced pluripotent cells and gene editing.

Keywords: Adeno-associated virus, Gene therapy, Clinical trials

1. Introduction

Gene therapy is currently one of the most promising technologies for the treatment and/or cure of several genetic diseases. Furthermore, it has the potential to battle inherited disorders as well as acquired diseases. By inducing modification of the gene pool, gene therapy aims to permanently and non-invasively treat the disease. Among the gene modifications that the therapy allows, a gene could be added, by direct introduction of a gene copy, silenced, by administering shRNA or siRNA, or removed, by the ZFN technology. Therefore, the spectrum of diseases that could potentially benefit from this technology is expanding.

Even though the idea of gene transfer has been pursued for decades using an array of diverse delivery approaches, several setbacks hampered its success for some time. In 1999, the death of Jesse Gelsinger after receiving an adenoviral-based gene therapy for the treatment of severe combined immunodeficiency disorder forced the halt on gene therapy progress [1]. Following this tragic incident, a more serious regulatory scrutiny was established and the use of alternative viral and nonviral vectors was investigated. Among viral platforms for gene delivery, adeno-associated virus (AAV) emerged in 1965 and has attracted much attention since then because the virus is not pathogenic, does not induce significant immune response and/or toxicity to humans while it allows long-term transgene expression.

2. Emergence of rAAV as a therapeutic platform

Adeno-associated virus was first discovered in 1965 as a contamination of rhesus monkey kidney cell cultures that were infected with adenovirus stocks [2]. Initially, the virus was called defective as it was incapable of self-replicating in the absence of a helper virus, adenovirus or herpesvirus. Later, it was classified as a member of the Parvovirus family, genus Dependovirus.

Further investigation determined that it is a small virus (approximately 20 nm) composed of an icosahedral protein capsid, which contains single-stranded DNA of 4.7 kb. The viral genome is flanked at each end by inverted terminal repeats sequences of 145 bp called ITRs. These sequences self-assemble into hairpin structures, generating a double-stranded sequence, which serves as a template for replication. The viral genome encodes for two proteins: Rep and Cap. Rep is required for single-stranded DNA replication and packaging. Cap is necessary to form the viral capsid and transduce cells efficiently.

AAV has never been associated with a disease or pathology [3]. Furthermore, due to the homology between the Rep-binding element present on the ITR, and the rAAVS1 sequence found on human chromosome 19, the viral genome can result in integration into the human genome [4]. This last feature is important because it shows that the virus can facilitate long-term expression of the viral genome. Additionally, specific integration of AAV in a defined locus minimizes the risks of mutagenesis due to random insertions, as other vectors do.

However, several genetic modifications of AAV have been performed in order to guarantee further safety for its translation into the clinic. First, the gene required for viral replication, called Rep, and the element required for site-specific integration were eliminated from the AAV genome. Therefore, this AAV variant, called recombinant vector (rAAV), will exist in an extrachromosomal state with very low integration efficiency into the genomic DNA, reducing the possibility of inducing random mutagenesis. Second, packaging of the rAAV genomic DNA was modified, incorporating a self-complementary rAAV genome rather than a single-stranded DNA genome [5]. Self-complementary virus differentiates from the recombinant virus in its ability to refold into double-stranded DNA, bypassing the synthesis of the second strand. This substitution has the advantage of reducing the lag time prior to transgene expression and consequently, increasing the biological efficiency of gene delivery. However, it significantly reduces the size of the transgene that could be inserted into the rAAV genome, from 5 kb to 3 kb. Third, several capsid serotypes that carry the rAAV genome have been identified and isolated.

3. AAV capsid serotypes

Even though serotype 2 has been more extensively used and studied, other capsids are gaining more interest. The existence of a variety of serotypes makes rAAV gene therapy more attractive as they differ in infectivity rates and tissue specificity. For instance, a biodistribution analysis of different AAV capsid serotypes carrying the same luciferase reporter gene showed a broad dissemination of the virus in the mouse following intravenous administration [6]. In an attempt to study phylogenetic relationships among serotypes 1 to 12, their capsid amino acid sequences (NCBI reference sequences: NP_049542.1, YP_680426.1, NP_043941.1, NP_044927.1, YP_068409.1, AAB95450.1, YP_077178.1, YP_077180.1, AAS99264.1, AY631965.1, AY631966.1 and AX753364.1) were aligned using ClustalOmega [7] and JalView, version 2.8.2 (Figure 1). According to the degree of similarity that a residue has with the consensus residue for each column, a certain color is given. Intensive blue corresponds to more than 80% agreement, light blue to agreement between 60% and 80%, light grey to agreement between 40% and 60% and white for agreement lower or equal to 40%. Below the alignment, conservation, quality and consensus information are provided. Conservation graphic highlights alignment regions where physicochemical properties are conserved. The more intense the color, the more conserved the physicochemical property is in the column. Alignment quality indicates the likelihood of observing substitutions in a particular amino acidic position. Finally, the residue consensus provides the most common residues and their percentage for each column of the alignment.

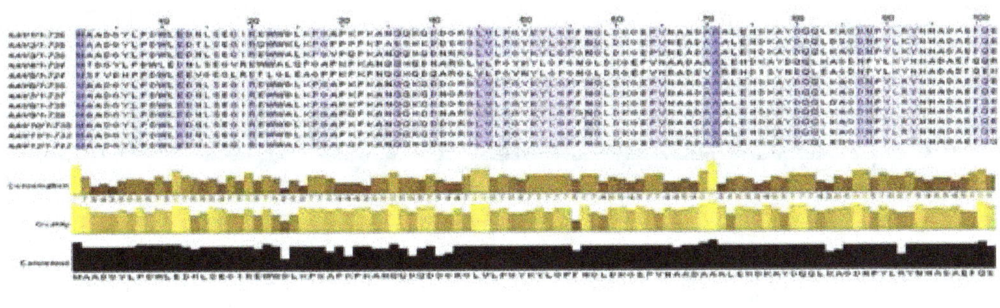

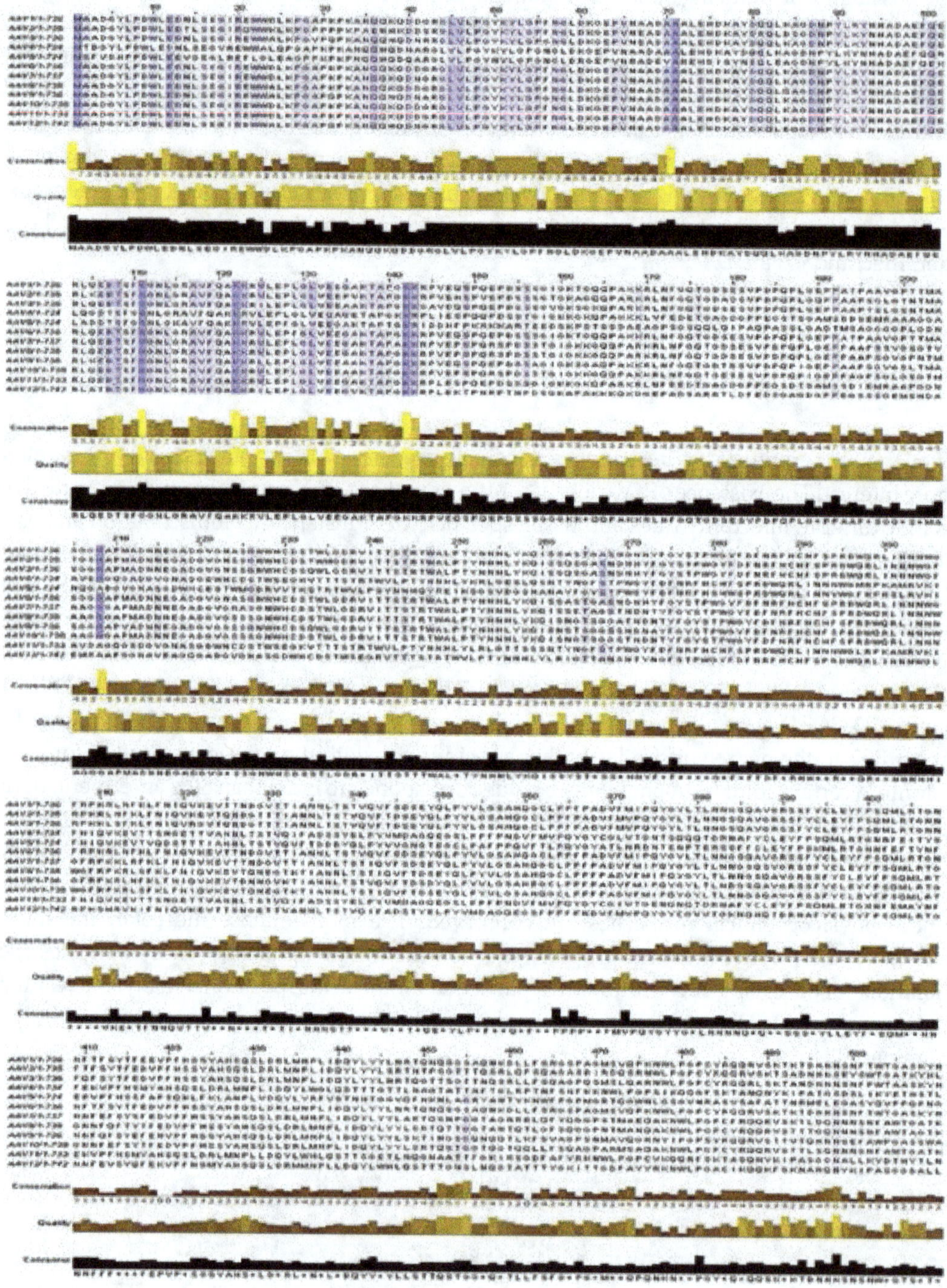

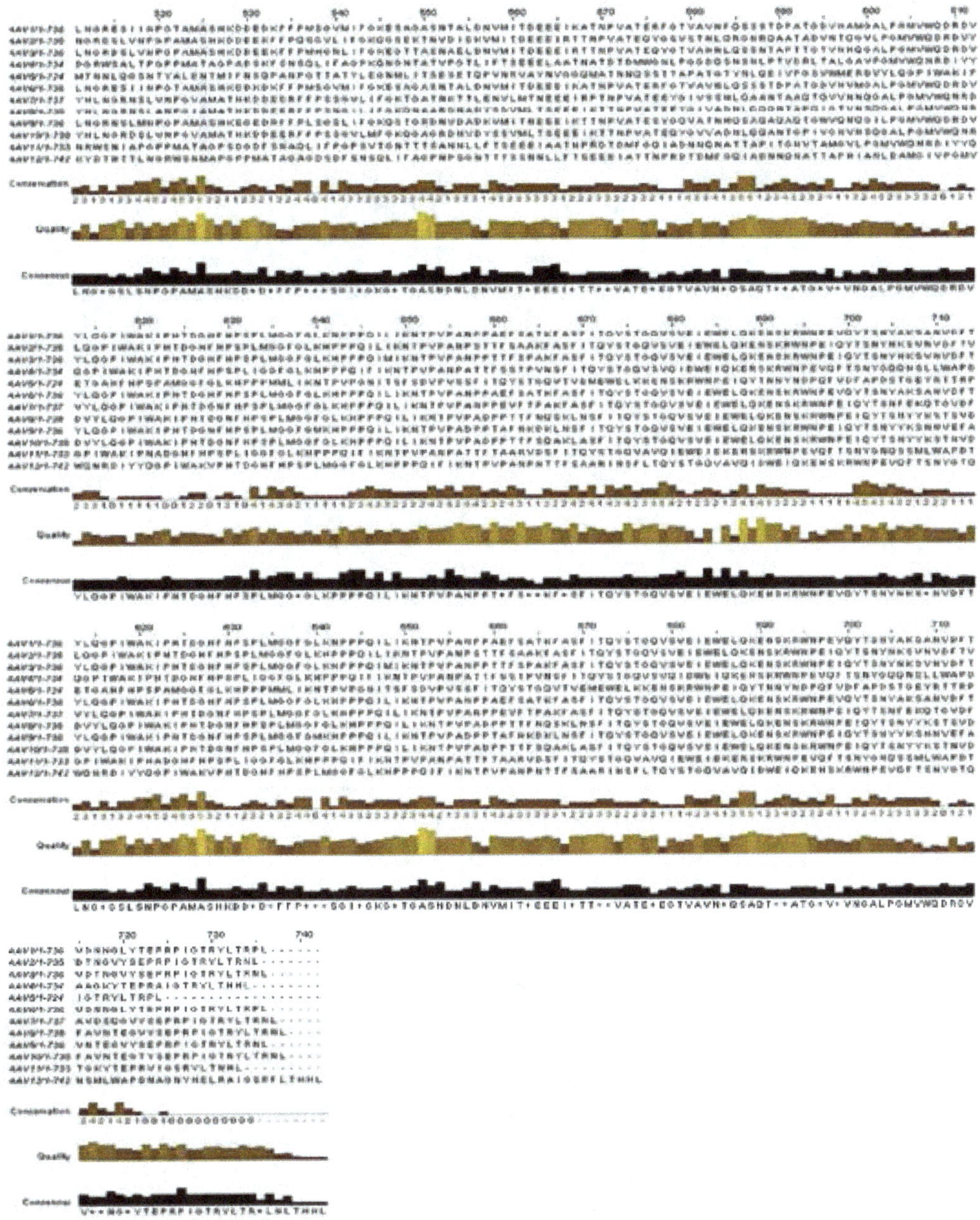

Figure 1. Multi-sequence alignment of AAV serotypes from 1-12 using ClustalOmega and JalView software.

Following the multisequence alignment, the percentage of sequence homology was determined by performing BLAST alignments of dual AAV sequences at the time (Figure 2a). Furthermore, the phylogenetic relationships among these AAV serotypes were determined by creating a neighbor-joining tree (Figure 2b), which uses the percent identity [8].

A

	AAV1	AAV2	AAV3	AAV4	AAV5	AAV6	AAV7	AAV8	AAV9	AAV10	AAV11	AAV12
AAV1	100%	83%	86%	64%	59%	99%	85%	84%	82%	85%	67%	61%
AAV2	83%	100%	87%	61%	58%	83%	82%	83%	82%	84%	63%	60%
AAV3	86%	87%	100%	63%	58%	87%	84%	85%	83%	85%	65%	61%
AAV4	64%	61%	63%	100%	53%	63%	64%	64%	63%	64%	82%	79%
AAV5	59%	58%	58%	53%	100%	59%	59%	58%	57%	57%	53%	53%
AAV6	99%	83%	87%	63%	59%	100%	85%	84%	82%	85%	66%	61%
AAV7	85%	82%	84%	64%	59%	85%	100%	88%	81%	88%	67%	62%
AAV8	84%	83%	85%	64%	58%	84%	88%	100%	85%	93%	66%	62%
AAV9	82%	82%	83%	63%	57%	82%	81%	85%	100%	86%	64%	60%
AAV10	85%	84%	85%	64%	57%	85%	88%	93%	86%	100%	67%	61%
AAV11	67%	63%	65%	82%	53%	66%	67%	66%	64%	67%	100%	84%
AAV12	61%	60%	61%	79%	53%	61%	62%	62%	60%	61%	84%	100%

B

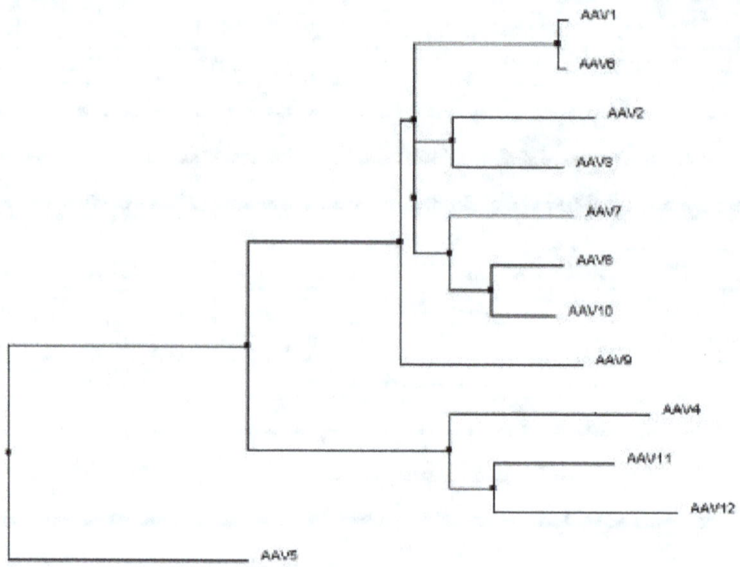

Figure 2. A, Blast alignment of dual combination of AAV serotypes to determine percentage of homology. **B**, Phylogenetic tree to determine phylogenetic relationships among the studied serotypes.

This tree shows that serotype AAV5 has the most divergent amino acid capsid sequence, sharing between 53% and 59% homology with the rest of the human serotypes that have been discovered so far (highlighted in orange). AAV4 also shows a considerable degree of divergence, when comparing sequences of AAV1 to 9 (between 53% and 64%). However, AAV4 shares a more recent common ancestor with serotypes 11 and 12. Furthermore, AAV1 and AAV6 share 99% homology, being the closest AAV serotypes in sequence. The most common AAV serotype, AAV2, is closer in amino acid sequence to all the AAV serotypes, especially AAV3, but greatly differs from serotypes AAV5, AAV4 and therefore, AAV11 and AAV12. Serotypes AAV8 and AAV10 are also very close between each other, sharing 93% amino acid sequence homology. These differences in sequences were observed in other studies, not only when analyzing the sequence similarities but also when studying antigenic reactivities [9]. Remarkably, the variabilities in amino acidic sequences were mainly localized in the looped-out domains that are exposed to the surface of the capsid, rather than evenly distributed along the capsid protein sequence [10]. More interesting, Gao et al. compared phylogenies from human and nonhuman primate AAV serotypes. They observed that human AAV4 and AAV5 serotypes were the most divergent, and after they emerged, the rest of the viruses were clustered in groups that included human serotypes (AAV1, AAV6, AAV2, AAV3 and AAV9), exclusive rhesus serotypes (AAV7) or a combination of both (AAV8). Considering that human AAV serotypes share a high similarity in sequences with nonhuman AAV serotypes, they are both well disseminated and are able to cross species barriers. Therefore, there is a possibility that AAV from nonhuman primates could be used for treating human diseases. This is the case of AAVrh10, a serotype isolated from rhesus macaques. This virus was found to be significantly more efficient in transducing neurons from different areas in a healthy dog brain as compared with AAV1 or AAV5, but to a similar extent with AAV9 [11]. More importantly, the rhesus serotype is currently being tested for safety and efficacy in the clinic for the treatment of CNS diseases, such as Battens (NCT01414985 and NCT01161576, clinicaltrials.gov) and MLD (NCT01801709, clinicaltrials.gov). Additionally, a new study is planning to test the safety of this virus for delivering human alpha 1-antitrypsin cDNA to individuals with alpha 1-antitrypsin deficiency (NCT02168686, clinicaltrials.gov); although they are not yet recruiting patients.

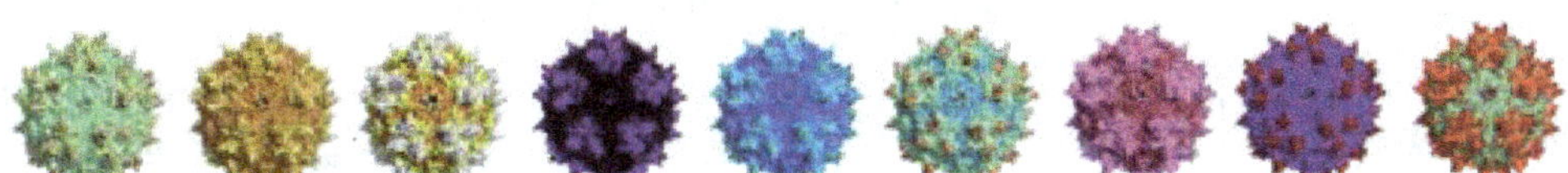

	AAV1	AAV2	AAV3	AAV4	AAV5	AAV6	AAV7	AAV8	AAV9
Mouse	Liver, heart, skeletal muscle	Liver, heart and muscle	Heart, Liver	Heart, lung, Liver	Liver	Liver, heart, skeletal muscle	Liver, skeletal muscle	Heart, Liver, brain, muscle	Liver, heart, brain, Lung, skeletal muscle

Figure 3. Biodistribution of AAV serotypes 1–9 in mouse.

According to the biodistribution study of AAV following tail vein injection into the mouse, AAV9 has the broadest tissue tropism, demonstrating robust transduction of all tested tissues other than the testes [6] (Figure 3). Moreover, it is the most efficient in reaching the brain, followed by AAV8. On the other hand, AAV7 showed strong tropism for the liver and to a lesser extent for the muscle. Meanwhile, AAV6 had more preference for the heart, in comparison to liver, lung and muscle. AAV4 was found in higher viral copies in the lung, followed by the heart. The rest of the serotypes transduced the selected tissues with lower efficiencies. AAV1 and AAV2 were more prone to reach the liver. In terms of infection kinetics, AAV7 and AAV9 were the fastest in targeting the tissue and showing expression of the reporter gene, luciferase. Meanwhile, AAV3 and AAV4 were the slowest ones. Additionally, among all the serotypes, AAV2, 3, 4 and 5 showed the lowest transduction efficiency.

The first AAV primary receptor that was identified was heparin sulfate proteoglycan (HSPG). It is the receptor that AAV2 and AAV3 bind when infecting cells (Figure 4). Even though AAV6 was shown to have moderate binding affinity for heparin, it does not have the two residues R585 and R588, that participate in AAV2 binding to HSPG. On the other hand, while sequence alignment comparison between AAV1 and AAV6 capsids revealed only a six–amino acid difference, AAV1 is not able to bind heparin. Mutagenesis analysis revealed that amino acid 531 was responsible for providing the heparin binding ability to AAV6 and not to AAV1 [12]. Furthermore, AAV1 binds both α2–3 and α2–6 *N*-linked sialic acid (SIA), same as AAV6. Interestingly, AAV5 also binds α2–3 SIA, although it only shares ~40% homology with capsid serotypes AAV1 and AAV6. Crystallography studies of AAV5 showed differences in the surface loop regions, specifically smaller HI loop and larger VR-VII loop, which are located on the depression wall at the icosahedral 2-fold axis and determine receptor binding, tissue transduction efficiency and antigenic reactivity [13].

AAV4 capsid serotype follows AAV5 in terms of low sequence similarity with the rest of the serotypes and between themselves (53% sequence homology). A study, in which sialic acids were removed from cell surfaces, by neuraminidase treatment, showed that both viruses require SIA for infectivity [14]. However, when cellular glycosylation was inhibited, only treatment with *O*-linked inhibitor decreased binding of AAV4 to cultured cells. Meanwhile, treatment with *N*-linked inhibitors of glycosylation blocked AAV5 binding to the cell surface. Resialylation experiments with neuraminidase-treated red blood cells further confirmed that AAV4 binding to SIA is through α2–3 *O*-linkage, rather than through α2–6 *N* linkage, which is the interaction that AAV5 establishes for the initial infection of a cell.

Still, currently, receptors for AAV7 and AAV8 are unknown. Glycan binding analysis on microarrays revealed that AAV7 and AAV8 did not bind to any of the glycans that commonly bind serotypes AAV1–6 [15]. However, similarly to AAV2 and AAV3, AAV8 and AAV9 interact with the 37/67 kDa laminin receptor (LamR), as a secondary receptor, for efficient internalization and transduction [16]. LamR participates in interactions of extracellular laminin1 with proteases and with the cell; therefore, it is widely distributed among human tissues. Even though, AAV2, 3, 8 and 9 serotypes mediate direct tissue transduction via interaction with the LamR molecule, they significantly differ in their tissue tropism. AAV8 and 9 are able to infect a broader spectrum of tissues, even the brain, compared to serotypes AAV2 and AAV3. This result suggests that the primary receptor or the combination of both receptors is required for viral biodistribution. At the UNC gene therapy center, the Asokan laboratory was able to identify that *N*-linked glycans with terminal galactosyl residues are involved in AAV9 tissue binding and transduction [17]. The high abundance of these glycans in various animal tissues could explain the broad tropism observed after AAV9 systemic administration.

Lastly, the brain is one of the most difficult tissues that AAV can access and infect following systemic administration. The presence of a mature blood–brain barrier constitutes a physical barrier to potential harmful molecules and infectious pathogens. Therefore, most of the AAV serotypes are not able to access the brain without direct intraparenchymal administration. However, AAV9 and AAV8 (to a lesser extent), have the capability to reach the brain following intravenous administration to neonatal or adult mice [18].

Furthermore, the rhesus serotypes AAV10 and AAV11 were found to be sequence homologous and structurally closest to the previously described serotypes AAV8 and AAV4, respectively [19].

AAV12, which was isolated from a simian adenovirus stock, showed 74% homology with AAV4 and 84% with AAVrh11. However, it does not bind SIA and appears to have strong affinity for human cancer cell lines [20].

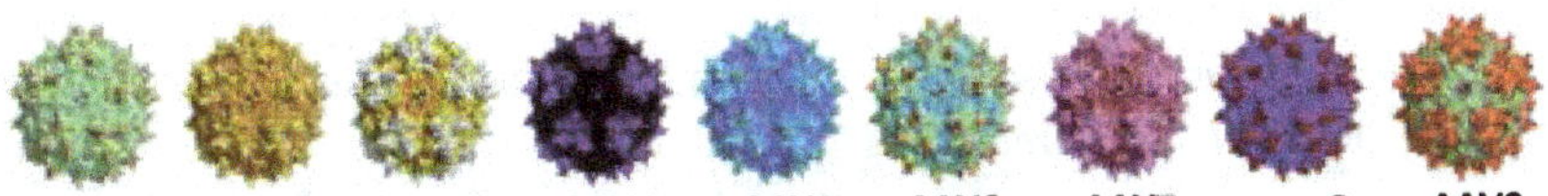

	rAAV1	rAAV2	rAAV3	rAAV4	rAAV5	rAAV6	rAAV7	rAAV8	rAAV9
Primary receptor	N-linked sialic acid	HSPG	HSPG	O-linked sialic acid	N-linked sialic acid	N-linked sialic acid; HSPG	unknown	unknown	N-linked galactose
Secondary receptor	unknown	FGFR1, HGFR, Integrins, CD9, LamR	FGFR1, HGFR, LamR	unknown	PDGFR	EGFR	unknown	LamR	LamR

Figure 4. Primary and secondary receptors used for AAV serotypes from 1 to 9 to infect and transduce cell types. HSPG, heparin sulfate proteoglycan; FGFR1 fibroblast growth factor receptor 1; PDGFRB, platelet-derived growth factor receptor beta; HGFR, met/hepatocyte growth factor receptor; EGFR, epidermal growth factor receptor; LamR, laminin receptor.

4. Preclinical studies of rAAV in large animal models

In an effort to translate the rAAV gene therapy to the clinic, preclinical studies for safety, efficient rAAV dosing and capsid transduction, transgene expression and immune responses towards the new transgene and/or the rAAV capsid were performed. In Figure 5, we summarize which serotype has been evaluated for targeting a certain disease in a large animal model, such as nonhuman primate, pig, cat, dog, rabbit and sheep. However, this section will be focused on preclinical studies using large animals for the treatment of hemophilia.

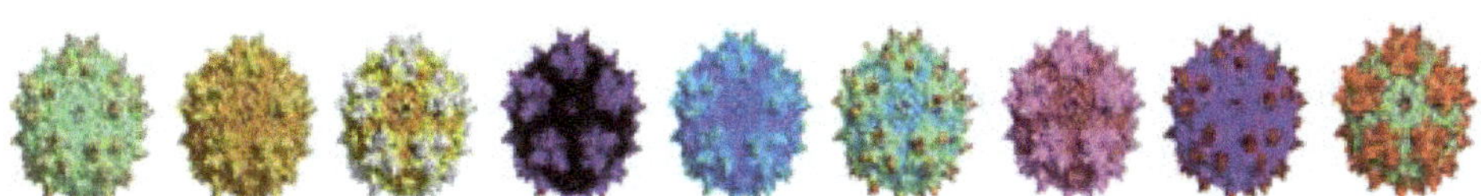

	AAV1	AAV2	AAV3	AAV4	AAV5	AAV6	AAV7	AAV8	AAV9
Large Animal	Heart, CNS and skeletal muscle	CNS, eye		Eye	CNS	Skeletal muscle and Heart, CNS		Eye, CNS	CNS, Heart and skeletal muscle

Figure 5. Diseases treated in large animal models with different AAV serotypes

5. rAAV targeting the liver for hemophilia treatment

Even though rAAV therapies for treating hemophilia in mice produced successful results, their translation into large animals, such as a dog or nonhuman primate, was not straightforward [21]. The vector efficacy does not completely follow a dose–response correlation in large animals, and it is drastically affected in the presence of an immunological response towards the viral capsids. Furthermore, in both mice and dogs, there is no direct correlation between the transgene copy numbers and the expression of the foreign protein. However, treatment of a large animal with the therapy was promising as FIX is a secreted protein and only 1%–2% normal factor IX levels is enough to correct the disease [21].

Therapies for hemophilia B were studied using different routes of rAAV gene therapy administration. Initially, intramuscular delivery of rAAV-CMV-cFIX to hemophilic dogs was pursued. A single administration of the virus generated a therapeutic FIX level in a dose-dependent manner [22]. However, the amount of antibody formation, and therefore, the success of the therapy, directly correlated with the increase in rAAV dose [23]. Considering that FIX is produced within the liver, delivery of the virus through the portal vein was also attempted. Several steps were performed in order to optimize the vector, such as the addition of a liver specific promoter, and testing different doses to determine the optimum for allowing normal levels of FIX in the dog through this route [24–26]. Mount et al. observed sustained levels of FIX between 4% and 12% at doses between 1.2×10^{12} and 3.4×10^{12} vg/kg for over 17 months in three out of four dogs [26]. The fourth dog experienced a transient correction of FIX levels for four weeks but eventually developed neutralizing antibodies against the transgene. In another study, delivery of a hyperfunctional FIX through rAAV-mediated transfer to the liver in hemophilic dogs resulted in 25% and 300% FIX levels for 1×10^{12} and 3×10^{12} vg/kg doses, respectively [27].

Studies performed with nonhuman primates generated variable outcomes, from no detection to detection up to 10% of FIX in the serum. Failure of the gene therapy was attributed to the preexistence of neutralizing antibodies against the transgene [28, 29]. However, direct administration of the rAAV vector to the liver induced some tolerance to the transgene [27, 28]. Another strategy to overcome the success of the therapy due to the presence of neutralizing antibodies consists of administration of the therapy to an early age of the animal, presumably because the immune system is not completely developed [30].

A comparison study of different administration routes for rAAV-FIX delivery on mice revealed that the same dose allowed 3-fold more transgene expression following intrahepatic rather than intramuscular or intravenous delivery [31]. Therefore, it seems that transgene delivery via rAAV virus is more successful when using the liver-directed gene route. When intrahepatic therapy was administered to dogs who suffered from hemophilia A, rAAV8 carrying the canine factor VII cDNA showed long-term correction of the phenotype, with no spontaneous bleeding episodes, no toxicity and no development of inhibitory antibodies towards the viral vector or the transgene [32]. Similarly, liver-directed rAAV-FIX therapy to dogs suffering from hemophilia B, significantly increased FIX activity to 4%–10% and remained stable for more than eight years [33]. However, direct injection of the virus to the muscle resulted in undetectable FIX levels in the dog due to the onset of an immune response.

6. Clinical trials using rAAV technology

Among the clinical trials reported in clinicaltrials.gov website, which cites ongoing studies all over the world, the United States is still the leading country conducting clinical trials with rAAV gene therapy. In 2010, 47 studies out of 70 were performed in the United States and in 2015, 44 total studies out of 66 have been sponsored by the same country. Since the first registered trial in 2004, a total of 14 studies have been completed, and three terminated prematurely. Furthermore, there are clinical trials in all phases as well as for traditional, not traditional and even recombinant serotypes (Figure 6). Worldwide, there are a total of more than 130 clinical trials testing rAAV gene therapy for the treatment of diseases (http://www.abedia.com/wiley/vectors.php).

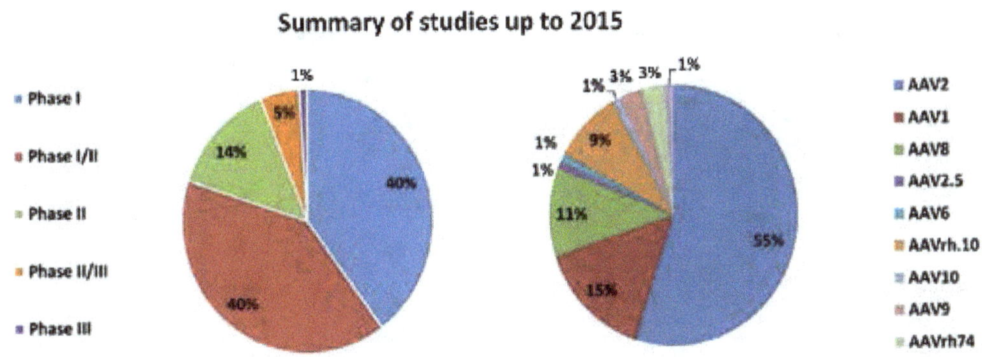

Figure 6. Statistics showing the clinical trials performed with rAAV gene therapy until 2015 according to clinicaltrials.gov. **A,** Classified according to the clinical phase. **B,** Classified according to the rAAV serotype used in the study.

7. rAAV serotypes used in clinical trials

Traditionally, the most common serotype used in clinical trials is AAV2. In 2010, sixty-two clinical trials were performed with rAAV2 vector; meanwhile, the number was reduced to thirty-six, almost half, in 2015 (89% vs. 54%) (Figure 7A). In addition, in 2010, three studies were performed with rAAV1, which increased to 10 in 2015 (4% vs 16%). Interestingly, more uncommon serotypes are acquiring an interest among the scientific community and the spectrum of serotypes being tested is increasing. Five years ago, five out of seventy clinical trials used serotypes other than rAAV1 and rAAV2. On the contrary, now in 2015, eighteen out of the current forty-nine trials are reported in clinicaltrials.org website (7% vs. 37%). For instance, the number of studies using serotype rAAV8 increased from two to seven in a five-year frame (Figure 7B).

The same results were found with the rhesus serotype rAAVrh10; initially, there was one study testing the virus; however, in 2015, six studies have taken place. To note, another rhesus rAAV serotype is being examined: rh74 for duchene muscular dystrophin. Serotypes rAAV5 and

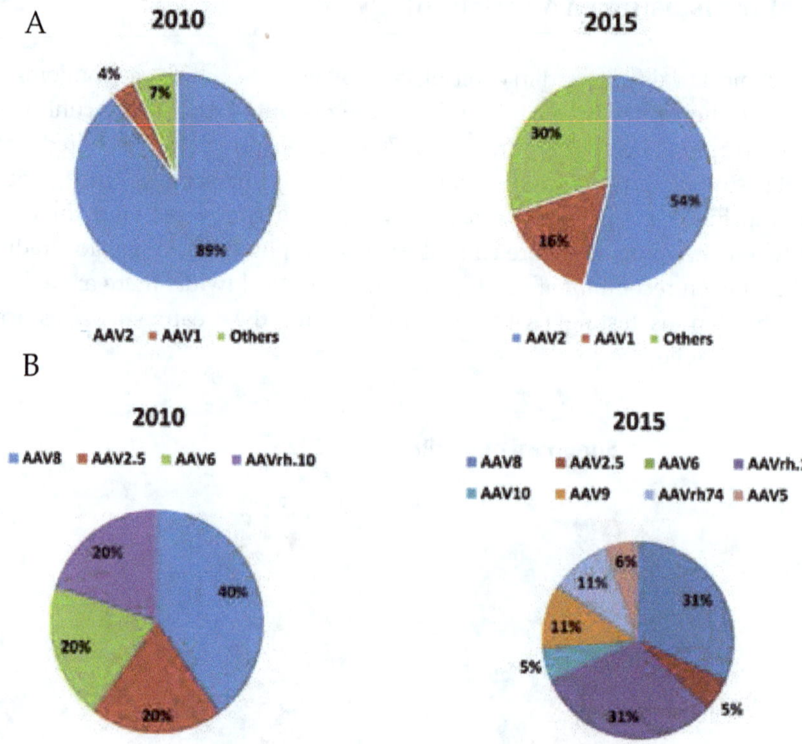

Figure 7. Statistics showing the clinical trials performed with rAAV gene therapy in 2010 and in 2015. **A,** Classified according to the use of traditional serotypes rAAV2 and rAAV1. **B,** Classified according the use of no traditional rAAV serotype.

rAAV9 also were introduced into the list of rAAV viruses in clinical trials. Similarly, phase I/ II rAAV10 trial for Sanfilippo type A syndrome started in 2011 and finished in 2014.

As Figure 8A shows, in 2010 a high percentage of the rAAV therapies were in phase I (62%) and a small percentage of the studies (17%) were testing phase I and II on the same trial. In 2015, the number of studies in phase I exclusively was reduced by 20%, compared to studies performed in 2010, and that extra 20% is testing safety and efficacy at the same time (phase I and II, 37%), probably due to the expensive costs of conducting a clinical trial.

Furthermore, the number of studies that were in phase III was reduced, as the therapies started to reach the market. For instance, in October 2012, Glybera became the first rAAV gene therapy to obtain marketing authorization from the European Commission.

Since their discovery in the 1960s as small DNA viruses contaminating cultures of simian and human adenoviruses [2, 34], AAV vectors have been tested in more than a hundred clinical trials. Completed and ongoing trials have consistently confirmed that rAAV vector delivery is safe, well tolerated by humans and efficient in transferring the therapeutic gene. Figure 8B summarizes the spectrum of diseases that have been tested with rAAV gene therapy in 2010

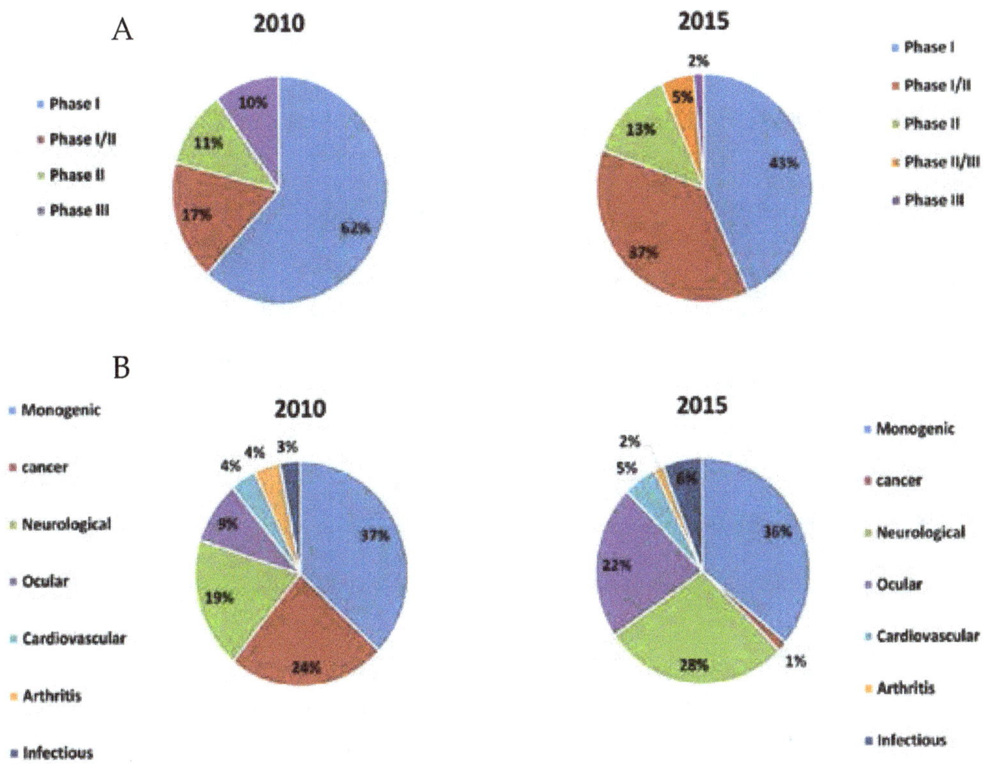

Figure 8. Statistics showing the clinical trials performed with rAAV gene therapy in 2010 and in 2015. **A,** Classified according to clinical phase. **B,** Classified according the treated disease.

and 2015. The statistics show that neurological and ocular diseases are gaining more interest, probably because they both constitute immunological privileged tissues. Figure 9 summarizes the diseases that are being treated with AAV technology, according to the serotype.

As an ocular AAV therapy, two clinical trials have tested rAAV2 therapy for the correction of Leber congenital amaurosis, an autosomal recessive disease that results in blindness. Specifically, patients who participated in these studies received the normal copy of the retinal pigment epithelium-specific 65 (RPE65) gene to correct for the deficient gene. One trial was performed in London and consisted of delivering the gene, the expression of which was driven by an endogenous RPE65 promoter, to adolescent patients [35]. On the other hand, the study performed in Philadelphia delivered the gene in the context of a constitutive promoter, to pediatric and adult patients [36, 37]. Pediatric patients treated in the US resulted in the best improvement in vision, followed by American adults. However, one out of three British patients manifested a visual function improvement. Another trial, sponsored by the University of Pennsylvania, conducted an open-label, dose-escalation phase I study on 15 patients aged between 11 and 30 years. The study examined safety and efficacy. Results showed no toxicity due to the therapy, although some adverse events were observed from the surgery procedure.

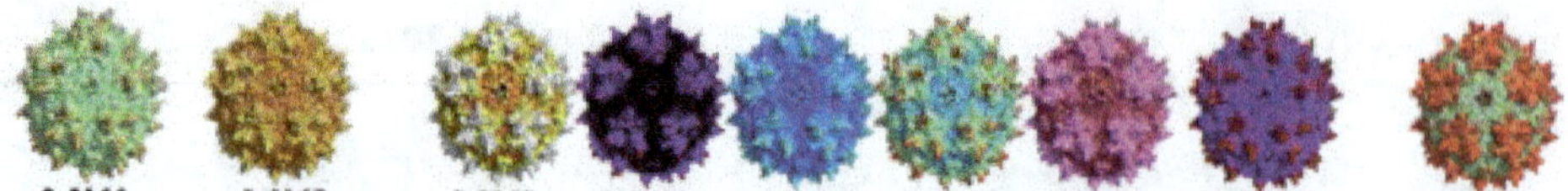

	AAV1	AAV2	AAV3	AAV4	AAV5	AAV6	AAV7	AAV8	AAV9
Condition to treat	Congenital heart failure, cardiomyopathies, Limb Girdle Muscular Dystrophy Type 2C, muscular dystrophies, α-1 antitrypsin deficiency and Lipoprotein Lipase Deficiency.	Aromatic L-amino acid decarboxylase, Parkinson's, age-related macular degeneration, retinal degenerative disorders Leber's congenital amaurosis and choroideremia, Squamous Cell Head and Neck Cancer, Alzheimer's, Hemophilia B and HIV infection			Hemophilia B			Hemophilia B, hepatitis C, X-linked Retinoschisis, Galactosialidosis	Spinal Muscular Atrophy 1, Pompe Disease

Figure 9. Diseases currently being tested in clinical trials with different rAAV serotypes.

Furthermore, visual function was improved in the 15 patients with a variable degree [38]. However, between 9 and 12 months of gene therapy administration, four of the fifteen patients experienced new pseudo-foveas in the retinal regions, for up to six years [39].

The company Sparks, which is sponsoring the studies in the US, is testing the technology developed at the Children's Hospital of Philadelphia in a phase 3 trial and expects to announce their results in 2015. If the results are promising, it could be the next rAAV gene therapy product to be launched in the market.

Among the brain diseases, Parkinson's treatment was attempted with rAAV gene therapy delivering different transgenes. Administration of glutamic acid decarboxylase (GAD) via rAAV2 produced modest efficacy improvements. Patients were injected with rAAV2 coding for GAD65 and GAD67 in the center of the subthalamic nucleus [40]. Six months following the injection, the unified Parkinson's disease rating scale decreased by 8.1 points, compared with a reduction of 4.7 points that the sham operation group evidenced. Six months later, clinical improvements were still being noticed. However, the results were modest and the protocol had some deviations. For instance, patients who showed no benefit on the primary endpoint were eliminated from the statistical analysis, arguing that the injections were off-target [41]. Administration of aromatic L-amino acid decarboxylase (AADC) gene was tested on a phase I trial that consisted of the treatment of 15 patients with moderate disease [42, 43]. The trial, sponsored by Genzyme, observed only a modest efficacy, results that were confirmed by a second study performed in Japan [44]. Similarly, phase I and II trials with the rAAV2-neurturin (CERE-120) vector from Ceregene failed to show statistically significant improvement in the rAAV-treated group compared with the group that received the sham surgery [45, 46]. As a conclusion of all these different trials, the technology is safe and is promising. However, efficacy is modest and does not justify the procedure. Further improvements could be performed, such as modification of the delivery vector, as rAAV1 and rAAV5 are more efficient in transducing the substantia nigra and caudate nucleus than rAAV2. Furthermore, viral dose increase should be considered [41]. On the other hand, long-term improvements were observed during the treatment of Canavan disease [47]. Patients were administered rAAV2 carrying the aspartoaculase gene directly to the brain parenchyma. Five years posttreatment, patients presented slower progression of brain atrophy, fewer frequent seizures and general clinical stabilization. Importantly, no serious adverse events were observed, even when one of the patients was a 3-month-old infant [48].

In a trial testing gene therapy for cardiac disease, patients received different doses (low, medium or high) of the sarcoplasmic reticulum Ca2+-ATPase (SERCA2a) gene via rAAV1 [49]. Six months following the percutaneous intracoronary infusion of the virus, several clinical parameters, such as walk test, peak maximum oxygen consumption, left ventricular end-systolic volume, cardiovascular events and time to clinical events were stabilized or even improved. Currently, a phase 2b trial is ongoing, which would test a larger patient population (NCT01643330).

The first clinical trial for rAAV gene therapy that reached the market was the product Glybera® (alipogene tiparvovec), an rAAV1 vector delivering a lipoprotein lipase variant (LPLS447X) for the treatment of lipoprotein lipase deficiency (LPLD). Lipoprotein lipase is a secreted enzyme produced by the skeletal muscle and adipose tissue. Its function involves the metabolism of triglycerides, chylomicrons and very low-density lipoproteins. Three clinical trials showed that Glybera is safe and efficient for the treatment of LPLD. In the first trial, two doses of rAAV1_LPLS447X were studied: low and high [50]. Nevertheless, none of the doses resulted in a permanent decrease in triglyceride levels. There was only a transient reduction, possibly due to the development of an immune response. The second clinical trial received the therapy in combination with an immunosuppressive regimen [51]. Similar to the first clinical trial, the effects of the therapy were only transient in the beginning. However, improvements were observed after two years posttreatment, such as tolerance to certain foods, changes in the blood lipid content and a decreased frequency of pancreatitis. Due to a discrepancy in the clinical outcomes and plasma triglycerides levels, a third trial was set with predetermined parameters to measure, as incidence frequency of abdominal pain, pancreatitis and chylomicron plasma clearance [52]. Five newly treated patients evidenced a reduction of the parameters and an improved quality of life for two years following administration.

These results, combined with the ones obtained from the reanalysis of 22 of the 27 previously treated patients, confirmed the therapeutic benefits of therapy and granted its approval to the market by the European Commission in November 2012.

8. Clinical trials for hemophilia B treatment

Hemophilia B is an X-linked recessive disorder, which originated from mutations within the gene that encodes the coagulation factor IX. Therefore, patients whose functional FIX levels are 1% of normal levels will bleed into the joint and muscle tissues. Bleeding in the brain could result in fatal death. If FIX levels are between 1% and 5%, the individual will experience a reduced number of bleeding incidents and a moderate phenotype of the disease. Any FIX levels above 5% will allow the person to have a normal life [53]. The only available treatment is protein replacement therapy, which requires regular intravenous injections and is expensive. Therefore, novel and permanent therapies/treatments are urgent. rAAV gene therapy currently constitutes a promising approach for the treatment of several diseases, including hemophilia B.

Based on animal studies that were described in the previous section, four clinical trials have been initiated. The first study administered rAAV carrying FIX gene into three patients by intramuscular injection. Despite the presence of preexistent high titer of neutralizing antibodies against capsid rAAV, strong transgene expression was observed in the muscle, even after 10 months of injection. However, levels of factor IX in circulation were less than 1–2% in most cases, even at the highest tested dose. Toxicity was not observed [54, 55].

The second trial conducted by the University of Pennsylvania infused the virus through the hepatic artery into seven patients. The rational in this protocol considered that FIX is a secreted protein and once it is produced and reaches the bloodstream; it can be distributed throughout the body.

Even though levels of FIX resulted higher than 5% after injecting an intermediate or high viral dose, the therapeutic effect was only transient (up to eight weeks), due to the development of a strong cytotoxic T response, which destroyed the transfected hepatocytes and thus hampered the production of FIX [56].

The third trial was designed in order to increase FIX expression production as well as to circumvent the possibility of a humoral response that could interfere with the success of the therapy [57]. To reach the first goal, they developed a codon optimized FIX gene that also delivered the gene in the context of self-complementary rAAV, which provides substantially higher levels of transgene expression rather than delivering the WT gene with single-stranded rAAV. In order to reduce antibody neutralization, the viral genome cassette was packed in rAAV8 capsid, as it has lower seroprevalence in humans and a high tropism for the liver. The virus was administered directly in the peripheral vein in six patients, and all of them developed 1–6% levels of factor IX expression in the first four months as well as for at least three years. There was no modification on the levels of neutralizing antibodies. However, transient elevations in serum liver enzymes, possibly as a result of a cellular immune response to the rAAV8 capsid, were observed in the three patients who received the high viral dose.

Recently, Baxter's laboratories launched a clinical trial to test the safety and efficacy of a self-complimentary rAAV8 vector carrying a mutant FIX sequence (BAX 335), created and preclinically tested at the UNC gene therapy center [58]. The FIX sequence had a single amino acid change at position 338, which substantially increased the levels of circulating FIX protein. A more effective rAAV delivery vehicle allowed the administration of lower viral doses with the same efficacy as previous tested virus, but without the associated toxicity. In this trial, sixteen adult patients were treated in different centers around the US. Updates on the trial were presented at the 8th Annual Congress of the European Association for Haemophilia and Allied Disorders this year in Finland. At this time, patients who received the highest dose did not develop inhibitory antibodies, reached FIX protein activity of 10% or more and did not manifest bleeding events. However, one of the patients experienced elevated levels of liver enzymes probably due to an immune response.

Nowadays, investigators are still developing better strategies to overcome the immunological response; currently, there are six trials evaluating safety and efficacy, including BAX 335.

9. rAAV and gene editing technology

Several genome editing tools have emerged recently in an attempt to correct the genetic cause(s) of a disease. These technologies rely on two components: a sequence-specific DNA-binding domain and a nuclease [59]. The procedure consists of several steps: (1) recognition of a targeted DNA sequence, (2) double stranded cut and (3) stimulation of a cellular repair mechanism to correct the DNA damage, which includes homologous recombination [60].

This technology allows for modifying a coding sequence, the epigenome, transcriptional activator/repressor as well as a regulatory element such as transcription factors, recombinases, transposases, and more. When targeting a particular gene, these technologies generate deletions, insertions or mutations of the gene, which may be useful to elucidate the gene function, or to generate cell lines with the null phenotype, or even to model a specific genetic condition for its study. Three different systems are currently available: zinc-finger nucleases (ZFN), TALEN nucleases and CRISPR/Cas9 [60].

Zinc-finger nucleases are a common type of DNA-binding motif found in eukaryotes and therefore, in the human genome. Usually, the DNA binding domain in the zinc-finger nuclease recognizes three base pairs in the DNA sequence. However, researchers have engineered the domain in order to detect and bind any defined DNA sequence of 9 to 18 bps in length, allowing the targeting of up to 68 billion bp of DNA [61].

Even though these technologies are very promising, an optimal delivery vehicle of the gene editing system needs to be developed. rAAV has the potential to deliver nucleases in vitro and in vivo and also has the potential to induce homologous recombination in the cell that infects, further enhancing the homologous recombination efficiency by 1000-fold [62–64].

In 2011, High et al. showed the generation of a ZFN system capable of cleaving F9 intron 1 and inducing homology-directed repair in the human hepatocyte Hep3B cell line. As proof of principle, the system induced up to 17% stable integration of a novel restriction enzyme site into the F9 locus. Furthermore, intraperitoneal administration of a ZFN system, which specifically targets F9, via rAAV8 delivery, in conjunction with an rAAV8 vector carrying a corrective F9 complementary DNA cassette into a humanized neonatal mouse model of hemophilia B, resulted in 1%–3% specific targeting of mouse liver. However, this mouse at two days old produced 2–3% normal F9 levels, enough amount to convert severe to mild hemophilia [65]. In 2013, they tested the same technology in a young adult mouse (8–10 weeks old), in which hepatocyte proliferation is slow as the liver already reached its maturity [66]. In theory, younger mice should show higher levels of gene correction, compared to older mice, as mice age affects the rate of homologous recombination, which is essential for genome editing to occur. In this publication, even though adult mice showed limited hepatocyte proliferation, following AAV injection, mice experienced a 5-fold increase in FIX expression, compared to the previous study. Moreover, when they tested the technology in even older mice, 7–8 months old, FIX levels were extremely low. Investigators argue that the discrepancies in FIX levels between neonate and adult mice could be attributable to the loss of rAAV vector genomes during liver development and/or different promoter activity. Furthermore, when they switched the use of homodimer nucleases to heterodimeric ZFN, nonspecific ZFN cleavage was observed without the loss of FIX expression.

Additionally, ZFN technology is currently being investigated in clinical trials for the treatment of HIV. Basically, the therapy consists of ex vivo permanent modification of patient T cells to knock down the HIV entry receptor CCR5 and autologous administration of the recombinant cells back to the patient. This clinical trial is sponsored by Sangamo Biosciences, the same company that collaborated with D. High for the in vivo targeting of hemophilia B mouse with rAAV-ZFN platform. In 2014, the company released an announcement for the first IND to test ZFN genome-editing platform in hemophilia A patients.

Even though these studies performed by Dr. High's laboratory and Sangamo Biosciences showed potential for in vivo gene editing via rAAV delivery, especially for diseases which do not allow ex vivo manipulation of target cells such as hemophilia B, the technology has several issues to address before being considered efficient and safe for treating human patients. First of all, we should consider all the challenges associated with rAAV delivery in vivo, such as the development of a cytotoxic T cell and/or neutralizing antibody responses and exclusively targeting of the tissue to correct with high efficiency. Furthermore, in order for this therapy to work efficiently, each cell needs to receive the two viruses at the same time, a condition that is possible but with a much lower probability to occur, and even if it takes place, the individual would be exposed to higher doses of rAAV8, which enhance the probability of inducing an immune response. Given that homologous recombination repair mainly takes place during the S phase of the cell cycle, gene editing is limited to be successful only in young patients, unless it is combined with molecules/drugs that boost cell division. Importantly, off-target double-stranded DNA breaks pose the possibility of inducing vector integration and/or undesired mutations and consequently, inducing oncogenesis, cell death and/or genetic diseases. This last possible issue could be solved by using self-inactivating viruses. Finally, the ZFN rAAV-mediated technology is still in the early phase of development, so far it has proven its potential for permanently correcting monogenetic diseases. However, considering that (1) rAAV gene therapy has shown great promise in the treatment of hemophilia B and (2) very low levels of FIX are enough to prevent bleeding and allow the person to have a normal life, in vivo gene editing technology seems too risky and unnecessary to pursue for the treatment of hemophilia diseases.

10. iPSC and rAAV

iPSC technologies have gained special interest since their discovery in 2006 by Takahashi and Yamanaka [67]. The generation of iPSC has several applications. One of the most important applications consists of the generation of: (1) pluripotent stem cells from a fully differentiated patient cell or (2) a specific human cell that is scarce or not accessible to the scientific population, from a healthy or diseased individual, following differentiation of the pluripotent stem cell. Moreover, sometimes, a personalized treatment is required or a diverse population cell sample is needed for testing the efficacy of a therapeutic technology, such as rAAV. For instance, the common practice is to reprogram patient-derived fibroblasts into a specific cell type that is affected by a disease. Some attempts have been performed to reprogram fibroblasts of patients suffering from retinal diseases into iPSC and finally differentiate the pluripotent stem cells into retinal pigment epithelial (RPE) cells that manifest the diseased phenotype [68, 69]. Following the validation of iPSC and then RPE cells, a panel of rAAV serotypes could be tested for their efficiency to transduce the cells and the most effective ones could be chosen for delivering the healthy gene copy in order to re-establish normal cellular phenotype [70].

Another approach for inducing iPSC development has been tried, but this time, using an rAAV system rather than a retrovirus. IPSC generated by Takahashi and Yamanaka's original protocol made use of retroviruses to deliver Oct3/4, Sox2, Klf4 and c-Myc. Even though the approach resulted in the generation of pluripotent stem cells from mouse embryonic or adult fibroblast cultures, still the efficiency was extremely low, the presence of c-Myc oncogene significantly increased the incidence of tumorigenicity and the use of retrovirus posed the threat of integration into the genome. Several new strategies have been developed, including the use of rAAV [69, 71]. Considering the advantages of using rAAV for gene delivery, such as long-term transgene expression for efficient reprogramming of mature cells as well as safety and efficacy as a gene delivery vehicle in the clinic; researchers have attempted their use in the reprogramming of fully differentiated fibroblasts as well as adipose-derived mesenchymal stem cells. However, both studies observed frequent rAAV integration into the host genome of iPSC cells when the iPSC were generated from nondividing cells. Integration events were independent of the rAAV vector, cell type and amount of virus. Both studies concluded that there is a certain degree of incompatibility between iPSC generation and the use of rAAV vectors, although reprogramming does not require an integration event. Furthermore, like retrovirus-mediated cell reprogramming, rAAV-mediated iPSC generation resulted in reprogramming transgene silencing, which affects the quality of the induced pluripotent stem cells that could be generated. Therefore, if the integration events are tightly controlled, which is feasible, and if the epigenetic mechanisms of rAAV silencing are discovered, rAAV technology could result in a safer mechanism for inducing pluripotent stem cells and consequently, increasing the chances of being applicable to the clinic.

Acknowledgements

This work was supported by NIH grants: R01AI072176, R01AR064369, R01DK084033, and P01HL1127611 (to RJS) and NIH grant T32-Grant: 5T32HL007149-39 (to MV), and support from the Alpha-1 Foundation.

Author details

Melisa A. Vance*, Angela Mitchell and Richard J. Samulski

*Address all correspondence to: melisa_vance@med.unc.edu

Gene Therapy Center, School of Medicine, University of North Carolina at Chapel Hill, Chapel Hill, NC, USA

References

[1] Sibbald, B., Death but one unintended consequence of gene-therapy trial. CMAJ, 2001. 164(11): p. 1612.

[2] Atchison, R.W., B.C. Casto, and W.M. Hammon, Adenovirus-associated defective virus particles. Science, 1965. 149(3685): p. 754–756.

[3] Mueller, C. and T.R. Flotte, Clinical gene therapy using recombinant adeno-associated virus vectors. Gene Ther, 2008. 15(11): p. 858–863.

[4] Kotin, R.M., R.M. Linden, and K.I. Berns, Characterization of a preferred site on human chromosome 19q for integration of adeno-associated virus DNA by non-homologous recombination. EMBO J, 1992. 11(13): p. 5071–5078.

[5] McCarty, D.M., P.E. Monahan, and R.J. Samulski, Self-complementary recombinant adeno-associated virus (scrAAV) vectors promote efficient transduction independently of DNA synthesis. Gene Ther, 2001. 8(16): p. 1248–1254.

[6] Zincarelli, C., et al., Analysis of rAAV serotypes 1–9 mediated gene expression and tropism in mice after systemic injection. Mol Ther, 2008. 16(6): p. 1073–1080.

[7] Sievers, F., et al., Fast, scalable generation of high-quality protein multiple sequence alignments using Clustal Omega. Mol Syst Biol, 2011. 7: p. 539.

[8] Saitou, N. and M. Nei, The neighbor-joining method: a new method for reconstructing phylogenetic trees. Mol Biol Evol, 1987. 4(4): p. 406–425.

[9] Gao, G., et al., Clades of Adeno-associated viruses are widely disseminated in human tissues. J Virol, 2004. 78(12): p. 6381–6388.

[10] Gao, G., et al., Adeno-associated viruses undergo substantial evolution in primates during natural infections. Proc Natl Acad Sci U S A, 2003. 100(10): p. 6081–6086.

[11] Swain, G.P., et al., Adeno-associated virus serotypes 9 and rh10 mediate strong neuronal transduction of the dog brain. Gene Ther, 2014. 21(1): p. 28–36.

[12] Wu, Z., et al., Single amino acid changes can influence titer, heparin binding, and tissue tropism in different adeno-associated virus serotypes. J Virol, 2006. 80(22): p. 11393–11397.

[13] Govindasamy, L., et al., Structural insights into adeno-associated virus serotype 5. J Virol, 2013. 87(20): p. 11187–11199.

[14] Kaludov, N., et al., Adeno-associated virus serotype 4 (rAAV4) and rAAV5 both require sialic acid binding for hemagglutination and efficient transduction but differ in sialic acid linkage specificity. J Virol, 2001. 75(15): p. 6884–6893.

[15] Mietzsch, M., et al., Differential adeno-associated virus serotype-specific interaction patterns with synthetic heparins and other glycans. J Virol, 2014. 88(5): p. 2991–3003.

[16] Akache, B., et al., The 37/67-kilodalton laminin receptor is a receptor for adeno-associated virus serotypes 8, 2, 3, and 9. J Virol, 2006. 80(19): p. 9831–9836.

[17] Shen, S., et al., Terminal N-linked galactose is the primary receptor for adeno-associated virus 9. J Biol Chem, 2011. 286(15): p. 13532–13540.

[18] Foust, K.D., et al., Intravascular rAAV9 preferentially targets neonatal neurons and adult astrocytes. Nat Biotechnol, 2009. 27(1): p. 59–65.

[19] Vandenberghe Luk H., M.J.R., Gao Gaung-Ping, Calcedo Roberto and James M. Wilson, The proposed rAAV serotypes 10 and 11 serologically cross-react with rAAV8 and rAAV4. Molecular Therapy 2006. 13: p. S47.

[20] Schmidt, M., et al., Adeno-associated virus type 12 (rAAV12): a novel rAAV serotype with sialic acid- and heparan sulfate proteoglycan-independent transduction activity. J Virol, 2008. 82(3): p. 1399–1406.

[21] Sarkar, R., et al., Long-term efficacy of adeno-associated virus serotypes 8 and 9 in hemophilia a dogs and mice. Hum Gene Ther, 2006. 17(4): p. 427–439.

[22] Herzog, R.W., et al., Long-term correction of canine hemophilia B by gene transfer of blood coagulation factor IX mediated by adeno-associated viral vector. Nat Med, 1999. 5(1): p. 56–63.

[23] Herzog, R.W., et al., Influence of vector dose on factor IX-specific T and B cell responses in muscle-directed gene therapy. Hum Gene Ther, 2002. 13(11): p. 1281–1291.

[24] Snyder, R.O., et al., Correction of hemophilia B in canine and murine models using recombinant adeno-associated viral vectors. Nat Med, 1999. 5(1): p. 64–70.

[25] Wang, L., et al., Sustained expression of therapeutic level of factor IX in hemophilia B dogs by rAAV-mediated gene therapy in liver. Mol Ther, 2000. 1(2): p. 154–158.

[26] Mount, J.D., et al., Sustained phenotypic correction of hemophilia B dogs with a factor IX null mutation by liver-directed gene therapy. Blood, 2002. 99(8): p. 2670–2676.

[27] Crudele, J.M., et al., rAAV liver expression of FIX-Padua prevents and eradicates FIX inhibitor without increasing thrombogenicity in hemophilia B dogs and mice. Blood, 2015. 125(10): p. 1553–1561.

[28] Jiang, H., et al., Effects of transient immunosuppression on adenoassociated, virus-mediated, liver-directed gene transfer in rhesus macaques and implications for human gene therapy. Blood, 2006. 108(10): p. 3321–3328.

[29] Nathwani, A.C., et al., Sustained high-level expression of human factor IX (hFIX) after liver-targeted delivery of recombinant adeno-associated virus encoding the hFIX gene in rhesus macaques. Blood, 2002. 100(5): p. 1662–1669.

[30] Mattar, C.N., et al., Stable human FIX expression after 0.9G intrauterine gene transfer of self-complementary adeno-associated viral vector 5 and 8 in macaques. Mol Ther, 2011. 19(11): p. 1950–1960.

[31] Nathwani, A.C., et al., Factors influencing in vivo transduction by recombinant adeno-associated viral vectors expressing the human factor IX cDNA. Blood, 2001. 97(5): p. 1258–1265.

[32] Margaritis, P., et al., Successful treatment of canine hemophilia by continuous expression of canine FVIIa. Blood, 2009. 113(16): p. 3682–3689.

[33] Niemeyer, G.P., et al., Long-term correction of inhibitor-prone hemophilia B dogs treated with liver-directed rAAV2-mediated factor IX gene therapy. Blood, 2009. 113(4): p. 797–806.

[34] Hoggan, M.D., N.R. Blacklow, and W.P. Rowe, Studies of small DNA viruses found in various adenovirus preparations: physical, biological, and immunological characteristics. Proc Natl Acad Sci U S A, 1966. 55(6): p. 1467–1474.

[35] Bainbridge, J.W., et al., Effect of gene therapy on visual function in Leber's congenital amaurosis. N Engl J Med, 2008. 358(21): p. 2231–2239.

[36] Maguire, A.M., et al., Age-dependent effects of RPE65 gene therapy for Leber's congenital amaurosis: a phase 1 dose-escalation trial. Lancet, 2009. 374(9701): p. 1597–1605.

[37] Simonelli, F., et al., Gene therapy for Leber's congenital amaurosis is safe and effective through 1.5 years after vector administration. Mol Ther, 2010. 18(3): p. 643–650.

[38] Jacobson, S.G., et al., Gene therapy for Leber congenital amaurosis caused by RPE65 mutations: safety and efficacy in 15 children and adults followed up to 3 years. Arch Ophthalmol, 2012. 130(1): p. 9–24.

[39] Cideciyan, A.V., et al., Pseudo-fovea formation after gene therapy for RPE65-LCA. Invest Ophthalmol Vis Sci, 2015. 56(1): p. 526–537.

[40] LeWitt, P.A., et al., rAAV2-GAD gene therapy for advanced Parkinson's disease: a double-blind, sham-surgery controlled, randomised trial. Lancet Neurol, 2011. 10(4): p. 309–319.

[41] Bartus, R.T., M.S. Weinberg, and R.J. Samulski, Parkinson's disease gene therapy: success by design meets failure by efficacy. Mol Ther, 2014. 22(3): p. 487–497.

[42] Eberling, J.L., et al., Results from a phase I safety trial of hAADC gene therapy for Parkinson disease. Neurology, 2008. 70(21): p. 1980–1983.

[43] Christine, C.W., et al., Safety and tolerability of putaminal AADC gene therapy for Parkinson disease. Neurology, 2009. 73(20): p. 1662–1669.

[44] Muramatsu, S., et al., A phase I study of aromatic L-amino acid decarboxylase gene therapy for Parkinson's disease. Mol Ther, 2010. 18(9): p. 1731–1735.

[45] Bartus, R.T., et al., Advancing neurotrophic factors as treatments for age-related neurodegenerative diseases: developing and demonstrating "clinical proof-of-concept" for rAAV-neurturin (CERE-120) in Parkinson's disease. Neurobiol Aging, 2013. 34(1): p. 35–61.

[46] Marks, W.J., Jr., et al., Gene delivery of rAAV2-neurturin for Parkinson's disease: a double-blind, randomised, controlled trial. Lancet Neurol, 2010. 9(12): p. 1164–1172.

[47] Leone, P., et al., Long-term follow-up after gene therapy for Canavan disease. Sci Transl Med, 2012. 4(165): p. 165ra163.

[48] Ahmed, S.S., et al., A single intravenous rAAV injection as late as P20 achieves efficacious and sustained CNS gene therapy in Canavan mice. Mol Ther, 2013. 21(12): p. 2136–2147.

[49] Jessup, M., et al., Calcium upregulation by percutaneous administration of gene therapy in cardiac disease (CUPID): a phase 2 trial of intracoronary gene therapy of sarcoplasmic reticulum Ca2+-ATPase in patients with advanced heart failure. Circulation, 2011. 124(3): p. 304–313.

[50] Stroes, E.S., et al., Intramuscular administration of rAAV1-lipoprotein lipase S447X lowers triglycerides in lipoprotein lipase-deficient patients. Arterioscler Thromb Vasc Biol, 2008. 28(12): p. 2303–2304.

[51] Gaudet, D., et al., Efficacy and long-term safety of alipogene tiparvovec (rAAV1-LPLS447X) gene therapy for lipoprotein lipase deficiency: an open-label trial. Gene Ther, 2013. 20(4): p. 361–369.

[52] Carpentier, A.C., et al., Effect of alipogene tiparvovec (rAAV1-LPL(S447X)) on post-prandial chylomicron metabolism in lipoprotein lipase-deficient patients. J Clin Endocrinol Metab, 2012. 97(5): p. 1635–1644.

[53] Coppola, A., et al., Treatment of hemophilia: a review of current advances and ongoing issues. J Blood Med, 2010. 1: p. 183–195.

[54] Manno, C.S., et al., rAAV-mediated factor IX gene transfer to skeletal muscle in patients with severe hemophilia B. Blood, 2003. 101(8): p. 2963–2972.

[55] Kay, M.A., et al., Evidence for gene transfer and expression of factor IX in haemophilia B patients treated with an rAAV vector. Nat Genet, 2000. 24(3): p. 257–261.

[56] Manno, C.S., et al., Successful transduction of liver in hemophilia by rAAV-Factor IX and limitations imposed by the host immune response. Nat Med, 2006. 12(3): p. 342–347.

[57] Nathwani, A.C., et al., Adenovirus-associated virus vector-mediated gene transfer in hemophilia B. N Engl J Med, 2011. 365(25): p. 2357–2365.

[58] Monahan, P.E., et al., Employing a gain-of-function factor IX variant R338L to advance the efficacy and safety of hemophilia B human gene therapy: preclinical evaluation supporting an ongoing adeno-associated virus clinical trial. Hum Gene Ther, 2015. 26(2): p. 69–81.

[59] Laufer, B.I. and S.M. Singh, Strategies for precision modulation of gene expression by epigenome editing: an overview. Epigenetics Chromatin, 2015. 8: p. 34.

[60] Gaj, T., C.A. Gersbach, and C.F. Barbas, 3rd, ZFN, TALEN, and CRISPR/Cas-based methods for genome engineering. Trends Biotechnol, 2013. 31(7): p. 397–405.

[61] Beerli, R.R., B. Dreier, and C.F. Barbas, 3rd, Positive and negative regulation of endogenous genes by designed transcription factors. Proc Natl Acad Sci U S A, 2000. 97(4): p. 1495–1500.

[62] Russell, D.W. and R.K. Hirata, Human gene targeting by viral vectors. Nat Genet, 1998. 18(4): p. 325–330.

[63] Hirsch, M.L., Adeno-associated virus inverted terminal repeats stimulate gene editing. Gene Ther, 2015. 22(2): p. 190–195.

[64] Hirsch, M.L. and R.J. Samulski, rAAV-mediated gene editing via double-strand break repair. Methods Mol Biol, 2014. 1114: p. 291–307.

[65] Li, H., et al., In vivo genome editing restores haemostasis in a mouse model of haemophilia. Nature, 2011. 475(7355): p. 217–221.

[66] Anguela, X.M., et al., Robust ZFN-mediated genome editing in adult hemophilic mice. Blood, 2013. 122(19): p. 3283–3287.

[67] Takahashi, K. and S. Yamanaka, Induction of pluripotent stem cells from mouse embryonic and adult fibroblast cultures by defined factors. Cell, 2006. 126(4): p. 663–676.

[68] Li, Y., et al., Gene therapy in patient-specific stem cell lines and a preclinical model of retinitis pigmentosa with membrane frizzled-related protein defects. Mol Ther, 2014. 22(9): p. 1688–1697.

[69] Chen, M.J., et al., Reprogramming adipose tissue-derived mesenchymal stem cells into pluripotent stem cells by a mutant adeno-associated viral vector. Hum Gene Ther Methods, 2014. 25(1): p. 72–82.

[70] Cereso, N., et al., Proof of concept for rAAV2/5-mediated gene therapy in iPSC-derived retinal pigment epithelium of a choroideremia patient. Mol Ther Methods Clin Dev, 2014. 1: p. 14011.

[71] Weltner, J., et al., Induced pluripotent stem cell clones reprogrammed via recombinant adeno-associated virus-mediated transduction contain integrated vector sequences. J Virol, 2012. 86(8): p. 4463–4467.

7

First Insights into Non-invasive Administration Routes for Non-viral Gene Therapy

Ilia Villate-Beitia, Gustavo Puras, Jon Zarate,
Mireia Agirre, Edilberto Ojeda and Jose Luis Pedraz

Abstract

Gene delivery has attracted increasing interest as a highly promising therapeutic method to treat various diseases, including both genetic and acquired disorders. However, its clinical application is still hampered by the lack of safe and effective gene delivery techniques, as well as by the need of non-invasive routes of administration in gene delivery platforms. Among the different approaches used to transport nucleic acids into target cells, non-viral vectors represent promising and safer alternatives to viruses. Non-invasive administration routes are currently being studied, such as intranasal administration to target the brain, topical retinal administration for ocular diseases and aerosolized formulations for inhalation for the treatment of pulmonary diseases. Reasonable evidence suggests that future gene delivery systems might be based on effective non-viral vectors administered through non-invasive routes, which would constitute a safe, easy to produce, cheap and customizable alternative to the current viral gene delivery platforms. In this review, after briefly introducing the basis of gene therapy, we discuss the up-to-date and possible future strategies to improve DNA transfection efficiency using non-viral vectors and focusing on the non-invasive routes of administration.

Keywords: Gene therapy, non-viral vector, intra- and extracellular barriers, non-invasive routes of administration

1. Introduction

1.1. Concept and historical evolution of gene therapy

Gene therapy can be broadly defined as the introduction of genetic material into target cells in order to modify and control protein expression for therapeutic or experimental purposes [1]. Nowadays, the culmination of the Human Genome Project along with recent advances in molecular biology have provided a better understanding of cellular and pathogenic processes, and several genes have been identified as targets for therapeutic approaches. Additionally, the constant advance in the development of gene carriers for the delivery of nucleic acids into target cells has led to conceiving new therapeutic strategies for the treatment of pathologies by genetic and cell-based approaches, collectively known as gene therapy [1].

Researchers have been working for decades to bring gene therapy to the clinic, but very few patients have received an effective gene-therapy treatment. The potential of gene therapy in medical applications was recognized soon after the discovery of DNA as genetic material, and the concept of gene therapy arose during the 1960s and 1970s [2]. The first success of gene therapy on humans arrived in 1990, it was performed by researchers at the National Institute of Health, and the treated disease was a form of severe combined immune deficiency (SCID) due to defects in the gene encoding adenosine deaminase (ADA) [3]. However, a fatal event in 1991 raised serious concerns about gene therapy. An eighteen-year-old boy died as a result of his voluntary participation in a gene therapy trial, becoming the first known human victim of this technology [4]. The Food and Drug Administration (FDA) investigation concluded that the scientists involved in the trial did not foresee serious side effects or fatality and that they did not follow the federal rules to ensure the safety of the participants [4]. This tragic case caused a severe setback in the research field of gene therapy.

According to data updated to June 2014 and presented by *The Journal of Gene Medicine* [5], since the onset of the first gene therapy clinical trial in 1989, more than 2000 new clinical trials for gene therapy have been approved globally (Figure 1). As shown in Figure 2, these trials address the most challenging diseases of today, that is, cancer (64.1% of approved trials), monogenic diseases (9.1%) such as cystic fibrosis, infectious diseases (8.2%) and cardiovascular diseases (7.8%). Although in a lesser extent, neurological diseases (1.8%) and ocular diseases (1.6%) are also subject to clinical trials with gene therapy. However, despite the intensive study during the last few years, at present only 0.1% of all the gene therapy products approved for clinical trials have arrived to the phase IV (Figure 3). In 2012, the European Medicine Agency approved for the first time a gene therapy product, Glybera, an adeno-associated viral vector engineered to express lipoprotein lipase in the muscle for the treatment of lipoprotein lipase deficiency [5].

1.2. The need of carriers

One of the main reasons why gene therapy clinical trials are still few in number is the lack of suitable and safe approaches to deliver the genetic material to target cells. The success of gene therapy critically depends on suitable transfection vectors, which should be able to: (i) protect nucleic acids against degradation by blood and interstitial nucleases, (ii) promote internalization of the genetic material into target cells and (iii) release the nucleic acids once inside the cell to the correct site [1]. Furthermore, an ideal gene delivery system should be effective, specific, long-lasting, safe, easy to use and as inexpensive as possible [6]. Broadly, gene delivery vectors are mainly classified into two categories: viral vectors and non-viral vectors. According to data updated to June 2014 and presented by *The Journal of Gene Medicine* [7], among the over 2,000 clinical trials for gene therapy approved globally nowadays, 70% correspond to trials using viral vectors. As shown in Figure 4, there is a 17.7% of the gene therapy clinical trials that use naked DNA, and 5.3% of trials use lipofection [7].

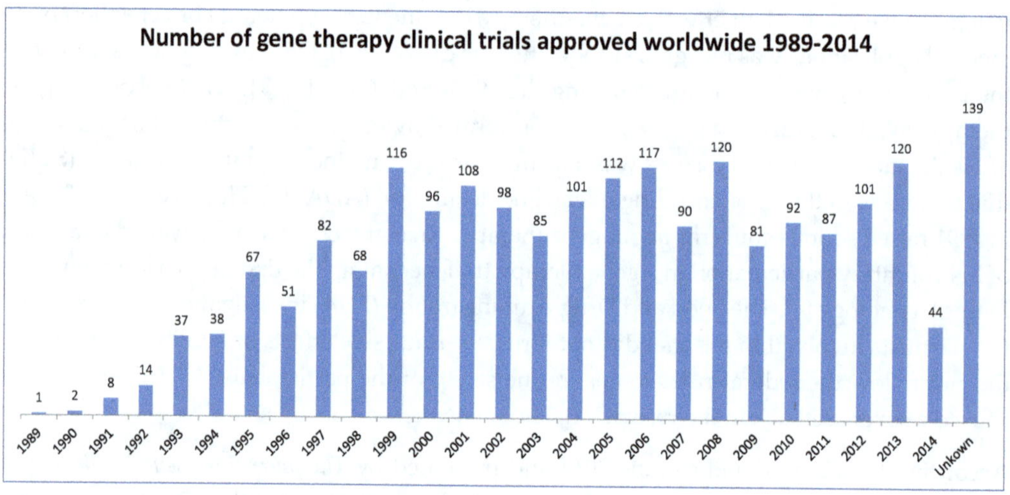

Figure 1. Number of gene therapy clinical trials approved worldwide 1989-2014 (adapted from http://www.wiley.co.uk/genmed/clinical).

Despite the still absolute predominance of viral-vector-based gene delivery platforms – which is due to their higher transfection efficiency – in clinical trials, non-viral vectors represent promising and safer alternatives to viruses. In addition, non-invasive routes of administration for gene delivery systems are currently being studied, such as intranasal administration to target the brain, topical administration on the surface of the eye to treat retinal inherited diseases and aerosolized formulations for inhalation for the treatment of pulmonary diseases. There is reasonable hope to suggest that future gene delivery systems might be based on effective non-viral vectors administered through non-invasive routes and that they would constitute a safe, easy to produce, cheap and customizable alternative to gene delivery platforms. Moreover, it is increasingly accepted that future gene delivery platforms may be based on multifunctional vectors specifically tailored for different applications [1].

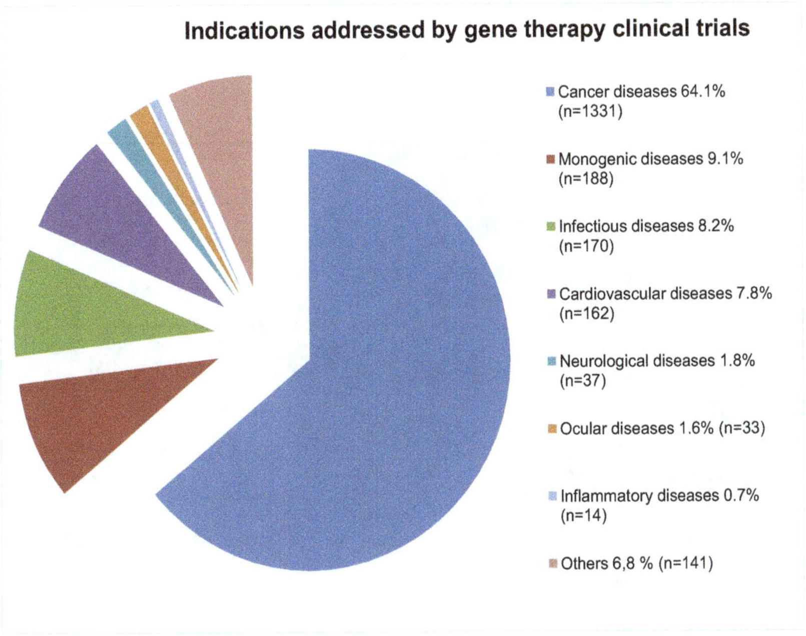

Figure 2. Indications addressed by gene therapy clinical trials (adapted from http://www.wiley.co.uk/genmed/clinical).

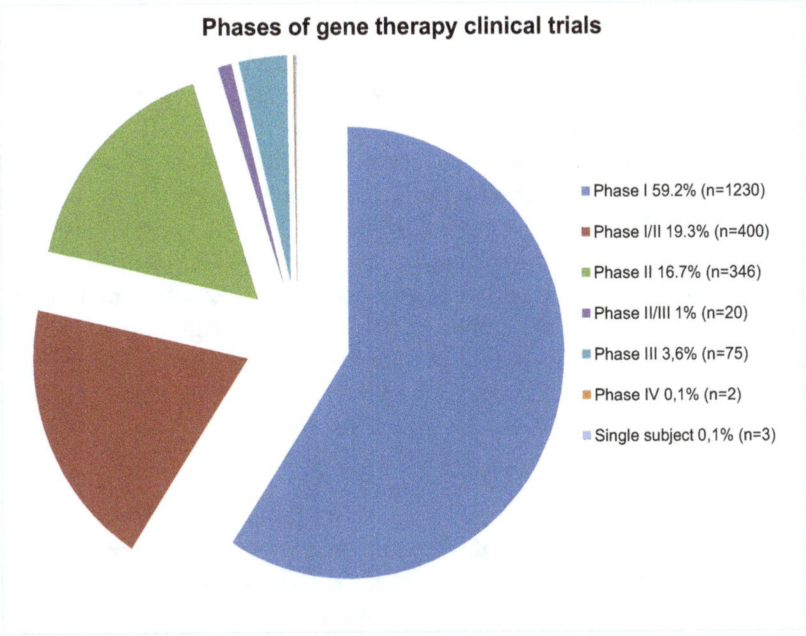

Figure 3. Phases of gene therapy clinical trials (adapted from http://www.wiley.co.uk/genmed/clinical).

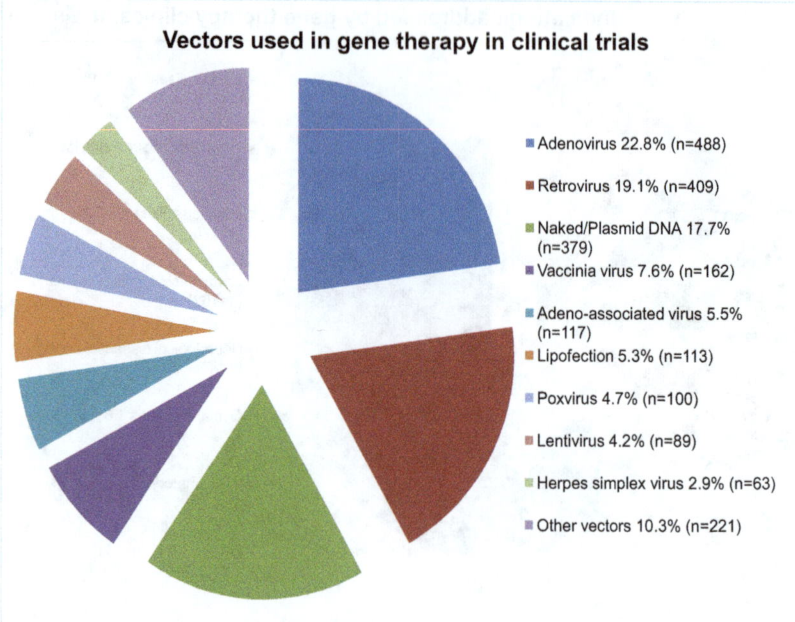

Figure 4. Vectors used in gene therapy in clinical trials (adapted from http://www.wiley.co.uk/genmed/clinical).

1.2.1. Viral vectors

In this review we will focus on non-viral-vector-based strategies for gene delivery platforms, but we will briefly discuss the most relevant aspects of viral gene therapy. Viruses are highly evolved biological machines that efficiently gain access into host cells, deliver their genetic material to cells and exploit the cellular machinery to facilitate their replication [8]. Therefore, viruses represent an excellent platform for the development of recombinant vectors containing foreign genes for gene delivery purposes [1]. However, viral vectors also present many impediments such as the low carrying capacity, the expensive and complex production and, most importantly, safety issues, since they can induce oncogenesis when randomly integrated in the host genome. In addition, the human immune system recognizes and combats viruses, shortening their effectiveness [1]. Table 1 summarizes the principal viral vectors used in gene therapy, as well as their main utilities and impediments. Viral vectors are, therefore, powerful tools but present important drawbacks for clinical use in humans.

1.2.2. Non-viral vectors

Non-viral vectors have emerged as a safer, cheaper and easier-to-produce alternative to viral vectors. In fact, non-viral vectors can be produced on a large scale with high reproducibility and acceptable costs, they are relatively stable to storage, they can be administered repeatedly with no or little immune response and the dimension of the genetic material they can carry is practically unlimited [1,9]. Nevertheless, the employment of non-viral gene delivery vectors is still strongly limited by their lower transfection efficiency as compared to viral vectors [1].

Viral vector	Integrative/ Episomal	Utility	Impediments
Adenovirus	Episomal	- Very efficient transfection in most tissues	- Induces inflammatory response
Adeno-associated virus (AAV)	Episomal (>90%)	- Not inducing inflammatory response	- Limited nucleic acid carrying capacity (<5 kb)
Retrovirus	Integrative	- Persistent gene expression	- Only transfects dividing cells - Risk of insertional mutagenesis
Lentivirus	Integrative	- Broad tropism - Persistent gene expression	- Risk of insertional mutagenesis
Herpes Simplex Virus-1 (HSV-1)	Episomal	- Large nucleic acid carrying capacity (up to 150 kb)	- Induces inflammatory response

Table 1. Principal viral vectors used in gene therapy, advantages and drawbacks. (Based on [8])

Non-viral vectors can be classified into two main categories depending on whether they are based on physical methods or on chemical methods. We will briefly review the most commonly employed non-viral DNA delivery systems for each category.

1.2.2.1. Physical methods

Physical methods for gene delivery purposes usually employ physical force to create transient membrane holes to cross the cell membrane and enhance gene transfer [6,10]. No particulate system is used to introduce the genetic material into the target cells [6]. Needle injection, ballistic DNA injection, electroporation, sonoporation, photoporation, magnetofection and hydroporation are the most utilized physical methods at present [6,11].

1.2.2.2. Chemical methods

Depending on the chemical feature, those methods can be classified into three groups: cationic lipids, cationic polymers and inorganic nanoparticles. Chemical vectors based on cationic lipids and cationic polymers form condensed complexes with negatively charged DNA through electrostatic interactions [10]. The complexes protect DNA and facilitate cell uptake intracellular delivery [10]. The principal characteristics of the non-viral chemical vectors are the following:

- *Vectors based on cationic lipids*

As shown in Figure 4, cationic lipid-mediated gene transfer or lipofection represents the most commonly used non-viral gene delivery system. Cationic lipids share four common functional domains: (i) a hydrophilic head-group, which is responsible for the interaction with the DNA; (ii) a hydrophobic domain, which is usually derived from aliphatic hydrocarbon chains; (iii) a linker structure, which influences the flexibility, stability and biodegradability of the cationic lipid; and (iv) a backbone domain, which separates the polar head-group from the hydrophobic domain and it is usually a serinol or a glycerol group [12]. Changes in those domains can vary the transfection efficiency of different vectors elaborated with cationic lipids. The most employed cationic lipid formulations for gene delivery platforms are: (i) **liposomes** – vesicles made up of phospholipids; (ii) **niosomes** –non-ionic surfactant vesicles, with greater physic-chemical and storage stability than liposomes; and (iii) **solid lipid nanoparticles (SLN)** – particles with a solid lipid core, stabilized with surfactants [13].

- *Vectors based on cationic polymers*

Vectors based on cationic polymers are mostly spherical particles ranging in the size 1-1000 nm and they condense DNA into polyplexes preventing DNA from degradation [6]. The DNA can be entrapped in the polymeric matrix or can be adsorbed or conjugated on the surface of the nanoparticles [6]. The most popular cationic polymers employed for DNA delivery purposes are: (i) poly(ethylene imine) – PEI, which has an excellent buffering capacity; (ii) chitosan – a linear polysaccharide derived from the deacetylation of the natural chitin; (iii) cyclodextrins – a series of natural cyclic oligosaccharids; (iv) dendrimers – tree-shaped synthetic molecules up to a few nanometers in diameter that are formed with a regular branching structure; and (vi) Poly(L-lysine) – PLL, which can form nanometer-size complexes with polynucleotides thanks to the presence of protonable amine groups on the lysine moiety [6,13,14].

- *Vectors based on inorganic nanoparticles*

Inorganic nanoparticles are nanostructures varying in size, shape and porosity, and calcium phosphate, silica, gold, and several magnetic compounds are the most studied [6,15]. Inorganic particles can be easily prepared and surface-functionalized. They exhibit good storage stability and are not subject to microbial attack [6,16].

In summary, non-viral vectors for gene delivery represent a safer alternative to conventional viral vectors. However, although tremendous progress has been made in this field in recent years, the clinical application of non-viral-vector-based gene therapy is still hampered by the lack of effective gene delivery techniques. In the present review, we will discuss the up-to-date and possible future strategies to improve DNA transfer efficacy using non-viral vectors and focusing on non-invasive routes of administration. First, the intracellular barriers that non-viral vectors have to overcome and the strategies to improve the transfection efficiency in this regard will be described. Second, we will review the extracellular barriers that hamper an efficient gene delivery, as well as the invasive and the alternative non-invasive routes of administration that elude those barriers. Finally, challenges for non-viral vectors to reach clinical trials will be discussed, focusing on the transfection efficiency, the targeting and the duration of the transfected gene expression.

2. Intracellular barriers and strategies to improve transfection efficiency

A key factor conditioning transfection efficiency is the ability of the gene delivery system to overcome the intracellular and extracellular barriers. In this section, we will describe the main intracellular barriers that gene delivery systems must overcome to reach an efficient transfection and the different strategies used for this purpose. Intracellular barriers involve all the obstacles that a gene delivery system must overcome from cell surface association to nuclear entry in target cells. The knowledge of the molecular features that command all these processes for the non-viral vectors and the overcoming of these hurdles are mandatory issues that need to be deeply considered in order to design efficient gene delivery methods. In this section, we will review the cellular uptake pathways and intracellular trafficking of non-viral vectors and we will discuss the existing methods to enhance the endosomal escape and the nuclear entry, which are the principal strategies to achieve an efficient transfection.

2.1. Cellular uptake pathways

Cell surface association is the first intracellular barrier that non-viral gene delivery platforms need to overcome and it can directly influence the next intracellular fates of the non-viral complexes [17]. Cell-binding interactions of non-viral vectors can be receptor-independent or receptor-mediated. Receptor-independent cell surface association occurs by electrophilic attraction between the positively charged non-viral complexes (i.e. cationic lipoplexes and cationic polyplexes) and the negatively charged cell surface proteoglycans [18]. This binding method can efficiently transfect many cell types *in vitro*, but therapeutic potential *in vivo* requires additional refinement. In fact, in order to specifically deliver a gene into a target tissue *in vivo*, non-specific cell binding would require very high and potentially toxic doses of the non-viral vector. The addition of cell-specific ligands or antibodies to the vectors reduces this problem, allowing the use of lower and safer vector doses and promoting tissue targeting [18]. For instance, transferrin (Tf), which is an iron-transporting protein, has been used to achieve brain delivery in view that the Tf receptor is expressed in neurons and in the capillary endothelial cells of the brain-blood-barrier (BBB) [19]. Ligand choice not only depends on the cell type being targeted, but it is also important to consider the type of cell entry pathway that will be induced after ligation. As discussed in the following section, the endocytic pathway used by the vector can depend on the targeting ligand.

Once bound to the cell surface, non-viral vectors need to cross the plasma membrane to enter the cell and initiate the intracellular trafficking to enter the nucleus. The cellular uptake of macromolecules and solutes into membrane-bound vesicles derived by the invagination and pinching off of pieces of the plasma membrane is known as endocytosis [20]. There are four principal endocytic pathways: clathrin-mediated endocytosis (CME), caveolae-mediated endocytosis (CvME), phagocytosis and macropinocytosis [17,21]. These endocytic pathways are described below.

2.1.1. Clathrin-mediated endocytosis

Clathrin-mediated endocytosis (CME) is a highly regulated and energy-dependent process, and it constitutes the major and best characterized endocytic pathway [20]. The first step in

CME is the strong binding of a ligand to a specific cell surface receptor. This triggers the localized accumulation of clathrin structures on the cytoplasmic surface of the plasma membrane, which helps to deform the membrane into a coated pit with a size about 100-150 nm [22]. As the clathrin lattice formation continues, the coated pits become deeply invaginated and they finally pinch off from the plasma membrane to form intracellular clathrin-coated vesicles (CCVs) [20]. The clathrin coats then depolymerize, resulting in early endosomes. A kind of GTPase named dynamin is necessary for the vesicle fission from the plasma membrane [23]. Cholesterol seems to be also important for CCV formation because its depletion impedes the coated pits to pinch off from the plasma membrane [24].

In the next step of the CME pathway, the endocyted vesicles internalized from the plasma membrane are integrated into late endosomes and those then deliver their cargos to lysosomes [25]. During maturation from early to late endosomes, proton pumps located on the endosome membrane produce the acidification of the compartment, and there is a further reduction to pH 5 in the progression from late endosomes to lysosomes [20]. The acid pH in endosomes seems to cause the dissociation of the ligands from their receptors. Most authors state that, in the absence of an endosomal escape mechanism, non-viral vector/DNA complexes are retained and degraded in the lysosomes due to the acid environment and the enzymatic activity in these compartments. The final result is that DNA molecules have little or almost no access to the nucleus [20].

Some authors suggest that in some cases, depending on the formulation of the non-viral vector, the CME pathway might be the most suitable to achieve a high transfection efficiency because the lysosomal activity facilitates the cytosolic release of nanoparticles and enhances the nuclear entry of DNA [26]. Depending on the composition of the vector, the most appropriate internalization mechanism may be modulated [26]. Therefore, it is crucial to have a comprehensive understanding of the cellular internalization pathways of non-viral gene delivery systems.

2.1.2. Caveolae-mediated endocytosis

Caveolae-mediated endocytosis (CvME) begins in membrane microdomains called caveolae, which are small, hydrophobic, and cholesterol- and sphingolipid-rich smooth invaginations [17,20]. As well as CME, CvME is a type of receptor-mediated and dynamin-dependent pathway in which cholesterol also plays an important role [27]. The main difference between the clathrin- and the caveolae-mediated pathways is that in CvME there are no endosomes. Instead, internalized molecules go into intracellular vesicles called caveosomes, which do not fuse with lysosomes and, therefore, the potential degradation process of the DNA is avoided in this pathway [17]. In fact, CvME is generally considered a non-acidic and non-digestive internalization pathway, meaning that the internalized molecules can be directly transported into their intracellular target sites without being degraded in lysosomes [17,28]. Nevertheless, this issue is still under debate because some authors have recently reported that sometimes caveosomes join the classical endocytic pathway, in which they eventually fuse with lysosomes [29]. Therefore, in this regard further evidence is needed in order to understand the relationship between caveosomes and lysosomes.

2.1.3. Phagocytosis

Phagocytosis is a special type of endocytic pathway that is primarily used by professional phagocytes such as macrophages, monocytes, neutrophils and dendritic cells, although other cells might use it too [17]. Cup-like membrane extensions larger than 1 μm mediate the phagocytic pathway, and it is usually employed by cells to internalize large particles such as bacteria or dead cells, although large lipoplexes and polyplexes can also be internalized through this pathway [17].

Phagocytosis usually involves three steps that are common to all molecules internalized through this pathway, including non-viral vectors. First, non-viral vector/DNA complexes are recognized by opsonins and, therefore, opsonized, in the bloodstream. Second, the opsonized complexes bind to the surface of macrophages through the interaction between macrophage receptors and the constant fragment of particle-adsorbed immunoglobulins [17]. Antibodies lacking the constant fragment can be employed in non-viral gene delivery systems to prevent their recognition and clearance by macrophages *in vivo* [30].

Finally, the union of the molecule or non-viral/DNA complex to the macrophage receptors activates Rho-family GTPases, which trigger actin assembly and cell surface extension formation [17]. The complexes are ingested by the macrophages when the surface extension zippers up around them [20]. The vesicles internalized in the cells though the phagocytic pathway are called phagosomes and they usually have a diameter of 0.5–1.0 μm [20]. The phagosomes carrying the internalized complexes form mature phagolysosomes when they fuse with lysosomes, where the complexes undergo an acidification process [20]. In view of the fact that the intracellular fate of the phagocytic pathway is the fusion with lysosomes, the nucleic acids carried in the non-viral vector complexes will probably be degraded in this internalization pathway [31].

2.1.4. Macropinocytosis

Macropinocytosis is an internalization pathway based on fluid-phase endocytosis, since it non-specifically takes up a large amount of fluid-phase contents [17]. Similarly to the phagocytic pathway, macropinocytosis also happens through the formation of actin-directed membrane protuberances. Nevertheless, here the protrusions do not zipper up the ligand-coated particle. Alternatively, as shown in Figure 5, in the macropinocytic pathway the protuberances fuse with the plasma membrane. Macropinosomes are also different from clathrin-coated vesicles (CCVs) and caveosomes, since macropinosomes have no coat structures and, even if they are heterogeneous in size, they use to be larger than 0.2 μm in diameter [32]. As well as the other endocytic pathways, macropinocytosis also depends on small GTPase proteins since they are necessary for the vesicle fission from the plasma membrane [17].

The connection between macropinosomes and lysosomes remains still unknown. In some studies, early macropinosomes have been reported to show the same markers as early endosomes, and late macropinosomes have been reported to present lysosome markers [17]. However, macropinosomes have been shown to present different intracellular fates depending on the cell type, even if the explanation of this event remains unclear, and they do not always fuse with lysosomes [17].

2.2. Endosomal escape mechanisms

As mentioned before, most non-viral vectors are internalized in the cells mainly through the clathrin-mediated endocytic pathway. The major problem here is the intracellular fate of the endosomes that fuse with lysosomes and this can potentially lead to the degradation of the nucleic acids. In order to avoid this effect, while taking advantage of the CME pathway for cellular uptake, several attempts have been made to promote the early endosomal escape of non-viral gene delivery systems.

Many pathogens, mainly viruses and bacteria, have evolved different mechanisms to promote endosomal escape when internalized in cells. Several endosomal escape agents derive from virus (i.e. haemagglutinin protein of influenza virus) and bacteria (i.e. diphtheria toxin), and some derive from plants (i.e, ricin), human (i.e. fibroblast growth factors) or animals (i.e. melittin form bee venom) too [33]. The understanding of the mechanism used by pathogens allows to design and to ameliorate endosomal escape strategies applicable to non-viral gene delivery systems. Nowadays, several synthetic peptides with specific sequences and length are designed (i.e. the amphiphatic Sweet Arrow Peptide), as well as specific chemical agents (i.e. the polymer polyethylenimine PEI) for endosomal escape induction [33]. In the following paragraphs, the principal endosomal escape mechanisms are described.

2.2.1. Pore formation in the endosomal membrane

Pore formation is based on the interplay between a membrane tension that enlarges the pore and a line tension that closes the pore. Some peptides have a high affinity for the edge of the pore, and binding of those peptides to the edge of the pore produces a reduction of the line tension [33].

Some studies have reported that the union of cationic amphiphilic peptides to the lipid bilayer produces a strong internal membrane tension able to create pores in the lipid membrane [33].

2.2.2. pH-buffering effect (the proton sponge effect)

In this endosomal escape mechanism, the low pH of the endosomal environment leads to the protonation of the entrapped agents with a high buffering capacity. Protonation causes an influx of ions (H^+ and Cl^-) and water into endosomes, resulting in osmotic swelling and endosome rupture [33].

The proton-sponge effect has been observed in certain cationic polymers with a high H^+ buffering capacity over a wide pH range [34]. These polymers usually contain protonable secondary or tertiary amine groups with pKa close to endosomal/lysosomal pH. As explained before, during the maturation of endosomes, the membrane-bound ATPase proton pumps actively translocate protons from the cytosol into endosomes, causing the acidification of the endosomal compartments. At this point, cationic polymers with high buffering capacity become protonated and resist the acidification of endosomes, which results in more protons pumped into the endosome in an attempt to decrease the pH [34]. The proton pumping action is followed by passive chloride ions entry, increasing ionic concentration and, consequently, water influx [34]. The high osmotic pressure produces the swelling and the rupture of endosomes, releasing their contents to the cytosol [34]. Histidine-rich molecules show a buffering effect upon protonation [33] and histidine can be included in non-viral vectors to enhance transfection efficiency by facilitating endosomal escape.

2.2.3. The flip-flop mechanism

This endosomal escape mechanism can be useful for endocytozed lipoplexes. Lipoplexes are endocytozed and become entrapped inside the early endosomes. There is an electrostatic interaction between the cationic lipoplexes and the anionic lipids of the endosomal membrane [34]. The anionic lipids of the endosomal membrane laterally diffuse into the lipoplexes and form charge-neutralized ion pair with cationic lipids of the lipoplexes, resulting in the nucleic acids being displaced from the lipoplexes and released in the cytoplasm [34].

2.2.4. Fusion in the endosomal membrane

This mechanism of endosomal escape is based on the destabilization of the endosomal membrane by water soluble and partly hydrophobic, and/or polybasic peptides known as cell-penetration peptides or CPPs. CPPs were originally derived from viruses, and they constitute short sequences of amino acids (10-30 residues) that use to be cationic and/or amphiphatic [34]. The main features of CPPs are their abilities to penetrate the cell membrane at low molecular concentrations without causing significant membrane damage and to internalize electrostatically or covalently bound biologically active cargoes (including proteins, peptides and nucleic acids) with high efficiency and low toxicity [35]. CPPs either form complexes with nucleic acids, through electrostatic interaction, or can be incorporated into polymeric and lipidic delivery systems [34]. To date, the internalization mechanism of CPPs still remains controversial, since there is evidence for both energy-independent and endocytic processes for cellular uptake of CPPs. Nowadays, it is generally accepted that endocytosis is the major internalization mechanism for most CPPs. However, it seems plausible that several CPPs utilize two or more cellular uptake pathways depending on the experimental conditions [35]. Further research would be needed in order to elucidate the exact uptake mechanisms and to identify the precise factors influencing these processes.

There are different criteria to categorize CPPs into different families. In general, CPPs can be classified into two categories [36]: (i) Cationic peptides that usually contain arginine and lysine residues; and (ii) amphiphatic peptides that consist of both hydrophobic and hydrophilic segments. Two examples of CPPs currently used to improve transfection efficiency of non-viral gene delivery platforms are the transcriptional activator protein or TAT (which belongs to the first category and was the first CPP identified, derived from the transcription activating factor of human immunodeficiency virus 1 (HIV-1)) [33,37] and the Sweet Arrow Peptide or SAP (which belongs to the second category and is a proline-rich amphipathic peptide of synthetic origin) [38].

2.2.5. Photochemical disruption of the endosomal membrane

Photochemical internalization (PCI) is a light-directed delivery technology that utilizes photosensitizers to facilitate the transport of membrane-impermeable macromolecules from endocytic vesicles into the cytoplasm [34]. Photosensitizers are usually amphiphilic compounds that can bind and localize in the plasma membrane. In this mechanism, photosensitizers bind to and localize in the plasma membrane, and they can be taken up by endocytosis together with the non-viral gene delivery systems. Photosensitizers are confined to the endosomal membrane and remain inactive until they are triggered by light with specific wavelengths matching their absorption spectra [39]. Once activated, they induce the formation of highly reactive oxygen species, causing the rupture of endosomes' and lysosomes' membrane. As a result, macromolecules that are trapped inside the endosomes/lysosomes can be liberated into the cytosol [34].

In general, the enhancement of endosomal escape is believed to be a crucial factor in non-viral-vector-based DNA delivery platforms. Different strategies for endosomal escape have different characteristics. A safe endosomal escape agent applicable in the clinic should have low immunogenicity and toxicity, high efficiency, ease of use and production, modular attachment of targeting ligands and the potential for cost-effective large-scale manufacture [33].

2.3. Nuclear import

In the previous section, we have seen several strategies suitable for non-viral gene delivery to avoid endosomal degradation of the DNA and to enhance its release to the cytoplasm. However, in order to achieve an effective transfection, the DNA molecules have to enter the nucleus. Here, we will discuss the principal strategies to transport DNA to the nucleus once released in the cytoplasm.

To enter the nucleus, molecules must pass through nuclear pore complexes (NPCs), which are multimeric structures with a central channel of 9 nm that prevents molecules with a molecular weight higher than 45 kDa from passively diffusing into the nucleus [40]. In the case of naked DNA, molecules smaller than 300 bp can passively diffuse into the nucleus, but larger DNA molecules, even when condensed by a non-viral vector, are excluded from the nucleus except when cells are undergoing mitosis [40-42]. During cell division, the integrity of the nuclear membrane is lost, which allows the nuclear entry of DNA-vector complexes within the daughter cells [21,40]. This is the case in the *in vitro* transfection with dividing cells, but *in vivo* transfection often targets slow dividing or terminally differentiated cells [21,40]. Therefore, the nuclear envelope cannot be neglected in *in vivo* situations, and there is considerable interest in improving the nuclear import efficiency of non-viral vectors [21,40].

Classically, proteins that are destined for the nucleus contain a nuclear localization signal (NLS), which is abundant in basic amino acids and it can be recognized by cytoplasmic proteins known as importins [17] that mediate energy-dependent transport through the NPC [40,43]. The same approach can be used to enhance non-viral gene delivery to the nucleus [21]. An NLS-containing vector can be added to the DNA-vector formulation or an NLS sequence can be directly bound to the DNA in order to promote its transport to the nucleus by the importins

[40]. In addition, highly basic polymers such as polylysine and protamine, the highly basic sequence of which resembles typical NLS sequences, have been used as potential agents to enhance nuclear targeting when complexed with DNA [40].

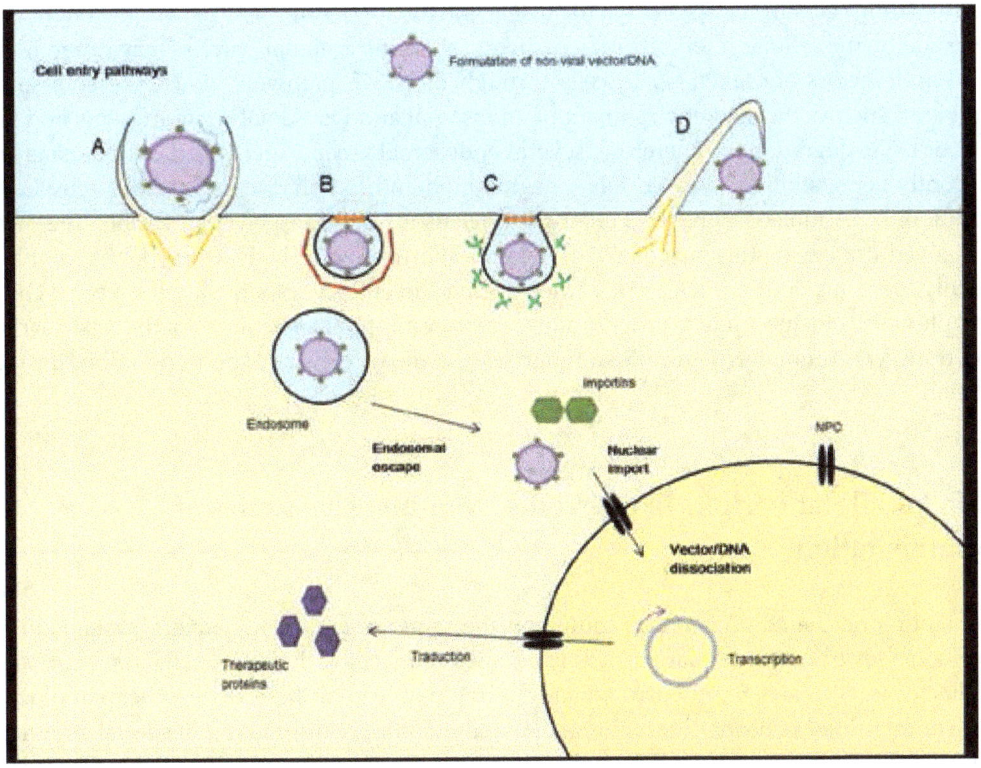

Figure 5. Cell entry pathways and intracellular trafficking of non-viral gene delivery systems. A) Phagocytosis. B) Clathrin-mediated endocytosis (CME). C) Caveolae-mediated endocytosis (CvME). D) Macropinocytosis. Internalized vector/DNA complexes following the CME pathway escape from endosomes and can be transported into the nucleus by the importins if they contain an NLS. When vector and DNA dissociate from each other, the transgene is expressed in the target cells. Yellow filaments represent actin; red chain represents clathrin coat; green filaments represent caveolin dimers; orange little circles represent the small GTPase dynein; blue filaments represent opsonins. (Adapted from [23; 24])

Finally, it should be considered that, once inside the nucleus, the non-viral vector itself may constitute a barrier to transgene expression. In fact, the agent used to condense the DNA could potentially interfere with the access of the cellular transcription machinery to the transgene promoter, thereby reducing or preventing its expression [40]. Still, premature release of DNA from the vector may expose the DNA to enzymatic degradation before expression can occur [40,44]. For liposomal-based vectors, DNA displacement from the vector seems to be connected to endosomal escape, driven by the anionic lipids of the endosomal membrane that neutralize the charge of the cationic lipids in the liposomal formulation [40,45,46]. In contrast, polycation/DNA complexes appear to release from each other in the nucleus through exchange of the polycations in the complexes with the protein components of the surrounding proteins

[40,47,48]. However, it seems plausible that additional mechanisms other than competitive charge interactions may be involved in the dissociation of DNA from polycations, and a deeper understanding of chromatin remodelling mechanisms may shed further light on this issue.

In summary, non-viral vectors for DNA delivery systems must overcome several intracellular barriers from cell-surface association to nuclear entry and DNA release. Depending on the cell type and on the cellular internalization pathway, some intracellular barriers may differ. Most non-viral vectors are taken up in cells through the CME pathway, which presents some problems such as the acid environment of endosomal and lysosomal compartments and the risk of DNA degradation. Therefore, several endosomal escape agents and mechanisms are currently being studied to avoid DNA degradation and to enhance its cytosolic release. In addition, DNA molecules have to enter the nucleus for the transgene expression. The most employed strategy for this purpose is the incorporation of an NLS in the vector-DNA complex. Finally, once inside the nucleus or earlier during the endocytic pathway, the vector-DNA complex needs to dissociate in order to allow the transcriptional machinery of the cell to access the transgene promoter. Figure 5 summarizes the most relevant aspects described in this section.

3. Extracellular barriers to overcome. Non-invasive routes of administration

Depending on the administration route and the target organ, gene delivery systems must overcome several extracellular barriers *in vivo* before reaching the target cells. As mentioned earlier, cancer diseases represent 60% of all clinical trials in gene therapy; yet other pathologies such as infectious, neurodegenerative, ocular and pulmonary diseases merit special attention, which, in sum, represent 10% of clinical trials in gene therapy. The principal and most studied route of administration of non-viral gene delivery systems for those diseases is the intravenous administration. Here, vectors need to be properly designed in order to overcome all the hurdles this route presents. Moreover, when specific tissues need to be targeted, such as the brain, the eye or the lungs, additional extracellular barriers appear and vectors have to be able to surpass them too. In this section, we will review the principal systemic barriers following the intravenous administration of non-viral gene delivery systems, as well as the additional tissue-specific barriers DNA/vector complexes have to overcome. We will also describe several attempts that have been made in order to overcome those barriers using invasive and alternative non-invasive routes of administration. Many efforts are being conducted to achieve effective strategies for safe non-viral gene delivery platforms based on non-invasive administration routes.

3.1. Intravenous administration

For many cancer forms, and specially disseminated cancer diseases, treatment needs to be administered systemically. Thus, intravenously administered current gene delivery systems to treat cancer should be able to transport and deliver the genetic cargo into cancerous cells.

The principal challenge of systemically administered DNA is to resist the extracellular enzymatic degradation, since DNA is subject to enzymatic degradation from the point of entry. However, it is possible to considerably surmount this hurdle by condensing the negatively charged DNA with the positively charged non-viral vectors [13].

Secondly, the other major extracellular barrier in the systemic route is the non-specific binding of the non-viral vector/DNA complex, which has a net positive charge, with blood cells and serum proteins such as albumin, complements, immunoglobulins and fibronectin,which have a negative surface charge [49]. These interactions could potentially end in aggregation or dissociation of vector/DNA complexes, resulting in their rapid clearance and elimination by the reticuloendothelial systems [49].

A third obstacle in systemic delivery might be the colloidal instability of non-viral vector/DNA complex formulations in the extracellular environment, which can also result in the aggregation of the complexes [49]. Fourth, vascular system is an extracellular barrier to be considered since it limits the size of the nanoparticles that can pass through the endothelial cells, which are relatively small and have tight junctions [49].

Finally, the activation of the immune system by the foreign vector/DNA complexes is an extracellular issue to be taken into consideration as well. In fact, foreign synthetic vectors can also induce an inflammatory response and/or complement activation, and hydrophobic particles can be eliminated by mononuclear phagocytic system through opsonization [49].

In order to overcome all these systemic barriers, non-viral vectors should be structurally modified. Formulation of gene delivery vectors is a key factor in determining their bioavailability and transfection efficiency *in vivo* [49]. Some of the strategies that are being developed to improve the properties of nanoparticles in the extracellular environment are discussed below.

The most employed strategy to increase the stability of vector/DNA complexes is shielding the outer surface of complexes with poly(ethylene glycol) or PEG [50]. Because of its highly hydrophobic nature, PEG produces a steric barrier against nuclease degradation and aggregation of nanoparticles in blood circulation [49]. However, despite the promising results, some difficulties exist in conjugation of PEG to gene delivery systems. PEGylation could decrease binding ability of non-viral vectors to DNA causing instability of lipo- or polyplexes in blood circulation. It may also affect the binding of vector/DNA complexes to receptors on the cell membrane [51]. Moreover, PEGylation can induce accelerated blood clearance due to activation of splenic synthesis of anti-PEG IgM antibody after first injection, resulting in the opsonization of the subsequent doses [49]. The length and the degree of PEGylation can also affect the ability of DNA condensation and biodistribution of gene carriers *in vivo*, and the optimal PEG length and content depends on gene carrier systems [52].

Consequently, considerable research has been made with the aim of compensating the negative effect of PEGylation in non-viral gene delivery systems. As reported in a recent study, one possible solution is to replace PEG by some hydrophilic polymers such as poly(N-vinyl-2-pyrrolidone) (PVP), poly(4-acryloylmorpholine), or poly(N,N-dimethylacrylamide) [53]. Coating of nanoparticles with these polymers led to extended residence of the nanoparticles in blood circulation in rats, although they had a shorter half-life than the PEG-coated nanoparticles [53]. Other strategies include providing stability against serum compounds and enzymatic digestion using copolymers of poly(L-lysine) and poly(2-methyl-2-oxazoline) [54], the pH-sensitive shielding of DNA polyplexes or lipoplexes (e.g. with PEG-acetal-MAL or maleimide moiety) [55], the use of enzymatically cleavable PEG linkers (e.g. PEG-peptide-DOPE or PPD that is cleaved in a matrix metalloproteinase-rich environment) [56], or the production of reducible PEG nanoparticles (e.g. PEG and chitosan bound through disulphide bridges) [57].

Besides PEGylation, other chemical and structural modifications can be applied to gene delivery agents in order to overcome the systemic barriers. In the case of cationic lipid-based non-viral vectors, incorporation of cholesterol can stabilize lipoplexes against binding to red blood cells [49]. In the case of cationic polymer-based non-viral vectors, conjugation of lactose to chitosan polyplexes has shown excellent DNA binding ability, good protection of DNA from nuclease, and the suppression of self-aggregation and serum-induced aggregation [58]. Therefore, current research has focused on multifunctional and diverse non-viral gene carriers that can be adjusted for each particular condition.

3.2. Targeting specific tissues: additional extracellular barriers

When targeting specific tissues, vectors have to be able to surpass additional barriers as well. Here, we will focus on specific extracellular barriers present in gene delivery to the central nervous system (CNS), to the eye and to the lungs. The invasive and alternative non-invasive routes of administration that avoid those barriers will also be discussed.

3.2.1. Gene delivery to CNS

The CNS possesses particular anatomical and physiological properties that make gene delivery to CNS specially challenging. The CNS is protected by the blood-brain-barrier (BBB), which consists of tightly joined capillary endothelial cells [19], and it is considered to be impermeable for almost 100% of the macromolecular drugs and over 98% of small molecule drugs [59]. The spinal cord is part of the CNS and it is protected by the blood-cerebrospinal fluid barrier (BCSFB), which is constituted of choroid plexus epithelial cells and restricts the free diffusion of molecules into the cerebrospinal fluid (CSF) [19]. Transport into the CNS of essential nutrients, such as glucose and amino acids, occurs through specific receptors present in the BBB and the BSCFB [19]. Within the CNS, distinct cell types exist including neurons and different types of glial cells; neurons are particularly challenging to transfect and it is thought this is attributable to their post-mitotic nature, their complex structure and the complexity of neuronal networking [19].

Most of the strategies to cross the BBB upon systemic administration of non-viral vector/DNA complexes exploit receptor-mediated uptake of molecules such as transferrin (Tf), lactoferrin and insulin, since receptors of those molecules are expressed on many cell types, including neurons and the capillary endothelial cells of the BBB [19]. By attaching a ligand for those receptors to the non-viral delivery system, one can enhance the transport of the vector/DNA complex towards the CNS. Another strategy known as 'Molecular Trojan Horse' uses peptidomimetic monoclonal antibodies that are designed to target specific receptors on the BBB and induce receptor-mediated transcytosis of the non-viral delivery system into the CNS [60]. Other approaches investigated for CNS delivery of conventional pharmaceutics upon systemic administration include transient mechanical disruption of the BBB and RNAi-mediated knockdown of tight junction proteins [19].

The ultimate goal for CNS gene therapeutics is delivery by systemic route, which is the most acceptable for clinical use. Nevertheless, in view of the high amount of extracellular barriers that vectors must overcome, many studies have attempted different routes of administration. To date, several pre-clinical studies have essayed local administration to the brain, either by injection or by infusion. However, even if local administration to the brain eludes the extracellular barriers to access the CNS, the need for brain surgery to infuse a gene therapy vector clearly limits the clinical applicability for this approach.

Intranasal delivery offers a novel and non-invasive means by which non-viral gene delivery systems can gain access to the brain. The mechanisms by which intranasally delivered substances enter the CNS have not been fully elucidated, but an accumulating amount of evidence suggests that substances can reach the brain through a combination of perineuronal, perivascular and lymphatic transport pathways. In addition, the prevailing nose-to-brain pathway will largely depend on the region where the delivered agent is placed within the nasal cavity and the physicochemical properties of the therapeutic being administered [61]. It is currently accepted that the intranasally administered substance can reach the CNS by three main pathways: (i) direct paracellular or transcellular transport via the olfactory neurons or olfactory epithelial cells ('olfactory neural pathway'), (ii) transport via the trigeminal nerves ('trigeminal pathway') or (iii) indirectly, *via* blood vasculature and/or lymphatic system ('systemic pathway') [62]. The nasal mucosa is highly vascularized, and the blood vessels allow passage of drugs following nasal administration in nano-drug delivery systems; however, the substance that has been absorbed into the systemic circulation has to cross the BBB in order to reach the CNS [61]. Following olfactory and trigeminal nerve pathways, drug is delivered to the olfactory bulbs and to more caudal brain areas, respectively [63]. Within the brain, pulsatile flow in perivascular spaces has been postulated to allow for widespread transport of molecules within interstitial fluid to sites deep in parenchyma [63,64].

Advantages of intranasal administration include ease of administration (non-invasive), rapid dose absorption via highly vascularized mucosa, large nasal mucosa surface area for dose absorption, avoidance of the gastrointestinal tract, first-pass metabolism and fewer side effects, among others [65]. Moreover, intranasal administration confers improved convenience and compliance compared to other more invasive routes and it allows self-administration [65]. Disadvantages of this route include that nasal congestion could interfere with dose absorption, that the amount of dose that reaches the CNS varies with each agent and that the frequent use of this route leads to mucosal damage [65]. In addition, the administered formulation can undergo rapid clearance from nasal cavity by the mucociliary system [59,66]. This latter drawback can be overcome by adding a mucoadhesive substance to the formulations. For non-viral-vector-based gene delivery systems, chitosan is an attractive excipient that can confer both bio-adhesion and absorption properties, and it is the most widely investigated absorption enhancer material both in terms of efficiency and safety [63]. Chitosan is able to interact through its positively charged amino groups with the anionic counterpart present in the mucus layers, mainly sialic acid, and to affect permeability of the epithelial membrane by the transient opening of the tight junctions in the epithelial cells [67]. In a recent study, another substance, the non-ionic surfactant laureate sucrose ester has been also reported to be an effective intranasal absorption enhancer [68].

Recently, the first report that intranasal delivery of DNA nanoparticles can bypass the BBB and transfect and express the encoded protein in rat brain has been published, thereby affording a non-invasive approach for gene therapy in CNS disorders [63]. Authors demonstrated that intranasal delivery of unimolecularly compacted DNA nanoparticles, which consist of single molecules of plasmid DNA encoding enhanced green fluorescent protein (eGFP) compacted with 10 kDa commercial peptide (PEG-substituted lysine 30 mers or CK30PEG10k), successfully transfects cells and leads to the expression of the eGFP in the rat brain [63]. The results further suggest that the cells transfected within the brain are likely to be pericytes, and that the distribution of nasally administered substances occurs via perivascular transport [63]. Additionally, another recent study has reported brain (cortex and hippocampus) transfection upon intranasal administration of chitosan and polyethyleneimine (PEI)-coated magnetic micelles [69]. Even if those nanoparticles were able to reach the brain presumably because of a transient disruption of the BBB following mild traumatic brain injury, the results show that the intranasal route might be useful for targeting the brain. Although further optimization of the dose, dosing regimen and dose interval is needed to achieve appropriate levels of transgene expression [63], the promising results will certainly encourage the research in the field of intranasal administration of non-viral-vector-based gene delivery systems, which has clinical importance due to its non-invasive nature.

3.2.2. Gene delivery to the eye

The eye is an attractive target organ for gene therapy because of its unique characteristics. The tissue volume to be treated is small, the therapeutic concentration to be administered is relatively low and the diffusion of active products from the eye to the circulation is minimal [70]. In addition, the eye benefits from a relative immune privilege, minimizing the potential immune and inflammatory reactions that may follow the intraocular injections of foreign agents [70].

In general, gene delivery systems for eye diseases range from simple eye drops and ointments to more advanced bio- and nanotechnology-based systems such as muco-adhesive systems, polymers, liposomes and ocular inserts. Most of these technologies were developed for front-of-the-eye ophthalmic therapies and are not applicable as back-of-the-eye delivery systems [71].

When the systemic administration is used to target the eye, non-viral vector/DNA complexes must cross the blood-ocular-barrier (BOB) to reach the ocular tissue. This constitutes a real challenge, since the BOB is composed of tight epithelial junctions. Two principal strategies to overcome this barrier are the use of vectors smaller than 100 nm to allow intracellular passage across the BOB [72] and the use of ligand-equipped vectors that recognize specific receptors in the BOB [73]. Therefore, even if the intravenous route permits the delivery of larger volumes of the formulations as well as repeated administrations, the therapeutic effect achieved by this method is often limited by the factors restricting the access to the eye.

Invasive methods such as intravitreal injection, subconjuntival injection and subretinal injection can bypass some of those barriers, and intravitreal and subretinal injections are currently considered as the most effective and common methods of gene delivery to retinal ganglion cells and to inner layers of the retina, respectively. However, these methods are very invasive and repeated gene delivery to the eye using such methods can cause further damage of the eye like retinal detachment, haemorrhages, and sub- or pre-retinal fibrosis [71]. Therefore, non-invasive and effective methods for ocular gene delivery are needed. In this regard, topical administration in the form of eye drops is a non-invasive delivery method that can be performed repeatedly with minimal side effects [71].

However, the non-invasive route of administration is perhaps the most ambitious goal because the barriers associated with topical gene delivery to the posterior ocular tissue are the most challenging. First, vector/DNA complexes have to surpass the tear film, which is an aqueous layer covered by lipids and underlined by mucin that covers the corneal and conjuctival layers [71]. This tear film restricts the bioavailability of applied formulations because of the tear turnover rate and the lacrimal and nasolacrimal drainage [85]. Strategies to overcome this barrier include addition of viscosity enhancers such as cellulose derivatives or thermoreversible poloxamer gels [71] and, most importantly, the incorporation of muco-adhesive polymers such as chitosan and hyaluronic acid derivatives in gene delivery systems [74]. Second, ocular tissue barriers such as the cornea, conjunctiva, sclera and choroid, contain epithelial tight junctions, proteoglycan matrices and fibril collagen networks within their structures, which contribute to restrict the passage of vector/DNA complexes to the neuroretina [71]. Finally, the vitreous is an aqueous biogel composed of collagen, hyaluronan and proteoglycans that hinders transfection of the retinal cells [71]. Strategies to overcome those barriers include all the above-mentioned methods from the use of vectors of suitable dimensions to the use of specific ligands and muco-adhesive polymers [71].

The majority of success in ocular gene therapy research thus far was accomplished for applications involving the anterior part of the eye, using mainly viral-based delivery systems and invasive delivery methods. Interestingly, effective gene delivery to the retina and retinal pigment epithelium using non-viral vectors has been recently reported; however, in this study magnetic nanoparticles were administered invasively, through intravitreal and subretinal injections [75]. Rather than in gene delivery, significant advances have been made in drug delivery systems to target the posterior part of the eye using non-invasive administration routes. For instance, in a recent study, it was reported that surface-modified submicron-sized lipid emulsions could be promising vehicles of hydrophobic drug delivery to the ocular posterior segment [76]. In that study, researchers performed surface modification of the lipid emulsions using a positive charge inducer and the functional polymers chitosan and poloxamer 407. Authors suggested that poloxamer 407 increased the lipid emulsion retention time on the eye surface by its adhesive properties, therefore enhancing gene delivery to the ocular posterior segment. Additionally, another study has reported successful drug delivery to the posterior segment of the eye of rats and rabbits using annexin A5-associated liposomes [77]. Here, authors suggested that annexin A5 mediated endocytosis can enhance the delivery of associated lipidic drug delivery vehicles across biological barriers. Moreover, a novel study has reported the topical drug delivery to retinal pigment epithelium with microfluidizer produced small liposomes, which might be an attractive option for drug delivery to the posterior segment tissues of the eye [78]. It may be reasonable that some of the advances in drug delivery will be applicable for gene delivery systems as well, and they will probably inspire further strategies for non-invasive, non-viral gene therapy platforms aimed at targeting the posterior segment of the eye.

3.2.3. Gene delivery to the lungs

Pulmonary gene therapy is considered for the treatment of a variety of lung diseases like cystic fibrosis, asthma, emphysema and lung cancer [79]. Depending on the respiratory disease to be treated, the target cells in the lung can vary from epithelial cells, alveolar cells, macrophages, respiratory stem cells or endothelial cells [79]. Besides, the nucleic acid cargo needs to be delivered to cells in the target region of the lung. Nevertheless, this is severely limited by the pulmonary architecture, the presence of mucus, the clearance mechanisms and the activation of the immune system [79]. Inhalation, intranasal instillation, intratracheal instillation, and intratracheal intubation are techniques that can be used to administer materials of interest to the lungs. Considering the interest of non-invasive administration routes for clinical applications, aerosolized non-viral vector/DNA complexes for inhalation would be the ideal choice for lung gene therapy. There are many advantages to administering medications to the lungs as an aerosol, such as the high local concentration by delivery directly to the airways, and the pain- and needle-free delivery.

Respiratory secretions, which include mucus and alveolar fluid, are the most important extracellular barriers for lung gene delivery. Respiratory mucus is one of the most important defence mechanisms and it is mainly composed by a three-dimensional network of cross-linked mucin chains, which gives the mucus viscoelastic properties [79]. The major proteins in respiratory mucus are albumin, proteases, anti-proteases, immunoglobulins, lysozyme and lactoferrin, and the respiratory secretions of patients with cystic fibrosis or respiratory infections also contain huge amounts of DNA and actin [79]. The alveolar fluid is a thin continuous layer of pulmonary surfactant that covers the alveolar epithelium and it comprises phospholipids and specific surfactant-associated proteins [79].

Respiratory mucus can act as a barrier towards pulmonary gene delivery in several ways. The biopolymer network of mucus limits the diffusion of complexes by sterical obstruction or by binding the complexes [79]. Also, negatively charged and non-cross-linked macromolecules of mucus, as well as other components present in the mucus such as antibodies, can bind to the surface of vector/DNA complexes. These interactions may cause: (i) entrapment of the vector/DNA complexes in the mucus, (ii) aggregation of the complexes due to neutralization of their surface charges, (iii) release of the DNA cargo from the vector, and (iv) an inefficient cell binding of the complex due to shielding of their positive charges or their receptor binding ligands [79]. Finally, the mucus blanket is continuously removed via mucociliary transport or coughing. Therefore, the vector/DNA complex should be able to cross the mucus before they are cleared from the respiratory tract. The diffusion coefficient of the complexes in the mucus, the thickness of the mucus layer and the rate of mucus clearance will determine whether the vector/DNA complexes will reach the epithelial cells [79].

Regarding the alveolar fluid as a barrier towards pulmonary gene therapy, the presence of this surfactant layer can inhibit transfection of cationic lipid-based vector/DNA complexes [79]. It has been suggested that this inhibitory effect results from disintegration of the lipoplexes by the negatively charged lipids present in the surfactant layer, leading to accessibility of nucleases to the DNA cargo and thus its degradation and loss of function [80]. On the other hand, non-viral vectors based on cationic polymers such as PEI might be more resistant to detrimental effects by pulmonary surfactant [79].

Several strategies have been developed in order to overcome the extracellular barriers of lung gene delivery. Size and surface properties of non-viral vector/DNA complexes have a pivotal role in determining their behaviour in respiratory secretions. Most efforts have been conducted to increase the mobility of vector/DNA complexes in respiratory mucus and to avoid interactions of complexes with respiratory secretions.

There are different methods to increase non-viral vector/DNA complex mobility through the respiratory mucus. One straightforward mechanism consists of adding mucolytic agents that hydrolyze mucins present in the mucus [79]. Also, it has been demonstrated that N-acetylcysteine and its derivatives lower the viscosity and elasticity of mucus by reducing the disulphide bridges between the subunits of mucins [81]. As future directions, research is focusing on functionalized nanoparticles with mucolytic agents able to cut a way through the mucus, enhancing their transport across the extracellular matrix [79].

On the other hand, the principal strategy to avoid interactions between vector/DNA complexes and components of biological fluids is the shielding of the complexes by modification with biocompatible hydrophilic but biologically inert polymers [79]. Shielding of vector/DNA complexes may not only be important to reduce interaction with mucus and alveolar fluid components but also diminish clearance by alveolar macrophages. For instance, shielding the positive surface charges of vector/DNA complexes with neutral hydrophilic polymers such as polyethylene glycol (PEG) favours their physicochemical stability and their gene transfer capacity [79].

A number of challenges must be overcome before pulmonary gene therapy becomes a reality, such as the development of gene vectors that can more efficiently penetrate the mucus barrier [82]. However, real advances have been made in recent years, novel aerosol therapeutic modalities are currently being investigated for lung cancer, and inhaled gene therapy has already presented safety and effectiveness in cystic fibrosis [83].

As summarized in Figure 6, non-viral vector/DNA complexes have to overcome several extracellular barriers before binding the target cells and initiating the intracellular trafficking towards the nucleus, where transgene expression will occur. Intravenous injection is the most widely used administration route but it presents many hurdles that hamper effective gene delivery. Local administration routes are being explored in order to directly target the tissue of interest and avoid systemic barriers, but they often implicate invasive procedures (e.g. brain surgery). Many efforts are currently focused on the study of non-invasive routes of administration that can equally avoid the systemic barriers (e.g. intranasal administration). Besides, local administration into specific tissues such as the eye or the lungs, involve additional barriers that gene delivery systems have to elude. Surface modifications of the vector/DNA formulations are the most employed strategies to overcome both systemic and tissue-specific barriers. It is expected that future non-viral gene delivery systems will be based on multifunctional vectors and that they will allow a non-invasive administration of therapeutic genes into target tissues.

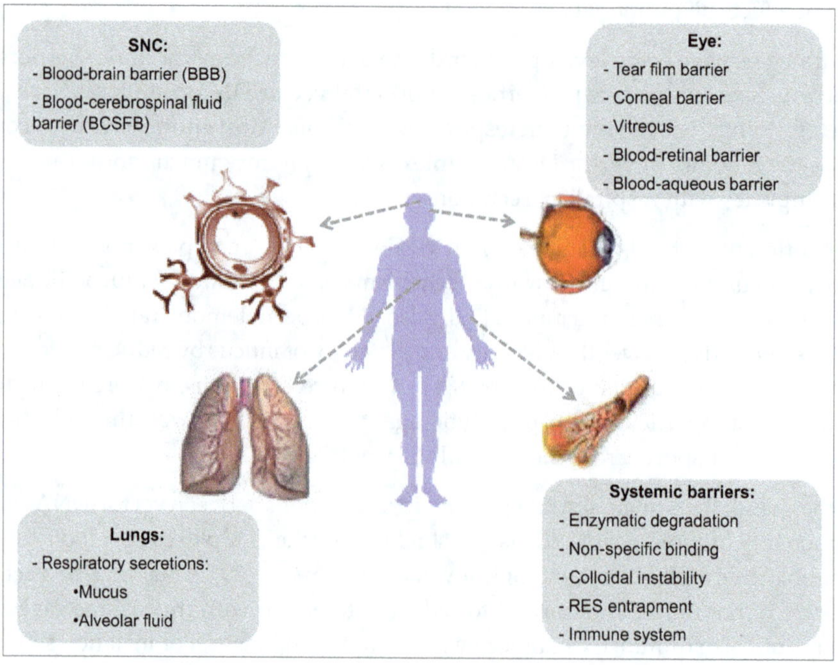

Figure 6. Overview of the systemic and tissue-specific (SNC, eye, lungs) extracellular barriers in non-viral gene therapy.

4. Challenges of non-viral gene therapy and future prospects

Non-viral gene therapy has emerged as a promising therapeutic approach for gene delivery. Even if this field is still far from clinical practice, much progress has been made in the last few years regarding both the optimization of the non-viral vector formulations and the exploration of alternative routes of administration. For transgene expression to occur, optimal non-viral vectors should not elicit an immune response and should be able, among other aspects, to protect the DNA cargo from degradation in circulation, to enable extravasation from the bloodstream, to traverse cellular membranes, to enhance endosomal escape and to facilitate DNA transport to the nucleus [84]. The comprehensive understanding of the extracellular and intracellular barriers that vector/DNA complexes have to overcome in order to achieve an efficient transfection, has allowed the development of several strategies to surpass all those barriers, most of them based on formulation modifications of the complexes and on the use of local routes of administration. Regarding this latter aspect, considerable evidence suggests that the optimization of non-invasive routes of administration may provide safer and more effective gene delivery platforms in the future; therefore, it might be relevant to guide some efforts in this direction.

The major limitation of non-viral gene delivery, as mentioned repeatedly, is the low transfection efficiency. Several strategies discussed along the chapter increase transfection efficiency by providing the nanoparticles the ability to overcome extra- and intracellular barriers. However, there are two other aspects that are also essential for developing optimal gene delivery platforms: *targeting* and *long-term expression* of the transgene. Both are crucial to bring non-viral gene delivery systems into the clinic, since they provide specificity and sustained effect of the treatment, respectively. Many efforts have been made in this regard; however, further research is still required. In addition, other aspects such as the toxicity of the nanoparticles and the manufacturing and regulatory issues have to be carefully considered. Here, we will briefly discuss the current strategies for targeting the desired cells or tissues and for achieving a long-term expression of the transgene. We will also highlight the importance of considering the toxicity, manufacturing and regulatory issues of the nanoparticle formulations.

4.1. Targeting

Targeting to the desired cells or tissue can be achieved by modifying either the vehicle (the non-viral vector) or the cargo (the plasmid DNA). The most employed strategy is the attachment to the non-viral vector specific ligands (such as transferrin for targeting the SNC) that recognize particular receptors present in the target cells or tissues. As discussed earlier, this approach has proved effective in several studies. Also, in cancer gene therapy, some strategies are based on the exploitation of the tumour-specific physiological changes (the tumour microenvironment) to specifically conduct the nanoparticles to cancer cells [85].

On the other hand, another possibility is to introduce modifications in the DNA cargo (instead of the vector) to achieve targeted expression of the transgene, this approach is known as "transcriptional targeting." This strategy is based on the use of DNA expression cassettes that contain regulatory regions that are recognized by transcription factors specifically present or selectively expressed by the target cell population [85]. In this strategy the DNA would, in theory, be delivered to all tissues, but the expression of the transgene would only occur in the cell populations where the particular transcription factors are present, that is, in the target cell populations [84]. The success of this method of targeting needs prior knowledge of a difference in transcription factor expression between the target and normal tissue [84].

Targeting is an essential requirement in gene delivery systems. Beneficial aspects of targeted gene delivery include, among others, increased bioavailability of the therapeutic product in the diseased tissue; reduced accumulation in healthy tissues and, hence, reduced side effects;

reduction of drug dosage and reduced dosing frequency, which enhances patient compliance. All these aspects help to increase the therapeutic efficacy and permit to reduce treatment costs [86].

4.2. Duration of gene expression

Long-term or sustained expression of the transgene delivery constitutes a real challenge in non-viral gene therapy, and it is a considerable limiting factor, since transient expression requires repeated dosing and makes the therapeutic effect unsustained. Transgene expression can decrease in time due to several factors, including destruction by nucleases, loss by recombination, distribution to non-nuclear compartments and/or recognition and subsequent silencing of foreign DNA [85]. In addition, in dividing cells the percentage of transfected cells decreases at each division, because while cells replicate, plasmids do not.

Strategies to increase duration of transgene expression have focused on plasmid DNA modifications rather than on vector modifications. Some of those strategies are aimed at integrating the transgenes into the host genome using viral integrases, site-specific recombinases and transposases, which are enzymes with capacity of inserting foreign DNA into the host genome [85]. However, this approach cannot be clinically applicable in humans because of its associated risks, such as the induction of insertional mutagenesis in the host cells.

A different strategy to achieve sustained transgene expression is the use of autonomously replicating plasmids or episomes, which does not require integration in the host genome and, hence, avoids insertional mutagenesis risks [85]. In addition, episomally replicating plasmids usually yield high levels of transgene expression. These strategies incorporate genes that encode necessary cofactors for transcription of the plasmid to the therapeutic plasmid DNA, making the transgene expression less dependent on host factors. Incorporation of viral DNA that allows the plasmid to replicate extrachromosomally is an efficient approach, but it presents a major drawback, since those replication-inducing viral DNA elements are associated with induction of immune response and risk of transformation and oncogenicity [85]. Alternatively, mammalian scaffold/matrix attachment regions (S/MARs) have been identified that can be incorporated to plasmid DNA instead of the aforementioned viral sequences. These sequences can also enhance episomal replication of the plasmids, probably by bringing the plasmids into contact with the host replication machinery [73]. Episomally replicating plasmids are especially important in cancer gene therapy, where maintenance and vertical transfer of the therapeutic plasmid will be essential because of the presence of dividing tumour cells [85].

Some other strategies for achieving sustained expression focus on the prevention of transgene silencing, since cellular gene silencing mechanisms can impede transgene expression [85].

Further modifications can be also applied to the therapeutic plasmid DNA in order to increase the strength or the specificity of the therapeutic transgene expression. For instance, positive feedback loops can be incorporated. To do this, a promoter that drives the expression of both the transgene and of a strong artificial transcriptional activator is used. This transcriptional activator is capable of interacting with appropriate binding sites within the promoter and, that way, upregulating transgene expression, as well as its own expression [85]. Technologies incorporating positive feedback loops are estimated to increase strength of weak but highly specific regulatory elements [85].

4.3. Toxicity, manufacturing and regulatory issues

Besides increasing transfection efficiency through targeting and other strategies, careful consideration of toxicity, manufacturing and regulatory issues of non-viral delivery systems is mandatory. Scalability and long-term storage requirements are essential factors to be taken into serious consideration when developing non-viral formulations for potential commercial application and introduction in clinical practice [19]. A generally accepted advantage of non-viral vectors is their ease of large-scale manufacture. However, this can become more complex as formulations increase in complexity, incorporating stabilizing components and bioactive targeting ligands.

Regarding toxicity of non-viral vectors, characteristics such as size, charge, surface functionalization, shape, and architecture may contribute to the toxicity profile of nanoparticles. Non-viral vectors are thought to cause toxicity through different mechanisms, including membrane destabilization and lysis, inducing oxidative stress, initiating inflammatory response, inducing global changes in gene expression profiles, among others [85]. Also, the properties of the biomaterials used can influence toxicity, depending on the rate of degradation and persistence in organs [19]. Persisting and accumulating biomaterials are more likely to induce an inflammatory response; also, products of the degradation of nanoparticles could potentially cause toxicity. However, knowledge about how non-viral vectors are disassembled and metabolically processed is still very scarce and further research is necessary in this regard [19].

To conclude, the concept of a unique universal non-viral vector is nowadays abandoned, and it is increasingly accepted that future non-viral gene delivery platforms will be based on multifunctional vectors specifically tailored for different applications [1]. However, there are some generally assumed features that all non-viral vectors should accomplish for efficient gene delivery. In short, three main factors should be taken into consideration when developing non-viral gene delivery platforms: (i) formulation components (of both the vector and the DNA) – the nanoparticle should be able to protect DNA over extra- and intracellular barriers and deliver the cargo into the nucleus of target cells; once inside the nucleus, the plasmids can be addressed to the nuclear matrix for episomal replication and sustained expression; (ii) manufacturing issues – non-viral vector formulations should have potential for scale-up; and (iii) safety and regulatory issues – formulations should be non-toxic, non-immunogenic and should have suitable storage conditions. Although non-viral vectors are still far from clinical practice, they represent a safer alternative to conventional viral vectors. Several formulations and strategies are under investigation with the aim of overcoming extra- and intracellular barriers, enhancing targeted transfection and, in general, increasing transfection efficiency. In addition, those formulations would ideally be suitable for administration through non-invasive routes, such as the intranasal administration to target the brain, topical ocular administration for the retina and aerosols for pulmonary diseases. Finally, the inclusion of novel functional modules within both the carrier and the DNA molecule will produce a range of non-viral vectors tailored for specific applications, including the safe and long-term expression of therapeutic genes in humans [40]. Therefore, reasonable hope suggests that next-generation gene delivery systems may be based on non-viral vector systems tailored for specific applications and suitable for non-invasive administration routes, representing an ideal platform to effectively shuttle the genetic material to target cells in a safe and controlled way.

Acknowledgements

This project was partially supported by the University of the Basque Country UPV/EHU (UFI 11/32), the Basque Government (Department of Education, University and Research, predoctoral PRE_2014_1_433 and BFI-2011-2226 grants), the National Council of Science and Technology (CONACYT), Mexico, Reg. # 217101 and the Spanish Ministry of Education (Grant SAF2013-42347-R). Authors also wish to thank the intellectual and technical assistance from the ICTS "NANBIOSIS", more specifically by the Drug Formulation Unit (U10) of the CIBER in Bioengineering, Biomaterials & Nanomedicine (CIBER-BBN) at the University of Basque Country (UPV/EHU).

Author details

Ilia Villate-Beitia[1,2], Gustavo Puras[1,2], Jon Zarate[1,2], Mireia Agirre[1,2], Edilberto Ojeda[1,2] and Jose Luis Pedraz[1,2*]

*Address all correspondence to: joseluis.pedraz@ehu.eus

1 NanoBioCel Group, Laboratory of Pharmaceutics, School of Pharmacy, University of the Basque Country (UPV/EHU), Vitoria-Gasteiz, Spain

2 Biomedical Research Networking Center in Bioengineering, Biomaterials and Nanomedicine (CIBER-BBN), Vitoria-Gasteiz, Spain

References

[1] Pezzoli D, Chiesa R, De Nardo L, Candiani G. We still have a long way to go to effectively deliver genes!. *J Appl Biomater Funct Mater* 2012;10(2) 82-91.

[2] Gene Therapy Net. http://www.genetherapynet.com/patient-information.html (accessed 7 January 2015).

[3] Kohn DB. Gene therapy for XSCID: the first success of gene therapy. *Pediatr Res* 2000;48(5) 578.

[4] Actionbioscience. http://www.actionbioscience.org/biotechnology/kolehmainen.html#primer (accessed 7 January 2015).

[5] European Medicines Agency, EMA. http://www.ema.europa.eu/ema/ (accessed 8 January 2015).

[6] Rodríguez-Gascón A, del Pozo-Rodriguez A, Solinis MA (2013). Non-viral delivery systems in gene therapy. In: Martin F. (ed.), *Gene Therapy – Tools and Potential Applications*. ISBN: 978-953-51-1014-9, InTech, DOI: 10.5772/52704. Available from: http://www.intechopen.com/books/gene-therapy-tools-and-potential-applications/non-viral-delivery-systems-in-gene-therapy (accessed 07 January 2015).

[7] Gene therapy clinical trials worldwide. *J Gene Med* http://www.wiley.com/legacy/wileychi/genmed/clinical/ (accessed 7 January 2015).

[8] Thomas CE, Ehrhardt A, Kay MA. Progress and problems with the use of viral vectors for gene therapy. *Nat Rev Genet* 2003;4(5) 346-358.

[9] Davis ME. Non-viral gene delivery systems. *Curr Opin Biotechnol* 2002;13(2) 128-131.

[10] Al-Dosari MS, Gao X. Nonviral gene delivery: principle, limitations, and recent progress. *AAPS J* 2009;11(4) 671-681.

[11] Kamimura K, Suda T, Zhang G, Liu D. Advances in gene delivery systems. *Pharmaceut Med* 2011;25(5) 293-306.

[12] Ojeda E, Puras G, Agirre M, Zarate J, Grijalvo S, Pons R, et al. Niosomes based on synthetic cationic lipids for gene delivery: the influence of polar head-groups on the transfection efficiency in HEK-293, ARPE-19 and MSC-D1 cells. *Org Biomol Chem* 2015;13(4) 1068-1081.

[13] Agirre M, Zarate J, Puras G, Rojas LA, Alemany R, Pedraz JL. Strategies for improving the systemic delivery of oncolytic adenoviruses and plasmids: potential application of non-viral carriers. In: Atta-ur-Rahman M, Choudhary I. (eds.), *Frontiers in Anti-Cancer Drug Discovery*. Bentham Science; 2013;2 190-225.

[14] Chawla V, Saraf SA, Saraf SK. Gene delivery: the non-viral vector advantage. *ACT-Biotechnol Res Commun* 2011;1(1) 1-7.

[15] Perez-Martinez FC, Carrion B, Cena V. The use of nanoparticles for gene therapy in the nervous system. *J Alzheimers Dis* 2012;31(4) 697-710.

[16] Guo X, Huang L. Recent advances in nonviral vectors for gene delivery. *Acc Chem Res* 2012;45(7) 971-979.

[17] Xiang S, Tong H, Shi Q, Fernandes JC, Jin T, Dai K, et al. Uptake mechanisms of non-viral gene delivery. *J Control Release* 2012;158(3) 371-378.

[18] Medina-Kauwe LK, Xie J, Hamm-Alvarez S. Intracellular trafficking of nonviral vectors. *Gene Ther* 2005;12(24) 1734-1751.

[19] O'Mahony AM, Godinho BM, Cryan JF, O'Driscoll CM. Non-viral nanosystems for gene and small interfering RNA delivery to the central nervous system: formulating the solution. *J Pharm Sci* 2013;102(10) 3469-3484.

[20] Khalil IA, Kogure K, Akita H, Harashima H. Uptake pathways and subsequent intracellular trafficking in nonviral gene delivery. *Pharmacol Rev* 2006;58(1) 32-45.

[21] Hillaireau H, Couvreur P. Nanocarriers' entry into the cell: relevance to drug delivery. *Cell Mol Life Sci* 2009;66(17) 2873-2896.

[22] Xu L, Huang CC, Huang W, Tang WH, Rait A, Yin YZ, et al. Systemic tumor-targeted gene delivery by anti-transferrin receptor scFv-immunoliposomes. *Mol Cancer Ther* 2002;1(5) 337-346.

[23] Rappoport JZ. Focusing on clathrin-mediated endocytosis. *Biochem J* 2008;412(3) 415-423.

[24] Subtil A, Gaidarov I, Kobylarz K, Lampson MA, Keen JH, McGraw TE. Acute cholesterol depletion inhibits clathrin-coated pit budding. *Proc Natl Acad Sci USA* 1999;96(12) 6775-6780.

[25] Luzio JP, Parkinson MD, Gray SR, Bright NA. The delivery of endocytosed cargo to lysosomes. *Biochem Soc Trans* 2009;37(Pt 5) 1019-1021.

[26] Delgado D, del Pozo-Rodriguez A, Solinis MA, Rodriguez-Gascon A. Understanding the mechanism of protamine in solid lipid nanoparticle-based lipofection: the importance of the entry pathway. *Eur J Pharm Biopharm* 2011;79(3) 495-502.

[27] Nichols B. Caveosomes and endocytosis of lipid rafts. *J Cell Sci* 2003;116(Pt 23) 4707-4714.

[28] Bengali Z, Rea JC, Shea LD. Gene expression and internalization following vector adsorption to immobilized proteins: dependence on protein identity and density. *J Gene Med* 2007;9(8) 668-678.

[29] Kiss AL, Botos E. Endocytosis via caveolae: alternative pathway with distinct cellular compartments to avoid lysosomal degradation? *J Cell Mol Med* 2009;13(7) 1228-1237.

[30] Ikeda Y, Taira K. Ligand-targeted delivery of therapeutic siRNA. *Pharm Res* 2006;23(8) 1631-1640.

[31] Wattiaux R, Laurent N, Wattiaux-De Coninck S, Jadot M. Endosomes, lysosomes: their implication in gene transfer. *Adv Drug Deliv Rev* 2000;41(2) 201-208.

[32] Swanson JA, Watts C. Macropinocytosis. *Trends Cell Biol* 1995;5(11) 424-428.

[33] Varkouhi AK, Scholte M, Storm G, Haisma HJ. Endosomal escape pathways for delivery of biologicals. *J Control Release* 2011;151(3) 220-228.

[34] Liang W, Lam J. Endosomal escape pathways for non-viral nucleic acid delivery systems. In: Ceresa B (ed.), ISBN: 978-953-51-0662-3, InTech;2012. DOI: 10.5772/46006.

Available from: http://www.intechopen.com/books/molecular-regulation-of-endocytosis/endosomal-escape-pathways-for-non-viral-nucleic-acid-delivery-systems (accessed 27 January 2015)

[35] Madani F, Lindberg S, Langel U, Futaki S, Graslund A. Mechanisms of cellular uptake of cell-penetrating peptides. *J Biophys* 2011;2011:414729.

[36] Patel LN, Zaro JL, Shen WC. Cell penetrating peptides: intracellular pathways and pharmaceutical perspectives. *Pharm Res* 2007;24(11) 1977-1992.

[37] Gupta B, Levchenko TS, Torchilin VP. Intracellular delivery of large molecules and small particles by cell-penetrating proteins and peptides. *Adv Drug Deliv Rev* 2005;57(4) 637-651.

[38] del Pozo-Rodriguez A, Pujals S, Delgado D, Solinis MA, Gascon AR, Giralt E, et al. A proline-rich peptide improves cell transfection of solid lipid nanoparticle-based non-viral vectors. *J Control Release* 2009;133(1) 52-59.

[39] Selbo PK, Weyergang A, Hogset A, Norum OJ, Berstad MB, Vikdal M, et al. Photochemical internalization provides time- and space-controlled endolysosomal escape of therapeutic molecules. *J Control Release* 2010;148(1) 2-12.

[40] Glover J, Glouchkova L, Lipps H, Jans D. Overcoming barriers to achieve safe, sustained and efficient non-viral gene therapy. In: Teixeira da Silva J.A., Shima K. (eds.), *Advances in Gene, Molecular and Cell Therapy*. Global Science Books; 2007. p126-140.

[41] Ludtke JJ, Zhang G, Sebestyen MG, Wolff JA. A nuclear localization signal can enhance both the nuclear transport and expression of 1 kb DNA. *J Cell Sci* 1999;112 (Pt 12)(Pt 12) 2033-2041.

[42] Lukacs GL, Haggie P, Seksek O, Lechardeur D, Freedman N, Verkman AS. Size-dependent DNA mobility in cytoplasm and nucleus. *J Biol Chem* 2000;275(3) 1625-1629.

[43] Jans DA, Hubner S. Regulation of protein transport to the nucleus: central role of phosphorylation. *Physiol Rev* 1996;76(3) 651-685.

[44] Lechardeur D, Sohn KJ, Haardt M, Joshi PB, Monck M, Graham RW, et al. Metabolic instability of plasmid DNA in the cytosol: a potential barrier to gene transfer. *Gene Ther* 1999;6(4) 482-497.

[45] Xu Y, Szoka FC,Jr. Mechanism of DNA release from cationic liposome/DNA complexes used in cell transfection. *Biochemistry* 1996;35(18) 5616-5623.

[46] Zelphati O, Szoka FC,Jr. Intracellular distribution and mechanism of delivery of oligonucleotides mediated by cationic lipids. *Pharm Res* 1996;13(9) 1367-1372.

[47] Cereghini S, Yaniv M. Assembly of transfected DNA into chromatin: structural changes in the origin-promoter-enhancer region upon replication. *EMBO J* 1984;3(6) 1243-1253.

[48] Masuda T, Akita H, Harashima H. Evaluation of nuclear transfer and transcription of plasmid DNA condensed with protamine by microinjection: the use of a nuclear transfer score. *FEBS Lett* 2005;579(10) 2143-2148.

[49] Parhiz H, Hashemi M, Ramezani M. Non-biological gene carriers designed for overcoming the major extra- and intracellular hurdles in gene delivery, an updated review. *Nanomed J* 2015;2(1) 1-20.

[50] Mishra S, Webster P, Davis ME. PEGylation significantly affects cellular uptake and intracellular trafficking of non-viral gene delivery particles. *Eur J Cell Biol* 2004;83(3) 97-111.

[51] Khargharia S, Kizzire K, Ericson MD, Baumhover NJ, Rice KG. PEG length and chemical linkage controls polyacridine peptide DNA polyplex pharmacokinetics, biodistribution, metabolic stability and in vivo gene expression. *J Control Release* 2013;170(3) 325-333.

[52] Amoozgar Z, Yeo Y. Recent advances in stealth coating of nanoparticle drug delivery systems. *Wiley Interdiscip Rev Nanomed Nanobiotechnol* 2012;4(2) 219-233.

[53] Ishihara T, Maeda T, Sakamoto H, Takasaki N, Shigyo M, Ishida T, et al. Evasion of the accelerated blood clearance phenomenon by coating of nanoparticles with various hydrophilic polymers. *Biomacromolecules* 2010;11(10) 2700-2706.

[54] von Erlach T, Zwicker S, Pidhatika B, Konradi R, Textor M, Hall H, et al. Formation and characterization of DNA-polymer-condensates based on poly(2-methyl-2-oxazoline) grafted poly(L-lysine) for non-viral delivery of therapeutic DNA. *Biomaterials* 2011;32(22) 5291-5303.

[55] Knorr V, Allmendinger L, Walker GF, Paintner FF, Wagner E. An acetal-based PEGylation reagent for pH-sensitive shielding of DNA polyplexes. *Bioconjug Chem* 2007;18(4) 1218-1225.

[56] Hatakeyama H, Akita H, Ito E, Hayashi Y, Oishi M, Nagasaki Y, et al. Systemic delivery of siRNA to tumors using a lipid nanoparticle containing a tumor-specific cleavable PEG-lipid. *Biomaterials* 2011;32(18) 4306-4316.

[57] Jia L, Li Z, Zhang D, Zhang Q, Shen J, Guo H, et al. Redox-responsive catiomer based on PEG-ss-chitosan oligosaccharide-ss-polyethylenimine copolymer for effective gene delivery. *Polym Chem* 2013;4 156-165.

[58] Hashimoto M, Morimoto M, Saimoto H, Shigemasa Y, Sato T. Lactosylated chitosan for DNA delivery into hepatocytes: the effect of lactosylation on the physicochemical properties and intracellular trafficking of pDNA/chitosan complexes. *Bioconjug Chem* 2006;17(2) 309-316.

[59] Kozlovskaya L, Abou-Kaoud M, Stepensky D. Quantitative analysis of drug delivery to the brain via nasal route. *J Control Release* 2014;189 133-140.

[60] Pardridge WM. Re-engineering biopharmaceuticals for delivery to brain with molecular Trojan horses. *Bioconjug Chem* 2008;19(7) 1327-1338.

[61] Dhuria SV, Hanson LR, Frey WH. Intranasal delivery to the central nervous system: mechanisms and experimental considerations. *J Pharm Sci* 2010;99(4) 1654-1673.

[62] Casettari L, Illum L. Chitosan in nasal delivery systems for therapeutic drugs. *J Control Release* 2014;190 189-200.

[63] Harmon BT, Aly AE, Padegimas L, Sesenoglu-Laird O, Cooper MJ, Waszczak BL. Intranasal administration of plasmid DNA nanoparticles yields successful transfection and expression of a reporter protein in rat brain. *Gene Ther* 2014;21(5) 514-521.

[64] Hadaczek P, Yamashita Y, Mirek H, Tamas L, Bohn MC, Noble C, et al. The "perivascular pump" driven by arterial pulsation is a powerful mechanism for the distribution of therapeutic molecules within the brain. *Mol Ther* 2006;14(1) 69-78.

[65] Parvathi M. Intranasal delivery to the brain: an overview. *IJPRC* 2012;2(3) 889-895.

[66] Illum L. Nasal drug delivery - recent developments and future prospects. *J Control Release* 2012;161(2) 254-263.

[67] Migliore MM, Vyas TK, Campbell RB, Amiji MM, Waszczak BL. Brain delivery of proteins by the intranasal route of administration: a comparison of cationic liposomes versus aqueous solution formulations. *J Pharm Sci* 2010;99(4) 1745-1761.

[68] Li Y, Li J, Zhang X, Ding J, Mao S. Non-ionic surfactants as novel intranasal absorption enhancers: in vitro and in vivo characterization. *Drug Deliv* 2014;27 1-8.

[69] Das M, Wang C, Bedi R, Mohapatra SS, Mohapatra S. Magnetic micelles for DNA delivery to rat brains after mild traumatic brain injury. *Nanomedicine* 2014;10(7) 1539-1548.

[70] Andrieu-Soler C, Bejjani RA, de Bizemont T, Normand N, BenEzra D, Behar-Cohen F. Ocular gene therapy: a review of nonviral strategies. *Mol Vis* 2006;12 1334-1347.

[71] Alqawlaq S, Huzil JT, Ivanova MV, Foldvari M. Challenges in neuroprotective nanomedicine development: progress towards noninvasive gene therapy of glaucoma. *Nanomedicine* (Lon) 2012;7(7) 1067-1083.

[72] Zhang Y, Schlachetzki F, Li JY, Boado RJ, Pardridge WM. Organ-specific gene expression in the rhesus monkey eye following intravenous non-viral gene transfer. *Mol Vis* 2003;9 465-472.

[73] Glover DJ, Lipps HJ, Jans DA. Towards safe, non-viral therapeutic gene expression in humans. *Nat Rev Genet* 2005;6(4) 299-310.

[74] Wadhwa S, Paliwal R, Paliwal SR, Vyas SP. Chitosan and its role in ocular therapeutics. *Mini Rev Med Chem* 2009;9(14) 1639-1647.

[75] Prow TW, Bhutto I, Kim SY, Grebe R, Merges C, McLeod DS, et al. Ocular nanoparticle toxicity and transfection of the retina and retinal pigment epithelium. *Nanomedicine* 2008;4(4) 340-349.

[76] Ying L, Tahara K, Takeuchi H. Drug delivery to the ocular posterior segment using lipid emulsion via eye drop administration: effect of emulsion formulations and surface modification. *Int J Pharm* 2013;453(2) 329-335.

[77] Davis BM, Normando EM, Guo L, Turner LA, Nizari S, O'Shea P, et al. Topical delivery of Avastin to the posterior segment of the eye in vivo using annexin A5-associated liposomes. *Small* 2014;10(8) 1575-1584.

[78] Lajunen T, Hisazumi K, Kanazawa T, Okada H, Seta Y, Yliperttula M, et al. Topical drug delivery to retinal pigment epithelium with microfluidizer produced small liposomes. *Eur J Pharm Sci* 2014;62 23-32.

[79] Sanders N, Rudolph C, Braeckmans K, De Smedt SC, Demeester J. Extracellular barriers in respiratory gene therapy. *Adv Drug Deliv Rev* 2009;61(2) 115-127.

[80] Ernst N, Ulrichskotter S, Schmalix WA, Radler J, Galneder R, Mayer E, et al. Interaction of liposomal and polycationic transfection complexes with pulmonary surfactant. *J Gene Med* 1999;1(5) 331-340.

[81] King M, Rubin BK. Pharmacological approaches to discovery and development of new mucolytic agents. *Adv Drug Deliv Rev* 2002;54(11) 1475-1490.

[82] Laube BL. The expanding role of aerosols in systemic drug delivery, gene therapy and vaccination: an update. *Transl Respir Med* 2014;2:3-0802-2-3. eCollection 2014.

[83] Zarogouldis P, Karamanos NK, Porpodis K, Domvri K, Huang H, Hohenforst-Schimdt W, et al. Vectors for inhaled gene therapy in lung cancer. Application for nano oncology and safety of bio nanotechnology. *Int J Mol Sci* 2012;13(9) 10828-10862.

[84] McCrudden CM, McCarthy HO. Cancer gene therapy – key biological concepts in the design of multifunctional non-viral delivery systems. In: Martín F. (ed.), *Gene Therapy – Tools and Potential Applications*. InTech; 2013. ISBN: 978-953-51-1014-9, InTech, DOI: 10.5772/54271. Available from: http://www.intechopen.com/books/gene-therapy-tools-and-potential-applications/cancer-gene-therapy-key-biological-concepts-in-the-design-of-multifunctional-non-viral-delivery-syst (accessed 17 February 2015)

[85] van Gaal EV, Hennink WE, Crommelin DJ, Mastrobattista E. Plasmid engineering for controlled and sustained gene expression for nonviral gene therapy. Pharm Res 2006;23(6) 1053-1074.

[86] Aneja MK, Geiger JP, Himmel A, Rudolph C. Targeted gene delivery to the lung. Expert Opin Drug Deliv 2009;6(6) 567-583.

8

Genetically Engineered Bacteria in Gene Therapy—Hopes and Challenges

Mustapha Chamekh

Abstract

The main concern of gene therapy is to target the gene of interest to intended cell tissues for optimizing treatment efficiency. Genetically engineered bacteria have been developed as shuttle vectors for localized delivery of therapeutics. Their success depends upon their tropism to target cells and the efficiency of the engaged delivery system. Bodies of evidence clearly indicate the great potential of recombinant bacteria in gene therapy, although most of the studies were just looking for proof-of-concept rather than a ready-to-use final product. This part will provide an overview of our current understanding of bacteria-based delivery of therapeutic genes and heterologous antigens for prophylactic strategies.

Keywords: Recombinant bacteria, Gene delivery, Gene therapy, Immunoprophylaxy

1. Introduction

1.1. Concept of genetically engineered microorganisms as delivery vectors

Although significant progress has been made in physical and chemical methods for gene delivery, these nonmicrobial strategies still present some drawbacks related to specificity and efficiency of gene transfer [1–6]. For example, new formulations of lipid nanoparticles have led to great improvement in gene stability and transfer, yet there remains a lack of a targeting system that would favor the gene transfer to particular cell tissues [7]. Live avirulent microbial vectors such as viruses and bacteria are a promising approach for gene delivery that may serve to fill in those blanks [8–14]. As such, microbial vectors are able to not only serve as cell factories for the production of the transgene but also as vehicles that deliver the transgene to specific cells for which they have a naturally high tropism. Gene transduction with recombinant viruses is generally based on the use of an expression cassette encompassing a transgene [8–11], while in bacteria, the classic approach of gene transfer is based on plasmid-encoded genes [12–14]. The gene of interest must be delivered to the cell's nucleus to allow an efficient manufacturing of the corresponding protein. DNA escape from intracellular bacteria to host cell cytosol may occur following their phagocytosis and lysosomal degradation within the cell. This is, however, not the case for intracellular bacteria that resist or subvert the phagolysosomal processing such as *Salmonella* or *Listeria* [15,16] and for extracellular bacteria that behave as commensals within a specific cellular niche. Commensal bacteria might be, however, of particular interest if the treatment strategy aims at delivering a gene product to targeted cell tissue through a potent delivery machinery. The delivery system used by avirulent vectors is therefore a critical point for optimizing the success of any therapy.

2. Bacteria as delivery vectors in gene therapy

Recombinant bacteria are being considered as an in vivo cell factory that could be used for the delivery of therapeutic genes to target cells. In this process known as "bactofection," a number of bacterial species have been developed as delivery vectors for their application in different therapeutic approaches.

2.1. Attenuated mutant bacteria

The most known bacteria for such purposes are *Salmonella typhimurium* strains that have proven to be useful in DNA vaccination approach. The strategy is based on the transformation of an attenuated strain with a plasmid DNA bearing the gene of interest. It has been shown that oral administration of such transformants into mice induced a robust immune response against gene-encoding antigen [17]. This study is the first to describe the possible transfer of a plasmid DNA from bacteria to host cells resulting in antigen processing and induction of specific immunity. This DNA vaccination approach has proven to be useful in prophylactic settings against tumor antigens. In the murine melanoma model, it has been shown that oral administration of attenuated *S. typhimurium* harboring gene sequences encoding tumoral peptide epitopes fused to murine ubiquitin gene could confer protection against tumor growth through the induction of a type I protective immunity [18]. This strategy of DNA delivery allowed an optimized antigen processing for vaccine development.

2.2. Naturally occurring nonpathogenic bacteria

The genus *Clostridium* comprises a group of nonpathogenic species that are strictly anaerobic and largely distributed in the environment. They are able to produce endospores that can selectively germinate under hypoxia. Given these characteristics, wild-type *Clostridium* has been used to target tumors that are known as poorly oxygenated tissues [19,20]. Various experimental studies have reported the usefulness of clostridia in cancer therapy [21–25]. The injection of either whole *Clostridium* or spores into tumor tissues resulted in tumor destruction as a consequence of the multiplication of bacteria within colonized tumors. Subsequently, more elaborate strategies were developed for the potential use of *Clostridium* as a carrier to deliver prodrug converting enzymes into tumor tissues. Following systemic administration of the prodrug, the latter can be locally activated by the enzyme within tumor tissues, hence promoting a targeted effect against cancer cells. Therefore, selective exposure of tumor tissues to the effect of the prodrug is a promising strategy that may have broad applications in clinical studies. Likewise, recombinant spores of *Clostridium* or *Bacillus subtilis* have been used as a model for surface expression of vaccine antigens. This is based on insertion into chromosomal DNA of bacteria of the gene of interest which is fused to a gene encoding a spore surface protein. This stable genetic construction has allowed an efficient assembly and expression of a variety of fused proteins on the surface of the forming spores. The strategy of recombinant spores has been mainly tested for the development of mucosal vaccines [26].

Gene therapy in cancer has been also investigated using a food-grade microorganism *Bifidobacterium infantis*, which is a nonpathogenic and anaerobic bacterium that can proliferate in the hypoxic environment of tumor tissues as well. *B. infantis* has been applied as a gene delivery system in various cancer models such as bladder cancer including melanoma [27] thanks to its specific targeting property to the anaerobic environment of tumor cells. This bacterium has been successfully used for antitumor suicide gene therapy in a murine model of renal cell carcinoma [27,28]. This strategy is based on the use of the herpes simplex virus thymidine kinase/ganciclovir system to selectively kill tumor cells. Recombinant bacteria bearing virus thymidine kinase gene can replicate within tumor tissue and locally express the enzyme which, in turn, catalyzes the nontoxic precursor ganciclovir to a toxic form resulting in tumor cell killing through termination of DNA replication.

Lactococcus lactis is another food-grade bacterium that has been engineered for gene therapy in inflammatory bowel diseases (IBD). As this bacteria tends to naturally colonize the intestinal epithelium, they were used as vectors for localized delivery of anti-inflammatory mediators. In murine model of induced colitis, oral administration of recombinant *L. lactis* expressing IL-10 [29], IL-27 [30] or anti-TNF nanobody [31] could reduce intestinal inflammation, thereby offering a safe and reliable strategy for the treatment of IBD.

3. Type III delivery system: A promising strategy for targeting intended cell tissues

A broad spectrum of pathogenic bacteria (*Salmonella, Shigella, Yersinia, Pseudomonas,...*) use the type III secretion system (TTSS) to deliver their effector molecules to the membrane or into the host cell's cytosol to subvert the signaling pathways [32,33]. Most of the effector proteins are produced and stored inside bacteria before their secretion by the TTSS upon contact with host cells [34]. This elaborate process allows the bacteria to optimize the function of delivered molecules and, therefore, to resist the host defense mechanisms and proliferate within their niche. The potential of TTSS in gene therapy has been investigated in various experimental models for localized delivery of vaccine antigens or therapeutic molecules.

3.1. Application in immunoprophylaxy

The first attempt in using the TTSS for the delivery of heterologous antigens for vaccine purposes was performed with attenuated *Salmonella*. It has been shown that recombinant *Salmonella* harboring a heterologous gene from pathogenic microorganisms fused to a *Salmonella* effector protein-encoding gene or to a small DNA sequence coding for bacterial signal peptide was able to deliver the hybrid protein into the host cytosol [35]. When injected into mice, these recombinant bacteria induced a protective cytotoxic T lymphocyte (CTLs) response against infection. Thus, the engagement of the hybrid protein by the TTSS allows their subsequent engagement by the major histocompatibility class-I pathway and generation of CTLs that are required for effective immunity against intracellular pathogens [36–38]. The use of the TTSS vaccination approach has been proven to work in different infectious models. In parasitic models of *Plasmodium berghei* infection, TTSS-dependent delivery of a dominant CD8 epitope by *Salmonella* conferred protection from infection in mice [39]. In a similar way, *Yersinia* has been used in vaccination studies in murine models to deliver antigens from a pathogenic protozoan parasite *Entamoeba histolytica* [40]. In this model, it has been shown that TTSS can mediate the delivery of high-molecular-weight antigen that induced significant protection against infection through promoting specific type 1 immune response.

The experimental approach of the bacterial TTSS in vaccination studies has been investigated in cancer models as well. Studies in mice indicated that oral administration of recombinant *Salmonella* expressing tumor antigens induced $CD8^+$ T cell-mediated control of tumor progression [41,42]. *Pseudomonas aeruginosa* was also evaluated as a live attenuated vector for TTSS delivery of antigen in antitumor vaccine experiments. Inoculation of recombinant *Pseudomonas* delivering ovalbumin to mice was shown to induce specific CD8+ T cell response that was associated with a significant resistance against ovalbumin-expressing tumor [43]. These experimental investigations underline the efficacy of this delivery system in antitumor immunoprophylaxy.

Besides their role in the delivery of heterologous antigens, bacterial vectors present major advantages over nonmicrobial adjuvant vaccines in that they are endowed with the ability to induce innate immunity through pathogen-associated molecular patterns (PAMPs). These specific microbial motifs include lipoproteins, lipopolysaccharides, single-strand RNA, and nonmethylated DNA sequences that can trigger the maturation process of antigen-presenting cells through binding to their specific Toll-like receptors and consequently induce the production of inflammatory cytokines [44]. This is particularly interesting for vaccination strategies aiming to optimize the protection efficacy [45].

3.2. Application in therapeutic development

Optimal efficiency of any microbial vector in gene therapy relies particularly on its ability to deliver a sufficient amount of the drug to targeted cell tissues while preserving healthy tissue.

The fact that *Shigella* specifically colonizes the colon and activates the TTSS upon contact with epithelial cells prompted their use as a candidate for localized delivery of anti-inflammatory mediators in inflammatory bowel diseases. Ulcerative colitis and Crohn's disease are characterized by the massive production of inflammatory cytokines such as TNF-α and IL-1β that mediate colon tissue destruction. Anti-inflammatory recombinant IL-10 was used successfully for treatment of IBD, although high doses and repeated administrations were necessary for minimal therapeutic efficacy [46–50]. *Bacteria* TTSS-mediated delivery of IL-10 may offer a good alternative of treatment targeting the colon. The proof-of-principle of this strategy was shown in inflammatory models of *Shigella* infection. When IL-10 was fused to a bacterial signal peptide, the hybrid protein was shown not only to be delivered by the TTSS of *Shigella* but also to be biologically active. Injection of IL-10 recombinant *Shigella* to mice induced a marked reduction of inflammatory symptoms as compared to wild-type *Shigella* and this was associated with a significant local reduction of TNF-α, a major inflammatory cytokine [51]. IL-1 receptor antagonist is a natural inhibitor that antagonizes the inflammatory potential of IL-1β. Imbalance between IL-1β and IL-1 receptor antagonist is associated with acute intestinal inflammation [52,53]. In keeping with this, it has been shown that delivery of recombinant IL-1 receptor antagonist in the intestine blocks IL-1β-mediated colitis in rabbits [54]. Localized delivery of IL-1 receptor antagonist by the TTSS of *Shigella* was shown to be as efficient as IL-10 in reducing the inflammatory symptoms within invaded tissues [51]. As outlined elsewhere, the treatment of experimental colitis could be partially achieved using IL-10 recombinant *Lactobacillus* that colonizes all the intestine. Nevertheless, *Shigella* may provide a useful alternative as a live vector thanks to its specific targeting to the site of IBD, the colon. Yet, due to safety concerns, this is possible only with the use of highly attenuated *Shigella* that can be biologically contained [55]. Furthermore, the efficiency of such an approach awaits additional insight into experimental intestinal models of *Shigella* [56,57]. Taken together, the use of bacterial TTSS for localized delivery of immunogenic antigens or therapeutic molecules may offer alternative options in improving the effectiveness of gene therapy.

4. Issues to overcome for better translating the generated proofs-of-concept to effective treatments in human

Bodies of evidence clearly indicate that bacterial vectors are a promising strategy for gene delivery. Many experimental investigations have shown proof-of-concept examples of the feasibility of such an approach, yet steps forward are still needed not only to translate these concepts into effective treatments for humans but also to find the perfect delivery system for each disease situation.

For safety reasons, nonpathogenic food-grade bacteria remain more attractive as live vectors for vaccine and therapeutic strategies. Some concerns exist, however, about targeting issues which is crucial for optimal efficiency. The best example is the potential use of *Lactobacillus lactis* for the delivery of IL-10 in the treatment of IBD. As this anti-inflammatory cytokine has a pleiotropic immunosuppressive effect, it is particularly crucial to target the inflammatory site while preserving healthy tissues. On the other hand, studies related to the potential application of some microbial vectors in gene therapy are on hold for safety issues. Although research on attenuated bacteria has led to significant progresses in gene therapy, there remain some limitations that preclude their use in immunocompromised populations as well as in infants. The challenge is how to emphasize the benefits while controlling the disadvantages of these microbial vectors. With this regard, recent studies highlighted new lines of development of TTSS-based delivery in avirulent vectors. Interestingly, the gene locus coding for TTSS of *Vibrio parahaemolyticus* has been cloned into a nonpathogenic *E. coli* K-12 strain and shown to be efficient in the delivery of heterologous peptides. The generation of a nonpathogenic *E. coli* displaying an active TTSS is an important step that opens the way for applicability of TTSS-dependent delivery of foreign molecules [58]. In the same way, it has been shown that bacterial minicells derived from aberrant cell division of a mutant strain of *S. typhimurium* may assemble functional TTSS. These nonreplicating nanoparticles were shown to deliver antigen by the TTSS and to promote Th1 immune response, thereby offering an alternative strategy of antigen delivery platform for vaccine and immunotherapeutic developments [59].

5. Perspectives

Recombinant bacteria have shown great potential in the preclinical trials. Their clinical potential relies on their safety and biological containment. Most of the studies were just looking for proof-of-concept rather than a final product that could be put directly to use. Given the global needs, future research challenges should focus on the balance between the optimization of gene therapy through effectiveness of gene delivery to target cells and the biological control of recombinant bacteria to ensure not only an appropriate shutoff mechanism but also to minimize the risks of insertional mutagenesis and aberrant genomic location of delivered genes.

Author details

Mustapha Chamekh*

Address all correspondence to: mchamekh@ulb.ac.be

Faculté de Médecine, Institut d'Immunologie Médicale, Université Libre de Bruxelles, Brussels, Belgium

References

[1] Alsaggar M, Liu DI. Physical methods for gene transfer. Adv. Genet. 2015, 89, 1-24.

[2] Jones CH, Chen CK, Ravikrishnan A, Rane S, Pfeifer BA. Overcoming nonviral gene delivery barriers: perspective and future. Mol. Pharm. 2013, 10, 4082–4098.

[3] Hsu CY, Uludag H. Nucleic-acid based gene therapeutics: delivery challenges and modular design of nonviral gene carriers and expression cassettes to overcome intracellular barriers for sustained targeted expression, J. Drug Target. 2012, 20, 301–328.

[4] Bergen JM, Pun SH. Analysis of the intracellular barriers encountered by nonviral gene carriers in a model of spatially controlled delivery to neurons. J. Gene Med. 2008, 10, 187–197.

[5] Wiethoff CM, Middaugh CR. Barriers to nonviral gene delivery. J. Pharm. Sci. 2003, 92, 203–217.

[6] Nishikawa M, Huang L. Nonviral vectors in the new millennium: delivery barriers in gene transfer. Hum. Gene Ther. 2001, 12, 861–870.

[7] Wang Y, Miao L, Satterlee A, Huang L. Delivery of oligonucleotides with lipid nanoparticles. Adv. Drug Deliv. Rev. 2015, doi: 10.1016/j.addr.2015.02.007.

[8] McConnel MJ, Imperial MJ. Biology of adenovirus and its use as a vector for gene therapy. Hum. Gene Ther. 2004, 15(11), 1022–1033.

[9] Dormond E, Perrier M, Kamen A. From the first to the third generation adenoviral vectors: What parameters governing the production yield. Biotech Adv. 2008, doi: 10.1016/j.biotechadv.2008.10.003.

[10] Gomez CE, Nàjera JL, Krupa M, Esteban M. The poxvirus vectors MVA and NYVAC as gene delivery systems for vaccine against infectious diseases and cancer. Curr. Gene Ther. 2008, 8(2), 97–120.

[11] Ferreira TB, Alves PM, Aunins JG, Carrondo MJ. Use of adenoviral vectors as veterinary vaccines. Gene Ther. 2005, 12, 73–83.

[12] Grillot-Courvalin C, Goussard S, Courvalin P. Bacteria as gene delivery vectors for mammalian cells. Curr. Opin. Biotech. 1999, 10, 477–481.

[13] Vassaux G, Nitcheu J, Jezzard S, Lemoine NR. Bacterial gene therapy strategies. J. Pathol. 2006, 208, 290–298.

[14] Chamekh M. Immunomodulation using genetically engineered bacteria for type III-mediated delivery of heterologous antigens and cytokines: potential application in vaccine and therapeutical developments. Immunopharmacol. Immunotoxicol. 2010, 32(1), 1–4.

[15] Dulcos S, Desjardins M. Subversion of young phagosome: the survival strategies of intracellular pathogens. Cell. Microbiol. 2000, 2(5), 365–377.

[16] Pizarro-Cerdà J, Cossart P. Subversion of cellular functions by *Listeria monocytogenes*. J. Pathol. 2006, 208(2), 215–223.

[17] Darji A, Guzman CA, Gerstel B, Wachholz P, Timmis KN, Wehland J, Chakraborty T, Weiss S. Oral somatic transgene vaccination using attenuated *S. typhimurium*. Cell. 1997, 91(6), 765–775.

[18] Xiang R, Lode HN, Chao TH, Ruehlmann JM, Dolman CS, Rodriguez F, Whitton JL, Overwijk WW, Restifo NP, Reisfeld RA. An autologous oral DNA vaccine protects against murine melanoma. Proc. Natl. Acad. Sci. U. S. A. 2000, 9(10), 5492–5497.

[19] Lambin P, Theys J, Landuyt W, Rijken P, van der Kogel A, van der Schueren E, Hodgkiss R, Fowler J, Nuyts S, de Bruijn E, Van Mellaert L, Anné J. Colonisation of *Clostridium* in the body is restricted to hypoxic and necrotic areas of tumours. Anaerobe 1998, 4, 183–188.

[20] Theys J, Landuyt AW, Nuyts S, Van Mellaert L, Lambin P, Anne J. *Clostridium* as a tumor-specific delivery system of therapeutic proteins. Cancer Detect. Prev. 2001, 25, 548–557.

[21] Van Mellaert L, Barbe S, Anne J. *Clostridium* spores as anti-tumour agents. Trends Microbiol. 2006, 14, 190–196.

[22] St Jean AT, Zhang M, Forbes NS. Bacterial therapies: completing the cancer treatment toolbox. Curr. Opin. Biotechnol. 2008, 19, 511–517.

[23] Wei MQ, Mengesha A, Good D, Anne J. Bacterial targeted tumor therapy—dawn of a new era. Cancer Lett. 2008, 259, 16–27.

[24] Zu C, Wang J. Tumor-colonizing bacteria: a potential tumor targeting therapy. Crit. Rev. Microbiol. 2014, 40, 225–235.

[25] Kubiak AM, Minton NP. The potential of clostridial spores as therapeutic delivery vehicles in tumour therapy. Res. Microbiol. 2015, doi: 10.1016/j.resmic.2014.12.006.

[26] Cutting SM, Hong HA, Baccigalupi L, Ricca E. Oral vaccine delivery by recombinant spore probiotics. Intern. Rev. Immunol. 2009, 28:487–505.

[27] Xiao X, Jin R, Li J, Bei Y, Wei T. The antitumor effect of suicide gene therapy using *Bifidobacterium infantis*-mediated herpes simplex virus thymidine kinase/ganciclovir in a nude mice model of renal cell carcinoma. Urology. 2014, doi: 10.1016/j.urology.2014.05.020.

[28] Yin X, Yu B, Tang Z, He B, Ren J, Xiao X, Tang W. *Bifidobacterium infantis*-mediated HSV-TK/GCV suicide gene therapy induces both extrinsic and intrinsic apoptosis in a rat model of bladder cancer. Cancer Gene Ther. 2013, 20(2), 77–81.

[29] Steidler L, Hans W, Schotte L, Neirynck S, Obermeier F, Falk W, Fiers W, Remaut E. Treatment of murine colitis by *Lactococcus lactis* secreting IL-10. Science. 2000, 289, 1352–1355.

[30] Hanson ML, Hixon JA, Li W, Felber BK, Anver MR, Stewart CA, Janelsins BM, Datta SK, Shen W, McLean MH, Durum SK. Oral delivery of IL-27 recombinant bacteria attenuates immune colitis in mice. Gastroenterology. 2014, 146(1), 210–221.

[31] Vandenbroucke K, de Haard H, Beirnaert E, Dreier T, Lauwereys M, Huyck L, Van Huysse J, Demetter P, Steidler L, Remaut E, Cuvelier C, Rottiers P. Orally administered *L. lactis* secreting an anti-TNF nanobody demonstrate efficacy in chronic colitis. Mucosal Immunol. 2010, 3(1), 49–56.

[32] Cornelis GR. The type III secretion injectisome. Nat. Rev. Microbiol. 2006, 4, 811–825.

[33] Galán JE, Lara-Tejero M, Marlovits TC, Wagner S. Bacterial type III secretion systems: specialized nanomachines for protein delivery into target cells. Annu Rev Microbiol. 2014, 68, 415–438.

[34] Parsot C. *Shigella* type III secretion effectors: how, where, when, for what purposes? Curr. Opin. Microbiol. 2009, 12(1), 110–116.

[35] Rüssmann H, Shams H, Poblete F, Fu Y, Galan JE, Donis RP. Delivery of epitopes by the *Salmonella* type III secretion system for vaccine development. Science. 1998, 281, 565–568.

[36] Rüssmann H, Igwe EI, Sauer J, Hardt WD, Bubert A, Geginat G. Protection against murine listeriosis by oral vaccination with recombinant *Salmonella* expressing hybrid *Yersinia* type III proteins. J. Immunol. 2001, 167, 357–365.

[37] Kotton CN, Lankowski AJ, Scott N, Sisul D, Chen LM, Raschke K, Borders G, Boaz M, Spentzou A, Galàn JE, Hohmann EL. Safety and immunogenicity of attenuated *Salmonella enterica* serovar *Typhimurium* delivering an HIV-1 Gag antigen via the *Salmonella* type III secretion system. Vaccine. 2006, 24, 6216–6224.

[38] Evans DT, Chen LM, Gillis J, Lin KC, Harty B, Mazzara GP, Donis RO, Mansfield KG, Lifson JD, Desrosiers RC, Galàn JE, Johnson RP. Mucosal priming of simian immunodeficiency virus-specific cytotoxic T-lymphocyte responses in rhesus macaques by the *Salmonella* type III secretion antigen delivery system. J. Virol. 2003, 77(4), 2400–2409.

[39] Tartz S, Rüssmann H, Kamanova J, Sebo P, Sturm A, Heussler V, Fleischer B, Jacobs T. Complete protection against *P. berghei* malaria upon heterologous prime/boost immunization against circumsporozoite protein employing *Salmonella* type III secretion system and *Bordetella* adenylate cyclase toxoid. Vaccine. 2008, 26(47), 5935–5944.

[40] Lotter H, Rüssmann H, Heesemann J, Tannich E. Attenuated recombinant *Yersinia* as live oral vaccine carrier to protect against amoebiasis. Intern. J. Med. Microbiol. 2008, 298, 79–86.

[41] Nishikawa H, Sato E, Briones G, Chen LM, Matsuo M, Nagata Y, Ritter G, Jäger E, Kondo S, Tawara I, Kato T, Shiku H, Old LJ, Galàn JE, Gnjatic S. In vivo antigen de-

livery by *a Salmonella typhimurium* type III secretion system for therapeutic cancer vaccines. J. Clin. Invest. 2006, 116, 1946–1954.

[42] Panthel K, Meinel KM, Sevil Domènech VE, Geginat G, Linkemann K, Busch DH, Rüssmann H. Prophylactic anti-tumor immunity against a murine fibrosarcoma triggered by the *Salmonella* type III secretion system. Microbes Infect. 2006, 8, 2539–2546.

[43] Epaulard O, Derouazi M, Margerit C, Marlu R, Filopon D, Polack B, Toussaint B. Optimization of a type III secretion system-based *Pseudomonas aeruginosa* live vector for antigen delivery. Clin. Vaccine Immunol. 2008, 15(2), 308–313.

[44] Kawai T, Akira S. Toll-like receptors and their crosstalk with other innate receptors in infection and immunity. Immunity. 2011, 27, 34(5), 637–650.

[45] Ishii KJ, Akira S. Toll or toll-free adjuvant path toward the optimal vaccine development. J Clin Immunol. 2007, 27(4), 363–371.

[46] O'Garra A, Barrat FJ, Castro AG, Vicari A, Hawrylowiks C. Strategies for use of IL-10 or its antagonist in human disease. Immunol. Rev. 2008, 223, 114–131.

[47] Herfarth HH, Mohanty SP, Rath HC, Tonkonogy S, Sartor RB. IL-10 suppresses experimental chronic, granulomatous inflammation induced by bacterial cell wall polymers. Gut. 1996, 38, 836–845.

[48] Van Deventer SJ, Elson CO, Fedorak RN. Multiple doses of intravenous IL-10 in steroid-refractory Crohn's disease. Crohn's Disease Study Group. Gastroenterology. 1997, 133, 383–389.

[49] Schreiber S, Fedoral RN, Nielsen OH, Wild J, Williams CN, Nikolaus S, Jacyna M, Lashner BA, Gangl A, Rutqeerts P, Isaacs K, Van Deventer SJ, Koningsberger JC, Cohard M, LeBeaut A, Hanauer SB. Safety and efficacy of recombinant human IL-10 in chronic active Crohn's disease: Crohn's Disease IL-10 Cooperative Study Group. Gastroenterology. 2000, 119, 1461–1472.

[50] Fedorak RN, Gangl A, Elson CO, Rutqeerts P, Schreiber S, Wild J, Hanauer SB, Kilian A, Cohard M, Lebeaut A, Feagan B. Recombinant human IL-10 in the treatment of patients with mild to moderately active Crohn's disease: the IL-10 Inflammatory Bowel Disease Cooperative Study Group. Gastroenterology. 2000. 119, 1473–1482.

[51] Chamekh M, Phalipon A, Quertainmont R, Salmon I, Sansonetti P, Allaoui A. Delivery of biologically active anti-inflammatory cytokines IL-10 and IL-1ra in vivo by the *Shigella* type III secretion system. J. Immunol. 2008, 180(6), 4292–4298.

[52] Andus T, Daig R, Vogel D. Imbalance of the IL-1 system in colonic mucosa: association with intestinal inflammation and IL-1 receptor antagonist genotype 2. Gut. 1997, 41, 651–657.

[53] Arondel J, Singer M, Matsukawa A, Zychlinsky A, Sansonetti PJ. Increased IL-1 and imbalance between IL-1 and IL-1 receptor antagonist during acute inflammation in experimental shigellosis. Infect. Immun. 1999, 67, 6056–6066.

[54] Cominelli F, Nast CC, Duchini A, Lee M. Recombinant interleukin-1 receptor antagonist blocks the proinflammatory activity of endogenous interleukin-1 in rabbit immune colitis. Gastroenterology 1992, 103, 65–77.

[55] Coster TS, Hoge CW, Van De Verg LL, Hartman AB, Oaks EV, Venkatesan MM, Cohen D, Robin G, Fontaine-Thompson A, Sansonetti PJ, Hale TL. Vaccination against shigellosis with attenuated *Shigella flexneri* 2a strain SC602. Infect. Immun. 1999, 67, 3437–3443.

[56] Singer M, Sansonetti PJ. IL-8 is a key chemokine regulating neutrophil recruitment in a new mouse model of *Shigella*-induced colitis. J. Immunol. 2004, 173(6), 4197–4206.

[57] Fernandez MI, Thuizat A, Pedron T, Neutra M, Phalipon A, Sansonetti PJ. A newborn mouse model for the study of intestinal pathogenesis of shigellosis. Cell. Microbiol. 2003, 5(7), 481–491.

[58] Akeda Y, Kimura T, Yamasaki A, Kodama T, Iida T, Honda T, Oishi K. Functional cloning *of Vibrio parahaemolyticus* type III secretion system 1 in *Escherichia coli* K-12 strain as a molecular syringe. Biochem Biophys Res Commun. 2012, 427(2), 242–247.

[59] Carleton HA, Lara-Tejero M, Liu X, Galán JE. Engineering the type III secretion system in non-replicating bacterial minicells for antigen delivery. Nat Commun. 2013, 4, 1590. doi: 10.1038/ncomms2594.

9

Encapsulation of Transgenic Cells for Gene Therapy

Wujie Zhang

Abstract

A major challenge to emerging cell-based medicine including gene therapy is the host immune rejection of transplanted donor cells or engineered tissue. One way to address this problem is to use drugs to achieve immunosuppression. However, suppressing the patient's immune system may put the patient at risk for many other diseases. An alternative is to encapsulate living cells in macro/microcapsules to achieve immunoisolation of the cells, thereby increasing cell viability in the patient's body following transplantation. The capsule's membrane protects the encapsulated cells from being damaged by both the host's immune system and mechanical stress while allowing free diffusion of nutrients and metabolic waste for the cells to survive. Moreover, the membrane could be designed to achieve controlled and/or sustained release of therapeutic products produced by the encapsulated transgenic cells to treat a variety of diseases such as cardiovascular disorders, anemia, wounds, bone fractures, and cancer.

Keywords: Cell microencapsulation, Encapsulation, Microcapsules, Gene therapy, Cell-based medicine

1. Introduction

Cell encapsulation is the process of entrapping cells into a matrix. In general, the matrix is spherical in shape and in the form of a polymeric hydrogel. Cell encapsulation technology has shown great promise for immunoisolation and controlled release of therapeutic products towards gene therapy. Figure 1 demonstrates the mechanism of encapsulated transgenic cells for gene therapy.

1.1. Encapsulation materials

Both natural and synthetic polymers have been utilized for cell encapsulation. Natural polymers that have been used include alginate, agarose, collagen, and hyaluronic acid, while synthetic polymers, including poly(vinyl alcohol), poly(lactic-co-glycolic acid), polyacrylates, HEMA-MMA-MAA, polyphosphazines, and polyepoxides, have been studied.[1] Natural polymers are more commonly used because of their biocompatibility and are easily accepted by the public. However, their product quality and characteristics can vary greatly between companies and batches compared to synthetic polymers. Alginate, agarose, and polylactide-co-glycolide (PLGA), the most commonly used encapsulation materials, are introduced here.

1.1.1. Alginate

Alginates, polysaccharides, are linear block polymers consisting of α-l-guluronic acid (G) and β-d-manuronic acid (M) blocks (Figure 2). Divalent cations, such as Ca^{2+}, Ba^{2+}, and Sr^{2+}, can link alginate molecules together (i.e. through ionic cross-linking) forming alginate hydrogel capsules while encapsulating cells inside. The G and M contents of the alginate molecules can affect the gel properties including mechanical strength, biocompatibility, and permeability.[2–6] Recently, it has also been shown that oligochitosan could be used as a cross-linker for polysaccharide-based gel formations.[7]

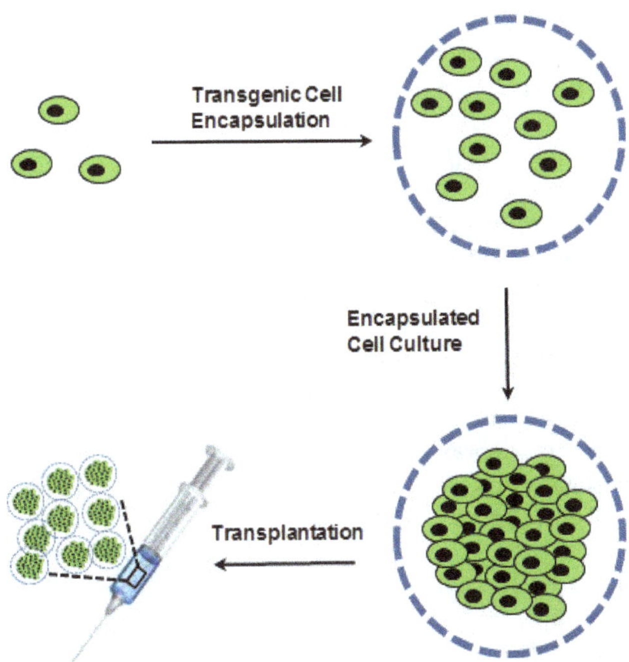

Figure 1. A conceptual schematic demonstrating cell encapsulation for gene therapy.

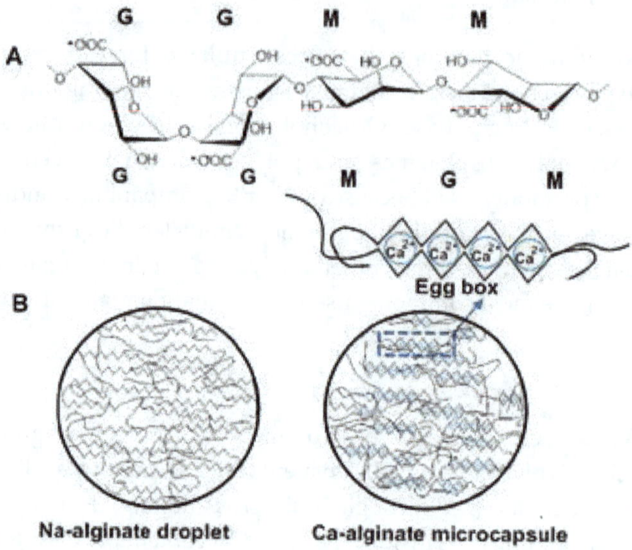

Figure 2. Chemical structure of alginate (A) and alginate-based hydrogel formation mechanism (B).

1.1.2. Agarose

Agarose, a thermal-responsive polymer, consists of β-d-galactopyranose and 3,6-anhydro-α-l-galactopyranose units which can undergo a sol–gel transition upon cooling (i.e. through thermal cross-linking) (Figure 3). Some agarose products have a transition temperature close to body temperature, making it a good candidate for cell encapsulation.[8]

1.1.3. Polylactide-co-Glycolide (PLGA)

PLGA polymers belong to aliphatic polyesters and are biodegradable (Figure 4). To prepare the capsules, PLGA is dissolved in methylene chloride, and then a second component is added to precipitate the polymer molecules (interfacial precipitation).[1,9]

1.2. Encapsulation technologies

Different technologies have been used for preparing macro/microcapsules, which include air-jet encapsulation, electrostatic spray, laminar jet breakup, and microfluidic channel/nozzle. Among them, electrostatic spray and microfluidic channel/nozzle are two of the most frequently used encapsulation approaches.[10]

1.2.1. Electrostatic spray method

The electrostatic spray method has a significant appeal due to its ease of operation, scale-up capabilities, negligible damage to cells, and allowance for sterile operation conditions.[10] The mechanism of cell encapsulation by using the electrostatic pray method is shown in Figure

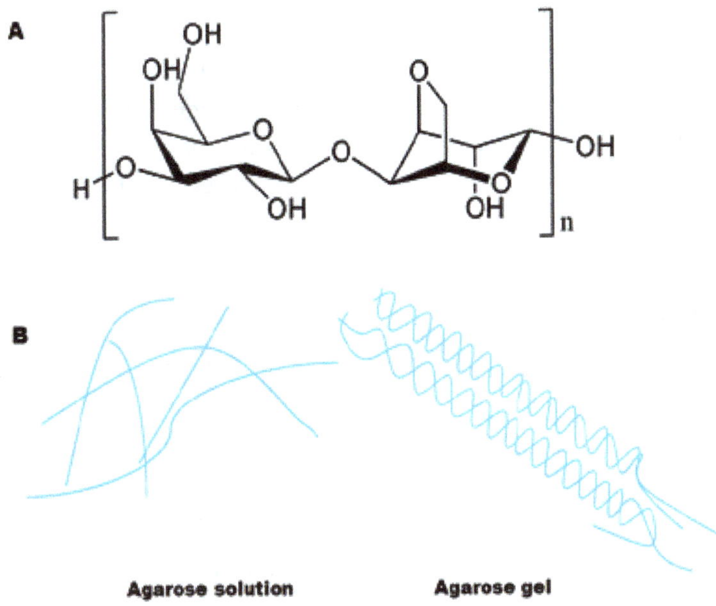

Figure 3. Chemical structure of agarose (A) and agarose-based hydrogel formation mechanism (B).

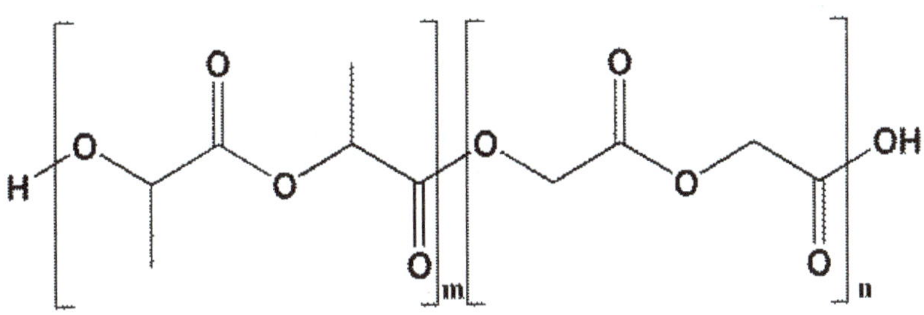

Figure 4. Chemical structure of PLGA.

5A. In general, a cell polymer mixture is extruded through a nozzle by using a pump or compressed air. The droplets are broken down into smaller ones under electrostatic force and/or other introduced forces (e.g. vibration). Once the droplets reach the gelling bath containing the cross-linkers, the cell-loaded hydrogel capsules form immediately through various forces, such as ionotropic reaction between divalent ions and alginate molecules. Moreover, the system could be modified to prepare the core-shell structure hydrogel capsules, as depicted in Figure 5B.[11]

1.2.2. Microfluidics channel/nozzle method

Microfluidics devices can be used to generate micrometer-scale droplets with a narrow size distribution and controlled morphology.[12–14] This method shows great promise for cell encapsulation, especially for single cell encapsulation.[15] In general, capsules are formed by allowing a core fluid to be surrounded by a flowing sheath stream.[16] Recently, these devices have also been successfully applied for the generation of cell-loaded core-shell capsules (Figure 6).[14] Besides the relatively low encapsulation efficiency, a significant drawback of the current microfluidic technologies is that the oil used for shearing may leave a residual adhesive oil layer on the capsule which affects subsequent coating processes.[10,17]

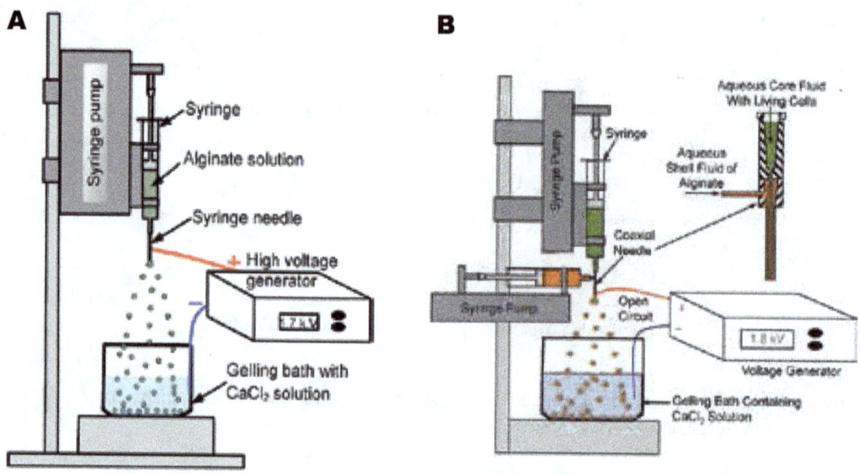

Figure 5. A sketch of the electrostatic spray device used for generating polymeric hydrogel capsules (A).[10] *Reproduced by permission of The American Society of Mechanical Engineering (ASME)*; A modified electrostatic spray setup for fabricating the core-shell structure hydrogel capsules (B).[11] *Reproduced by permission of The Royal Society of Chemistry.*

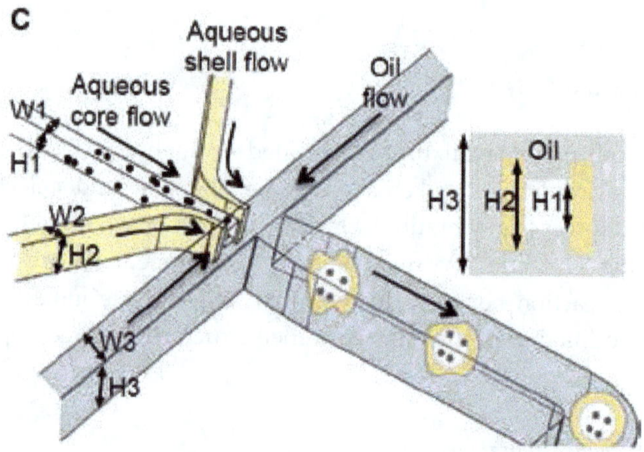

Figure 6. A sketch of the microfluidics device for generating core-shell hydrogel capsules. The core channel height (H1) is the lowest. H: height and W: width.[14] *Reproduced by permission of The Royal Society of Chemistry.*

2. Recent progress on transgenic cell encapsulation for gene therapy

Encapsulation of genetically modified cells has been conducted for the treatment of central nervous system diseases, cardiovascular disorders, mucopolysaccharidosis type VII (MPSVII) disease, wounds, bone fractures, and cancer.[18–30] Considering most genetically engineered cells are from allogeneic or xenogeneic sources, immunoisolation is a critical factor when using these cells.[5]

2.1. Bone-related diseases

Bone morphogenic protein-2 (BMP-2) is a member of the transforming growth factor-β (TGF-β) superfamily and has been widely reported to have osteoinductive activity. Ding *et al.* [31] studied the behaviour of BMP-2 gene-transfected bone marrow-derived mesenchymal stem cells in alginate-poly-l-lysine-alginate (APA) microcapsules. The results showed that encapsulated transfected cells could secrete BMP-2 proteins for at least 30 days and the APA microcapsules could be used for immunoisolation. Olabisi *et al.* [28] investigated microencapsulation of AdBMP-2-transduced MRC-5 cells (human diploid fetal lung fibroblasts) in poly(ethylene glycol) diacrylate (PEGDA) hydrogels. After injecting the encapsulated cells intramuscularly, the volume of the bone formed was about twice that of the control group (unencapsulated cells). Recently, rapid heterotrophic ossification by using cryopreserved PEGDA encapsulated BMP-2 expressing mesenchymal stem cells (MSCs) was also observed (as shown in Figure 7).[32] Additionally, human calcitonin delivered by microencapsulated recombinant myoblasts showed potential for allergenic gene therapy for postmenopausal osteoporosis. [33] Furthermore, transplantation of fibrin glue-compounding hepatocyte growth factor-transgenic MSCs is a promising novel method for avascular necrosis of the femoral head (ANFH) therapy.[34]

2.2. Cancer

Both mouse myoblasts (C2C12 cells) and human embryonic kidney 293 (HEK293) cells were engineered to continuously secrete angiostatin, and were encapsulated into alginate-based microcapsules for cancer treatment. The *in vivo* experimental results demonstrated the potential for angiostatin-mediated cancer therapy by using an encapsulated transgenic cell-based approach.[35,36] Considering immunotherapies have been proven to be alternative strategies for malignancy treatment[37], combined immunotherapy (an interleukin 2 fusion protein, sFvIL-2) and antiangiogenic therapy (angiostatin) were tested. It was shown that transplantation of angiostatin expression and sFvIL-2-expressing C2C12 cells encapsulated in APA microcapsules improved the survival rate of experimental animals.[38] Recently, microencapsulation of therapeutic antibodies producing cells in APA microcapsules was tested for cancer treatment. [39] Additionally, with the advancement of stem cell research, there is an increased potential for cancer therapy by using encapsulated stem cells.[40]

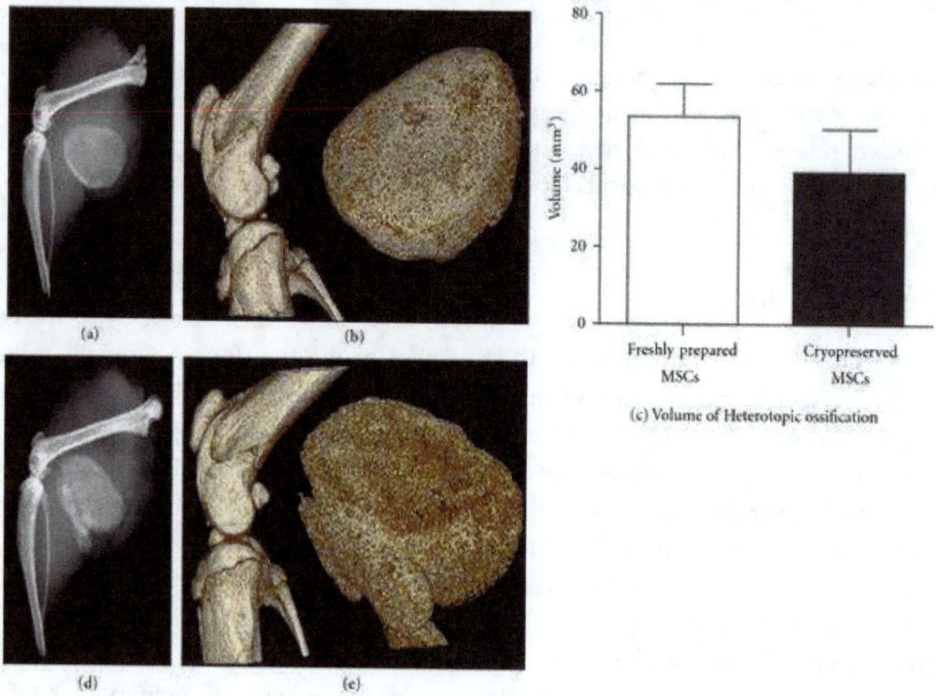

Figure 7. Microencapsulated BMP2-transduced MSCs in a mouse model for heterotopic ossification. X-ray and MicroCT images of the resulting heterotopic ossification for freshly prepared BMP2 microencapsulated MSCs (a and b) and for cryopreserved BMP2 microencapsulated MSCs (d and e).[32]

2.3. Neural diseases

Parkinson's disease (PD) belongs to a group of conditions called motor system disorders, resulting from the loss of dopamine-producing brain cells.[41] This disease could be amenable to gene product replacement strategies including implantation of encapsulated transgenic cells.[42] There are several publications regarding encapsulated cell biodelivery of glial cell line-derived neurotrophic factor (GDNF) for PD treatment; GDNF has been proven to have neuroprotective and neurotrophic properties on dopaminergic neurons.[26,43,44] Furthermore, encapsulated transgenic cells could be utilized in brain tumour treatment.[45,46]

Small capsules (<200 μm) have been developed for the delivery of gene products, secreted by encapsulated transgenic cells, to the brain, bypassing the blood–brain barrier (BBB). To date, several alginate-based microcapsule systems, Ca-alginate, APA, and alginate-chitosan-alginate (ACA), have been reported.[10,47,48] Encapsulation of transgenic cells has also been used for other disease treatments, such as mucopolysaccharidosis VII and myocardial infarction. Table 1 summarizes the recent gene therapy studies based on encapsulated transgenic cells, with the exception of bone-related and neural diseases and cancer treatment.

Disease	Therapeutic Product(s)	Cell Type	Encapsulation System	Ref.
Fabry disease	α-Galactosidase A	Chinese hamster ovary cells	Semipermeable Polymer Fiber	[49]
Mucopolysaccharidosis VII	β-Glucuronidase	Mouse 2A-50 fibroblasts	Alginate-poly-l-lysine	[50]
		Human amniotic epithelial cells	Polymer (polysulfon) Hollow fibers	[23]
Myocardial infarction and wound	Glucagon-like peptide-1	Human mesenchymal stem cells	CellBeads™	[51]
	Vascular endothelial growth factor	Chinese hamster ovary cells	Alginate-Poly-l-Lysine-Alginate Microcapsules	[27]
		Adipose stem cells	AP-PLL-brPEG microcapsules	[52]
		NIH3T3 cells	Alginate-barium microcapsules	[21]
		Human umbilical cord mesenchymal stromal cells	Alginate-barium microcapsules	[53]
		Human umbilical cord mesenchymal stem cells	Alginate-barium microcapsules	[54]
Polycythemic diseases	Erythropoietin	Mouse C2C12 myoblasts	Semipermeable polyethersulf hollow fibers	[55]
Hypertension and/or congestive heart failure	Atrial natriuretic peptide	Chinese hamster ovary cells	Polycaprolactone tubes	[56]
Acute skin flap ischemia	Basic fibroblast growth factor (FGF-2)	Mouse C2C12 myoblasts	Microporous polyethersulfone hollow fibers	[57]
Hemophilia B	Factor IX	Mouse C2C12 myoblasts mouse C2C12 myoblasts	Alginate-poly-l-lysine-alginate microcapsules	[58]
			Alginate-poly-l-lysine-alginate and alginate-poly-l-arginine-alginate microcapsules	[59]
Laron syndrome	Recombinant human IGF-1	Pig Sertoli cells	Alginate microcapsules	[60]

Table 1. Recent gene therapy studies by using encapsulated transgenic cells

3. Challenges and future direction

Recent clinical trials regarding gene therapy by using encapsulated transgenic cells are summarized in Table 2. For eventual clinical applications of encapsulated transgenic cells for gene therapy, however, there are still some issues that need to be addressed.[62,63]

1. **Protrusion of encapsulated cells**

Cell growth leads to protrusion of cells over time, which may cause the failure of immunoisolation following *in vivo* transplantation. Bhujbal *et al.* reported a novel multilayer immunoisolating encapsulation system aiming to prevent cell protrusion without compromising cell survival (Figure 8).[64]

2. **Scaling-up cell microencapsulation**

Cell encapsulation processes are usually performed at the lab scale. For successful clinical applications, massive production of encapsulated cells following good manufacturing practices (GMP) standardized procedures [65] for transplantation is critical. Different designs have been reported for scaling-up cell encapsulation. One design based on a 3D microfluidic approach, which contains a 3D air supply and multinozzle outlet, has been reported recently.[17]

3. **Monitor and control the encapsulated transgenic cells**

Once the therapy has reached its goal or when undesirable deleterious effects occur, noninvasive monitoring and deactivation/elimination of the encapsulated cells are critical for clinical practice.[63] Recently, Shen *et al.* [66] reported the encapsulation of recombinant cells by using a magnetized ferrofluid alginate for *in vivo* monitoring by magnetic resonance imaging (MRI). Moreover, magnetic field-controlled gene expression in encapsulated cells, coencapsulated with magnetic nanoparticles, has been reported. The cells were modified to produce therapeutic products under the control of a heat-inducible promoter. Heat induction could be achieved by elevating the temperatures of the capsules through coencapsulated magnetic nanoparticles subjected to a magnetic field (Figure 9).[67] Catena *et al.* reported an interesting and smart system which shows potential for monitoring encapsulated cells and selectively eliminating them at a specific moment by using the $SFG_{NES}TGL$ triple reporter system.[68]

Project	Therapeutic Product(s)	Target Disease(s)	Phase	Status
A study of encapsulated cell technology (ECT) implant for patients with late stage retinitis pigmentosa	Ciliary neurotrophic factor (CNTF)	Late-stage retinitis pigmentosa	II and III	Completed
A study of encapsulated cell technology (ECT) implant for	Ciliary neurotrophic factor (CNTF)	Early stage retinitis pigmentosa	II and III	Completed

Project	Therapeutic Product(s)	Target Disease(s)	Phase	Status
participants with early stage retinitis pigmentosa				
A Study of an Encapsulated Cell Technology (ECT) Implant for Patients With Atrophic Macular Degeneration	Ciliary neurotrophic factor (CNTF)	Macular degeneration	II	Completed
Pilot immunotherapy trial for recurrent malignant gliomas	Insulin-like growth factor receptor-1	Malignant glioma of brain	I	Completed
GLP-1 CellBeads® for the treatment of stroke patients with space-occupying intracerebral hemorrhage	Glucagon-like peptide-1	Intracerebral hemorrhage (ICH)	I and II	Terminated
CNTF implants for CNGB3 achromatopsia	Ciliary neurotrophic factor (CNTF)	Eye disease achromatopsia	I and II	Active
Retinal imaging of subjects implanted with ciliary neurotrophic factor (CNTF)-releasing encapsulated cell implant for early-stage retinitis pigmentosa	Ciliary neurotrophic factor (CNTF)	Early stage retinitis pigmentosa or Usher syndrome (type 2 or 3)	II	Recruiting
A phase 2 multicenter randomized clinical trial of CNTF FOR MacTel	Recombinant human ciliary neurotrophic factor	Macular telangiectasia type 2	II	Recruiting
MVX-ONCO-1 in patients with solid tumours	Irradiated autologous tumour cells	Solid tumour cancer	I	Recruiting
Study of the intravitreal implantation of NT-503-3 encapsulated cell technology (ECT) for the treatment of recurrent choroidal neovascularization (CNV) secondary to age-related macular degeneration (AMD)	Anti-VEGF therapy	Macular degeneration	I and II	Not yet recruiting
Encapsulated cell biodelivery of nerve growth factor to Alzheimer´s disease patients	Nerve growth factor (NGF)	Alzheimer's disease	I	Unknown

Table 2. Clinical trials of gene therapy involving encapsulated transgenic cells [61]

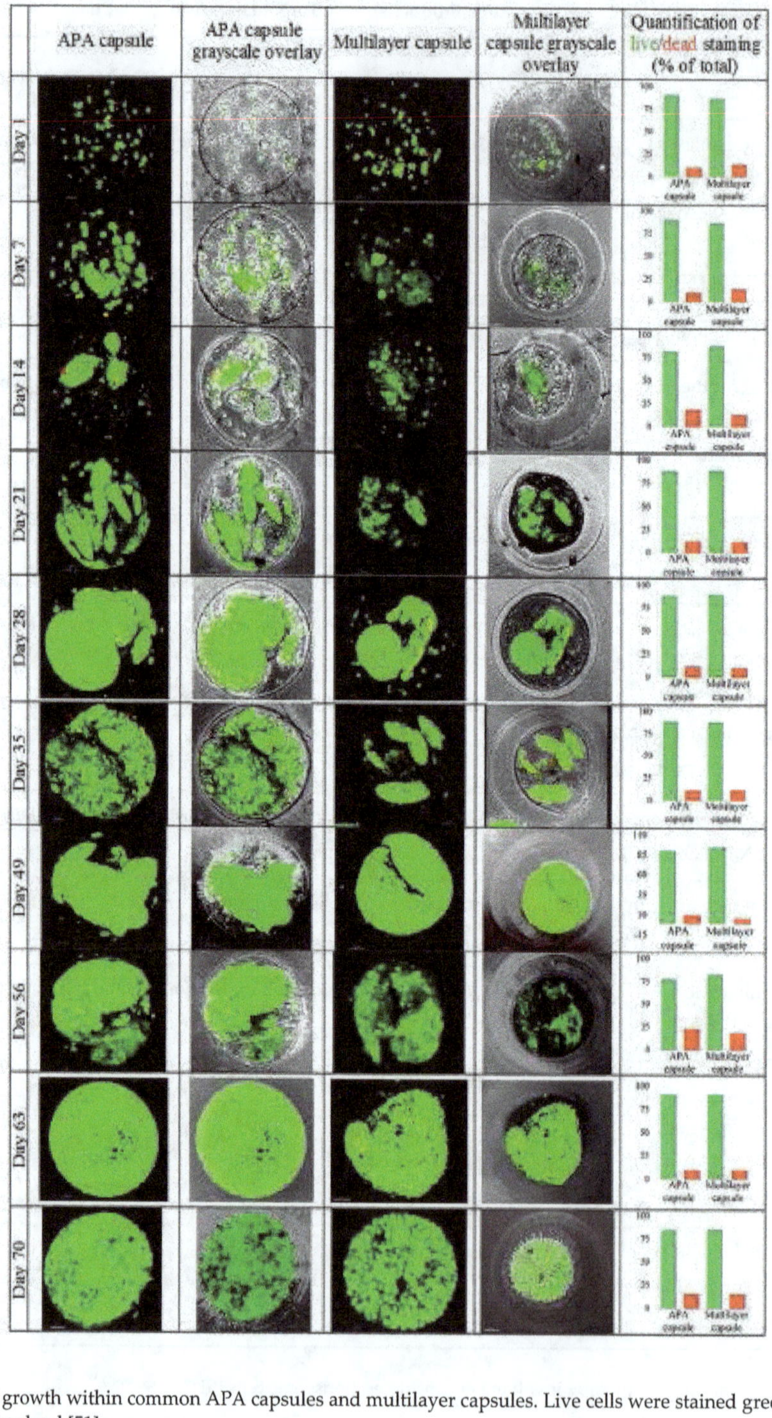

Figure 8. Cell growth within common APA capsules and multilayer capsules. Live cells were stained green while dead cells were stained red.[51]

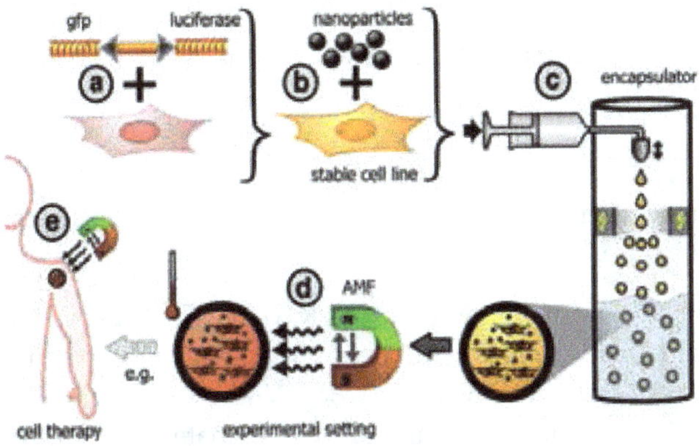

Figure 9. Schematic representation of the magnetic field-controlled gene expression in encapsulated cells.[67]

Acknowledgements

The author thanks Dr. Eryn Hassemer, Dr. Jung Lee, Alexander Dyble, Kendra Lehman, Rebecca Majewski, and Michael Wedemeyer for proofreading this book chapter. Also, the author thanks Dr. Jung Lee for drawing some of the figures. The author is grateful for funding provided by the Faculty Summer Development Grant at the Milwaukee School of Engineering.

Author details

Wujie Zhang*

Address all correspondence to: zhang@msoe.edu

BioMolecular Engineering Program, Department of Physics and Chemistry, Milwaukee School of Engineering, Milwaukee, WI, USA

References

[1] Olabisi RM. Cell microencapsulation with synthetic polymers. Journal of Biomedical Materials Research Part A. DOI: 10.1002/jbm.a.35205.

[2] de Vos P, Faas MM, Strand B, Calafiore R. Alginate-based microcapsules for immunoisolation of pancreatic islets. Biomaterials 2006, 27:5603–5617.

[3] Morch YA, Donati I, Strand BL, Skjak-Braek G. Effect of Ca2+, Ba2+, and Sr2+ on alginate microbeads. Biomacromolecules 2006, 7:1471–1480.

[4] Smidsrød O, Skjåk-Braek G. Alginate as immobilization matrix for cells. Trends in Biotechnology 1990, 8:71–78.

[5] Zhang W, He X. Microencapsulating and banking living cells for cell-based medicine. Journal of Healthcare Engineering 2011, 2:427–446.

[6] Zimmermann H, Zimmermann D, Reuss R, Feilen PJ, Manz B, Katsen A, Weber M, Ihmig FR, Ehrhart F, Gessner P, Behringer M, Steinbach A, Wegner LH, Sukhorukov VL, Vásquez JA, Schneider S, Weber MM, Volke F, Wolf R, Zimmermann U. Towards a medically approved technology for alginate-based microcapsules allowing long-term immunoisolated transplantation. Journal of Materials Science: Materials in Medicine 2005, 16:491–501.

[7] Zhang W, Mahuta KM, Mikulski BA, Harvestine JN, Crouse JZ, Lee JC, Kaltchev MG, Tritt CS. Novel pectin-based carriers for colonic drug delivery. Pharmaceutical Development and Technology 2014.doi:10.3109/10837450.2014.965327:1–4.

[8] Gasperini L, Mano JF, Reis RL. Natural polymers for the microencapsulation of cells. Journal of The Royal Society Interface 2014, 11:20140817.

[9] Abalovich A, Jatimliansky C, Diegex E, Arias M, Altamirano A, Amorena C, Martinez B, Nacucchio M. Pancreatic islets microencapsulation with polylactide-co-glycolide. Transplantation Proceedings 2001, 33:1977–1979.

[10] Zhang W, He X. Encapsulation of living cells in small (approximately 100 microm) alginate microcapsules by electrostatic spraying: a parametric study. Journal of Biomechanical Engineering 2009, 131:074515.

[11] Zhao S, Agarwal P, Rao W, Huang H, Zhang R, Liu Z, Yu J, Weisleder N, Zhang W, He X. Coaxial electrospray of liquid core-hydrogel shell microcapsules for encapsulation and miniaturized 3D culture of pluripotent stem cells. Integrative Biology (Camb) 2014, 6:874–884.

[12] Wan J. Microfluidic-based synthesis of hydrogel particles for cell microencapsulation and cell-based drug delivery. Polymers 2012, 4:1084–1108.

[13] Mazzitelli S, Capretto L, Quinci F, Piva R, Nastruzzi C. Preparation of cell-encapsulation devices in confined microenvironment. Advanced Drug Delivery Reviews 2013, 65:1533–1555.

[14] Agarwal P, Zhao S, Bielecki P, Rao W, Choi JK, Zhao Y, Yu J, Zhang W, He X. One-step microfluidic generation of pre-hatching embryo-like core-shell microcapsules for miniaturized 3D culture of pluripotent stem cells. Lab on a Chip 2013, 13:4525–4533.

[15] Wu L, Chen P, Dong Y, Feng X, Liu BF. Encapsulation of single cells on a microfluidic device integrating droplet generation with fluorescence-activated droplet sorting. Biomedical Microdevices 2013, 15:553–560.

[16] Kang A, Park J, Ju J, Jeong GS, Lee SH. Cell encapsulation via microtechnologies. Biomaterials 2014, 35:2651–2663.

[17] Tendulkar S, Mirmalek-Sani SH, Childers C, Saul J, Opara EC, Ramasubramanian MK. A three-dimensional microfluidic approach to scaling up microencapsulation of cells. Biomedical Microdevices 2012, 14:461–469.

[18] Bachoud-Lévi AC, Déglon N, Nguyen JP, Bloch J, Bourdet C, Winkel L, Rémy P, Goddard M, Lefaucheur JP, Brugières P, Baudic S, Cesaro P, Peschanski M, Aebischer P. Neuroprotective gene therapy for Huntington's disease using a polymer encapsulated BHK cell line engineered to secrete human CNTF. Human Gene Therapy 2000, 11:1723–1729.

[19] Gurruchaga H, Saenz Del Burgo L, Ciriza J, Orive G, Hernandez RM, Pedraz JL. Advances in cell encapsulation technology and its application in drug delivery. Expert Opinion Drug Delivery 2015. doi:10.1517/17425247.2015.1001362:1–17.

[20] Dvir-Ginzberg M, Konson A, Cohen S, Agbaria R. Entrapment of retroviral vector producer cells in three-dimensional alginate scaffolds for potential use in cancer gene therapy. Journal of Biomedical Materials Research Part B: Applied Biomaterials 2007, 80:59–66.

[21] Han YF, Han YQ, Pan YG, Chen YL, Chai JK. Transplantation of microencapsulated cells expressing VEGF improves angiogenesis in implanted xenogeneic acellular dermis on wound. Transplantation Proceedings 2010, 42:1935–1943.

[22] Murua A, Orive G, Hernandez RM, Pedraz JL. Epo delivery by genetically engineered C2C12 myoblasts immobilized in microcapsules. Advances in Experimental Medicine and Biology 2010, 670:54–67.

[23] Nakama H, Ohsugi K, Otsuki T, Date I, Kosuga M, Okuyama T, Sakuragawa N. Encapsulation cell therapy for mucopolysaccharidosis type VII using genetically engineered immortalized human The Tohoku Journal of Experimental Medicine 2006, 209:23–32.

[24] Salmons B, Gunzburg WH. Therapeutic application of cell microencapsulation in cancer. Advances in Experimental Medicine and Biology 2010, 670:92–103.

[25] Thanos CG, Bintz B, Emerich DF. Microencapsulated choroid plexus epithelial cell transplants for repair of the brain. Advances in Experimental Medicine and Biology 2010, 670:80–91.

[26] Yasuhara T, Date I. Intracerebral transplantation of genetically engineered cells for Parkinson's disease: toward clinical application. Cell Transplantation 2007, 16:125–132.

[27] Zhang H, Zhu SJ, Wang W, Wei YJ, Hu SS. Transplantation of microencapsulated genetically modified xenogeneic cells augments angiogenesis and improves heart function. Gene Therapy 2008, 15:40–48.

[28] Olabisi RM, Lazard ZW, Franco CL, Hall MA, Kwon SK, Sevick-Muraca EM, Hipp JA, Davis AR, Olmsted-Davis EA, West JL. Hydrogel microsphere encapsulation of a cell-based gene therapy system increases cell survival of injected cells, transgene expression, and bone volume in a model of heterotopic ossification. Tissue Engineering Part A 2010, 16:3727–3736.

[29] Awrey DE, Tse M, Hortelano G, Chang PL. Permeability of alginate microcapsules to secretory recombinant gene products. Biotechnology and Bioengineering 1996, 52:472–484.

[30] Sieving PA, Caruso RC, Tao W, Coleman HR, Thompson DJ, Fullmer KR, Bush RA. Ciliary neurotrophic factor (CNTF) for human retinal degeneration: phase I trial of CNTF delivered by encapsulated cell intraocular implants. Proceedings of the National Academy of Sciences of the United States of America 2006, 103:3896–3901.

[31] Ding HF, Liu R, Li BG, Lou JR, Dai KR, Tang TT. Biologic effect and immunoisolating behavior of BMP-2 gene-transfected bone marrow-derived mesenchymal stem cells in APA microcapsules. Biochemical and Biophysical Research Communications 2007, 362:923–927.

[32] Mumaw J, Jordan ET, Sonnet C, Olabisi RM, Olmsted-Davis EA, Davis AR, Peroni JF, West JL, West F, Lu Y, Stice SL. Rapid Heterotrophic Ossification with Cryopreserved Poly(ethylene glycol-) Microencapsulated BMP2-Expressing MSCs. International Journal of Biomaterials 2012, 2012:861794.

[33] Wang Y, Zeng B, Li X. Expression of human calcitonin by microencapsulated recombinant myoblasts. Biotechnology Letters 2006, 28:1453–1458.

[34] Wen Q, Zhou C, Luo W, Zhou M, Ma L. Pro-osteogenic effects of fibrin glue in treatment of avascular necrosis of the femoral head in vivo by hepatocyte growth factor-transgenic mesenchymal stem cells. Journal of Translational Medicine 2014, 12:114.

[35] Cirone P, Bourgeois JM, Chang PL. Antiangiogenic cancer therapy with microencapsulated cells. Human Gene Therapy 2003, 14:1065–1077.

[36] Visted T, Furmanek T, Sakariassen P, Foegler WB, Sim K, Westphal H, Bjerkvig R, Lund-Johansen M. Prospects for delivery of recombinant angiostatin by cell-encapsulation therapy. Human Gene Therapy 2003, 14:1429–1440.

[37] Schwenter F, Zarei S, Luy P, Padrun V, Bouche N, Lee JS, Mulligan RC, Morel P, Mach N. Cell encapsulation technology as a novel strategy for human anti-tumor immunotherapy. Cancer Gene Therapy 2011, 18:553–562.

[38] Cirone P, Bourgeois JM, Shen F, Chang PL. Combined immunotherapy and antiangiogenic therapy of cancer with microencapsulated cells. Human Gene Therapy 2004, 15:945–959.

[39] Saenz Del Burgo L, Compte M, Aceves M, Hernandez RM, Sanz L, Alvarez-Vallina L, Pedraz JL. Microencapsulation of therapeutic bispecific antibodies producing cells: immunotherapeutic organoids for cancer management. Journal of Drug Targeting 2015, 23:170–179.

[40] Shah K. Encapsulated stem cells for cancer therapy. Biomatter 2013, 3.

[41] http://www.ninds.nih.gov/disorders/parkinsons_disease/parkinsons_disease.htm on [Accessed: 2015-03-01]

[42] Ross CJ, Ralph M, Chang PL. Somatic Gene Therapy for a Neurodegenerative Disease Using Microencapsulated Recombinant Cells. Experimental Neurology 2000, 166:276–286.

[43] Lindvall O, Wahlberg LU. Encapsulated cell biodelivery of GDNF: a novel clinical strategy for neuroprotection and neuroregeneration in Parkinson's disease? Experimental Neurology 2008, 209:82–88.

[44] Kishima H, Poyot T, Bloch J, Dauguet J, Condé F, Dollé F, Hinnen F, Pralong W, Palfi S, Déglon N, Aebischer P. Encapsulated GDNF-producing C2C12 cells for Parkinson's disease: a pre-clinical study in chronic MPTP-treated baboons. Neurobiology Disease 2004, 16:428–439.

[45] Martinet O, Schreyer N, Reis ED, Joseph JM. Encapsulation of packaging cell line results in successful retroviral-mediated transfer of a suicide gene in vivo in an experimental model of glioblastoma. European Journal of Surgical Oncology 2003, 29:351–357.

[46] Visted T, Bjerkvig R, Enger PO. Cell encapsulation technology as a therapeutic strategy for CNS malignancies. Neuro-Oncology 2001, 3:201–210.

[47] Zhang W, Zhao S, Rao W, Snyder J, Choi JK, Wang J, Khan IA, Saleh NB, Mohler PJ, Yu J, Hund TJ, Tang C, He X. A novel core-shell microcapsule for encapsulation and 3D culture of embryonic stem cells. Journal of Materials Chemistry B Materials for Biology and Medicine 2013, 2013:1002–1009.

[48] Ross CJ, Chang PL. Development of small alginate microcapsules for recombinant gene product delivery to the rodent brain. Journal of Biomaterials Science, Polymer Edition 2002, 13:953–962.

[49] Naganawa Y, Ohsugi K, Kase R, Date I, Sakuraba H, Sakuragawa N. In vitro study of encapsulation therapy for Fabry disease using genetically engineered CHO cell line. Cell Transplantation 2002, 11:325–329.

[50] Ross CJ, Bastedo L, Maier SA, Sands MS, Chang PL. Treatment of a lysosomal storage disease, mucopolysaccharidosis VII, with microencapsulated recombinant cells. Human Gene Therapy 2000, 11:2117–2127.

[51] Houtgraaf JH, de Jong R, Monkhorst K, Tempel D, van de Kamp E, den Dekker WK, Kazemi K, Hoefer I, Pasterkamp G, Lewis AL, Stralford PW, Wallrapp C, Zijlstra F, Duckers HJ. Feasibility of intracoronary GLP-1 eluting CellBead infusion in acute myocardial infarction. Cell Transplantation 2013, 22:535–543.

[52] Paul A, Shao W, Abbasi S, Shum-Tim D, Prakash S. PAMAM dendrimer-baculovirus nanocomplex for microencapsulated adipose stem cell-gene therapy: in vitro and in vivo functional assessment. Molecular Pharmaceutics 2012, 9:2479–2488.

[53] Han Y, Tao R, Han Y, Sun T, Chai J, Xu G, Liu J. Microencapsulated VEGF gene-modified umbilical cord mesenchymal stromal cells promote the vascularization of tissue-engineered dermis: an experimental study. Cytotherapy 2014, 16:160–169.

[54] Han YF, Sun TJ, Han YQ, Tao R, Chai JK, Yin HN, Xu G, Liu J. Preparation of micro-encapsulated VEGF gene-modified human umbilical cord mesenchymal stem cells and in vitro culture. European Review for Medical and Pharmacological Sciences 2013, 17:217–223.

[55] Sommer B, Rinsch C, Payen E, Dalle B, Schneider B, Deglon N, Henri A, Beuzard Y, Aebischer P. Long-term doxycycline-regulated secretion of erythropoietin by encapsulated myoblasts. Molecular Therapy 2002, 6:155–161.

[56] Wang Z, Chen L, Wan C, Qu Y, Cornelissen G, Halberg F. In vitro circadian ANP secretion by gene transferring cells encapsulated in polycaprolactone tubes: gene chronotherapy. Peptides 2004, 25:1259–1267.

[57] Rinsch C, Quinodoz P, Pittet B, Alizadeh N, Baetens D, Montandon D, Aebischer P, Pepper MS. Delivery of FGF-2 but not VEGF by encapsulated genetically engineered myoblasts improves survival and vascularization in a model of acute skin flap ischemia. Gene Therapy 2001, 8:523–533.

[58] Hortelano G, Al-Hendy A, Ofosu FA, Chang PL. Delivery of human factor IX in mice by encapsulated recombinant myoblasts: a novel approach towards allogeneic gene therapy of hemophilia B. Blood 1996, 87:5095–5103.

[59] Van Raamsdonk JM, Ross CJ, Potter MA, Kurachi S, Kurachi K, Stafford DW, Chang PL. Treatment of hemophilia B in mice with nonautologous somatic gene therapeutics. Journal of Laboratory and Clinical Medicine 2002, 139:35–42.

[60] Luca G, Calvitti M, Mancuso F, Falabella G, Arato I, Bellucci C, List EO, Bellezza E, Angeli G, Lilli C, Bodo M, Becchetti E, Kopchick JJ, Cameron DF, Baroni T, Calafiore R. Reversal of experimental Laron Syndrome by xenotransplantation of microencapsulated porcine Sertoli cells. Journal of Controlled Release 2013, 165:75–81.

[61] clinicaltrials.gov. [Accessed: 2015-02-23]

[62] Murua A, Portero A, Orive G, Hernandez RM, de Castro M, Pedraz JL. Cell microencapsulation technology: towards clinical application. Journal of Controlled Release 2008, 132:76–83.

[63] Santos E, Pedraz JL, Hernandez RM, Orive G. Therapeutic cell encapsulation: ten steps towards clinical translation. Journal of Controlled Release 2013, 170:1–14.

[64] Bhujbal SV, de Haan B, Niclou SP, de Vos P. A novel multilayer immunoisolating encapsulation system overcoming protrusion of cells. Scientific Reports 2014, 4:6856.

[65] Villani S, Marazzi M, Bucco M, Faustini M, Klinger M, Gaetani P, Crovato F, Vigo D, Caviggioli F, Torre ML. Statistical approach in alginate membrane formulation for cell encapsulation in a GMP-based cell factory. Acta Biomaterialia 2008, 4:943–949.

[66] Shen F, Li AA, Gong YK, Somers S, Potter MA, Winnik FM, Chang PL. Encapsulation of recombinant cells with a novel magnetized alginate for magnetic resonance imaging. Human Gene Therapy 2005, 16:971–984.

[67] Ortner V, Kaspar C, Halter C, Tollner L, Mykhaylyk O, Walzer J, Gunzburg WH, Dangerfield JA, Hohenadl C, Czerny T. Magnetic field-controlled gene expression in encapsulated cells. Journal of Controlled Release 2012, 158:424–432.

[68] Catena R, Santos E, Orive G, Hernandez RM, Pedraz JL, Calvo A. Improvement of the monitoring and biosafety of encapsulated cells using the SFGNESTGL triple reporter system. Journal of Controlled Release 2010, 146:93–98.

Permissions

All chapters in this book were first published in GTPC, by InTech Open; hereby published with permission under the Creative Commons Attribution License or equivalent. Every chapter published in this book has been scrutinized by our experts. Their significance has been extensively debated. The topics covered herein carry significant findings which will fuel the growth of the discipline. They may even be implemented as practical applications or may be referred to as a beginning point for another development.

The contributors of this book come from diverse backgrounds, making this book a truly international effort. This book will bring forth new frontiers with its revolutionizing research information and detailed analysis of the nascent developments around the world.

We would like to thank all the contributing authors for lending their expertise to make the book truly unique. They have played a crucial role in the development of this book. Without their invaluable contributions this book wouldn't have been possible. They have made vital efforts to compile up to date information on the varied aspects of this subject to make this book a valuable addition to the collection of many professionals and students.

This book was conceptualized with the vision of imparting up-to-date information and advanced data in this field. To ensure the same, a matchless editorial board was set up. Every individual on the board went through rigorous rounds of assessment to prove their worth. After which they invested a large part of their time researching and compiling the most relevant data for our readers.

The editorial board has been involved in producing this book since its inception. They have spent rigorous hours researching and exploring the diverse topics which have resulted in the successful publishing of this book. They have passed on their knowledge of decades through this book. To expedite this challenging task, the publisher supported the team at every step. A small team of assistant editors was also appointed to further simplify the editing procedure and attain best results for the readers.

Apart from the editorial board, the designing team has also invested a significant amount of their time in understanding the subject and creating the most relevant covers. They scrutinized every image to scout for the most suitable representation of the subject and create an appropriate cover for the book.

The publishing team has been an ardent support to the editorial, designing and production team. Their endless efforts to recruit the best for this project, has resulted in the accomplishment of this book. They are a veteran in the field of academics and their pool of knowledge is as vast as their experience in printing. Their expertise and guidance has proved useful at every step. Their uncompromising quality standards have made this book an exceptional effort. Their encouragement from time to time has been an inspiration for everyone.

The publisher and the editorial board hope that this book will prove to be a valuable piece of knowledge for researchers, students, practitioners and scholars across the globe.

List of Contributors

Anjana Munshi and Preeti Khetarpal
Centre for Human Genetics, Central University of Punjab, Bathinda, India

Sneha Dadeech and M. Sai Babu
Department of Molecular Biology, Institute of Genetics and Hospital for Genetic Diseases, Osmania University, Hyderabad, India

Hakan Akbulut, Muge Ocal and Gizem Sonugur
Gene Therapy Research Unit, Department of Medical Oncology, Ankara University School of Medicine, Ankara, Turkey

Oleg E. Tolmachov and Tanya Tolmachova
Section of Molecular Medicine, National Heart and Lung Institute, Imperial College London, London, UK

Emma M. McErlean, Cian M. McCrudden and Helen O. McCarthy
School of Pharmacy, Queen's University Belfast, UK

Koichi Miyake, Noriko Miyake and Takashi Shimada
Department of Biochemistry and Molecular Biology, Division of Gene Therapy, Research Center for Advanced Medical Technology, Nippon Medical School, Japan

Melisa A. Vance, Angela Mitchell and Richard J. Samulski
Gene Therapy Center, School of Medicine, University of North Carolina at Chapel Hill, Chapel Hill, NC, USA

Ilia Villate-Beitia, Gustavo Puras, Jon Zarate, Mireia Agirre, Edilberto Ojeda and Jose Luis Pedraz
NanoBioCel Group, Laboratory of Pharmaceutics, School of Pharmacy, University of the Basque Country (UPV/EHU), Vitoria-Gasteiz, Spain
Biomedical Research Networking Center in Bioengineering, Biomaterials and Nanomedicine (CIBER-BBN), Vitoria-Gasteiz, Spain

Mustapha Chamekh
Faculté de Médecine, Institut d'Immunologie Médicale, Université Libre de Bruxelles, Brussels, Belgium

Wujie Zhang
BioMolecular Engineering Program, Department of Physics and Chemistry, Milwaukee School of Engineering, Milwaukee, WI, USA

Index

M

N

O

P

R

S

T

V

www.ingramcontent.com/pod-product-compliance
Lightning Source LLC
LaVergne TN
LVHW080632210926
848485LV00003B/247